Community Health Nursing

An Alliance for Health SECOND EDITION

THE PEDAGOGY

Community Health Nursing: An Alliance for Health, Second Edition, drives comprehension through various strategies that meet the learning needs of students, while also generating enthusiasm about the topic. This interactive approach addresses different learning styles, making this the ideal text to ensure mastery of key concepts. The pedagogical aids that appear in most chapters include the following:

Key Terms

Found in a list at the beginning of each chapter, these terms will create an expanded vocabulary. The "www" icon directs students to the companion website http://go.jblearning.com/holzemer to see these terms in an interactive glossary and use flashcards and word puzzles to nail the definitions.

KEY TERMS

Accreditation	Community health nursing	Nursing	Public health nursing
Assessment	*Healthy People*	Nursing of special interest	Public health nursing practice
Assurance	Home care services	Policy development	Reflective practice
Client	Justice		
Community			

Objectives

These objectives provide instructors and students with a snapshot of the key information they will encounter in each chapter. They serve as a checklist to help guide and focus study. Objectives can also be found on the companion website at http://go.jblearning.com/holzemer.

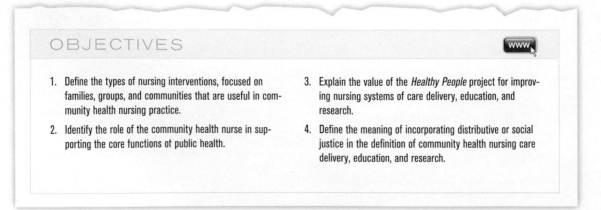

OBJECTIVES

1. Define the types of nursing interventions, focused on families, groups, and communities that are useful in community health nursing practice.

2. Identify the role of the community health nurse in supporting the core functions of public health.

3. Explain the value of the *Healthy People* project for improving nursing systems of care delivery, education, and research.

4. Define the meaning of incorporating distributive or social justice in the definition of community health nursing care delivery, education, and research.

Learning Activities

Review key concepts from each chapter with these questions at the end of each chapter. Questions can also be found at http://go.jblearning.com/holzemer, where students can submit their answers and instantly review their results.

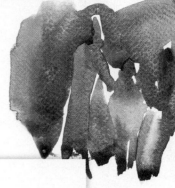

LEARNING ACTIVITIES www

1. Which of the following is the best example of a public health nursing intervention?
   A. Applying wet-to-dry dressings in the home, three times a week
   B. Developing a program for an aggregate that demonstrates a changing need for services in the community
   C. Answering an emergency crisis phone line for abused women
   D. Attending risk-reduction meetings for recovering alcoholic adolescents in a shelter

2. Which of the following nursing interventions is most important to implement, from a public health perspective?
   A. Installing handrails for senior adults in a nursing home
   B. Instructing neighbors in a community to create a "Safety Watch"
   C. Monitoring toxic emissions from a clean

5. The discoveries of John Snow helped to brin about an increase in which of the followin health-related ideas?
   A. A civic understanding and moral commitment to the betterment of people's lives through economic, socia and environmental reform
   B. A commitment of the government to reduce taxes on health care
   C. The need for health insurance for all citizens of London
   D. The understanding that there needed to be more control by the police in enforcing health laws

6. The focus of *Healthy People 2020* is related t which of the following ideas?
   A. Economic provision of low-cost health care for all citizens
   B. Development of objectives and outcomes intended to identify and

Additional Questions for Study

Students can work on these assignments individually or in a group after reading through the material. The "www" icon directs students to the companion website http://go.jblearning.com/holzemer to delve deeper into concepts by completing these exercises online.

ADDITIONAL QUESTIONS FOR STUDY

1. Visit the website of *Healthy People* and compare the goals of *Healthy People 2020* with those of *Health People 2000*. Write a brief paper describing what you see as the differences, if any, between these goals. What would you like to see incorporated into *Health People 2030*?

2. Identify a health-related problem in the community and examine the core functions of public health. For each aspect, explain how the core function relates to the problem.

3. Define the terms associated with the community health nursing paradigm. Compare your definitions with those of your classmates, and expand your definitions based on their ideas.

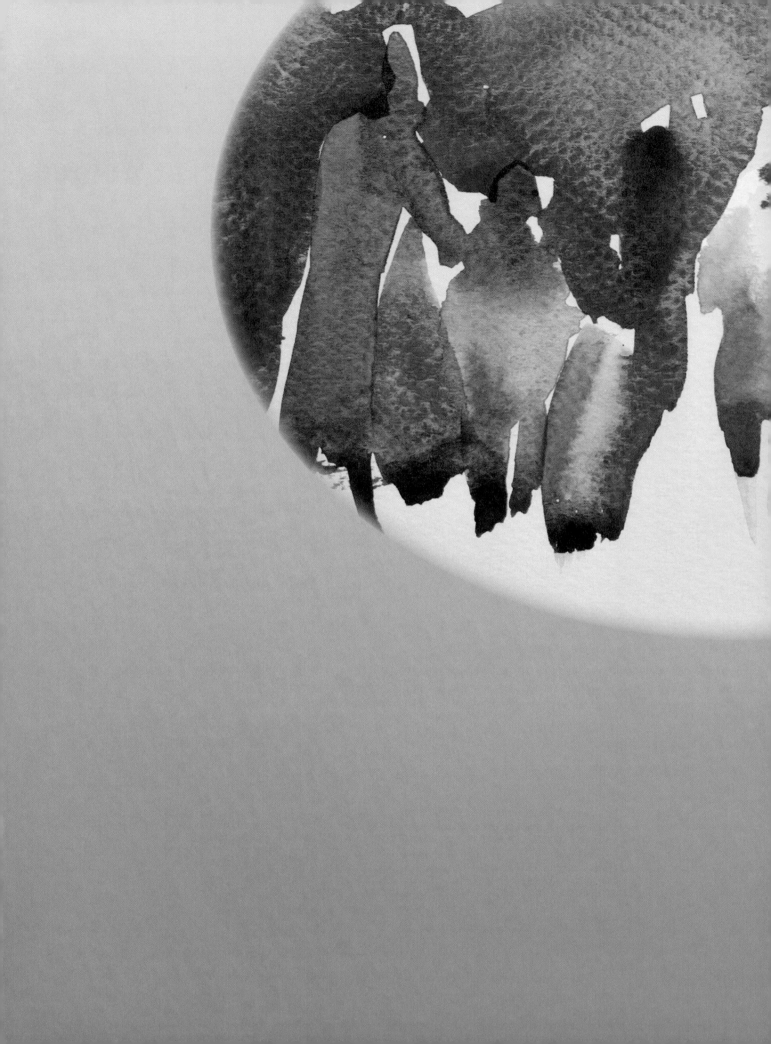

Edited by

Stephen Paul Holzemer, PhD, RN

Associate Dean and Associate Professor
Adelphi University School of Nursing
Garden City, New York

Marilyn Klainberg, EdD, RN

Associate Professor
Adelphi University School of Nursing
Garden City, New York

Community Health Nursing

An Alliance for Health SECOND EDITION

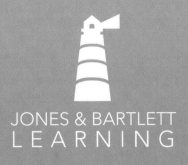

JONES & BARTLETT
LEARNING

World Headquarters
Jones & Bartlett Learning
5 Wall Street
Burlington, MA 01803
978-443-5000
info@jblearning.com
www.jblearning.com

Jones & Bartlett Learning books and products are available through most bookstores and online booksellers. To contact Jones & Bartlett Learning directly, call 800-832-0034, fax 978-443-8000, or visit our website, www.jblearning.com.

Substantial discounts on bulk quantities of Jones & Bartlett Learning publications are available to corporations, professional associations, and other qualified organizations. For details and specific discount information, contact the special sales department at Jones & Bartlett Learning via the above contact information or send an email to specialsales@jblearning.com.

Community Health Nursing: An Alliance for Health, Second Edition is an independent publication and has not been authorized, sponsored, or otherwise approved by the owners of the trademarks or service marks referenced in this product.

Some images in this book feature models. These models do not necessarily endorse, represent, or participate in the activities represented in the images.

The screenshots in this product are for educational and instructive purposes only. All trademarks displayed are the trademarks of the parties noted therein. Such use of trademarks is not an endorsement by said parties of Jones & Bartlett Learning, its products, or its services, nor should such use be deemed an endorsement by Jones & Bartlett Learning of said third party's products or services.

The authors, editors, and publisher have made every effort to provide accurate information. However, they are not responsible for errors, omissions, or for any outcomes related to the use of the contents of this book and take no responsibility for the use of the products and procedures described. Treatments and side effects described in this book may not be applicable to all people; likewise, some people may require a dose or experience a side effect that is not described herein. Drugs and medical devices are discussed that may have limited availability controlled by the Food and Drug Administration (FDA) for use only in a research study or clinical trial. Research, clinical practice, and government regulations often change the accepted standard in this field. When consideration is being given to use of any drug in the clinical setting, the health care provider or reader is responsible for determining FDA status of the drug, reading the package insert, and reviewing prescribing information for the most up-to-date recommendations on dose, precautions, and contraindications, and determining the appropriate usage for the product. This is especially important in the case of drugs that are new or seldom used.

Production Credits

Publisher: Kevin Sullivan
Acquisitions Editor: Amanda Harvey
Editorial Assistant: Sara Bempkins
Production Manager: Carolyn Rogers Pershouse
Senior Marketing Manager: Elena McAnespie
V.P., Manufacturing and Inventory Control: Therese Connell
Composition: Publishers' Design and Production Services, Inc.

Text Design: Timothy Dziewit
Cover Design: Scott Moden
Cover, Part Opener, and Chapter Opener Image: © SurlyaPhoto/ShutterStock, Inc.
Printing and Binding: Courier Companies
Cover Printing: Courier Companies

To order this product, use ISBN: 978-1-4496-5177-0

Library of Congress Cataloging-in-Publication Data
Community health nursing : an alliance for health / [edited by] Stephen P. Holzemer, Marilyn B. Klainberg. — 2nd ed.
 p. ; cm.
Includes bibliographical references and index.
ISBN 978-0-7637-8579-6 (pbk.)
I. Holzemer, Stephen P. (Stephen Paul) II. Klainberg, Marilyn B.
[DNLM: 1. Community Health Nursing. 2. Home Care Services. WY 106]
610.73'43—dc23
                                        2012027924
6048

Printed in the United States of America
16   15   14   13   12   10   9   8   7   6   5   4   3   2   1

CONTENTS

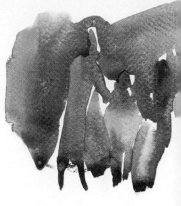

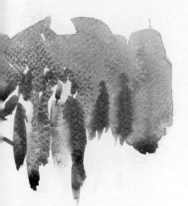

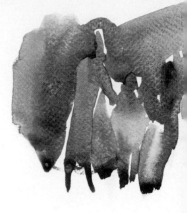

Chapter 7: Expertise of the Compassionate Nurse in Community-Based Care 145

Stephen Paul Holzemer and Anne Belcher

Section 3: Assessment and Diagnosis of Community-Based Needs 164

Chapter 8: Validity and Reliability in Epidemiology and Environmental Health 167

Patricia Eckardt and Patricia Facquet

Chapter 9: Inquiry and Health Promotion, Health Maintenance, and Health Restoration in the Community 195

Judith Aponte and Stephen Paul Holzemer

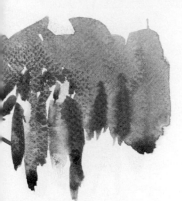

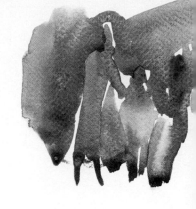

PREFACE

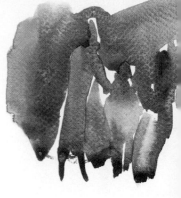

This book is intended to help prepare the nursing student to enter the profession of nursing with an understanding of the impact of health issues on the client and the community, whether it be a local or global community. It provides an introduction to the concepts of communication, ethics, management of care epidemiology, resources and resource allocation and their impact on the provision of care. It introduces the student to the Alliance Model in order to better understand the relationship between the client- or community-based needs, the system of care management, and the influence of resources allocations. The goal is to help the emerging professional with the knowledge to provide clients with relevant, safe care in a compassionate and realistic manner. The following chapters provide the basic concepts needed to prepare the student nurse with the role of the nurse in the community.

- Chapter 1 provides the student with an introduction to personal and professional nursing responsibilities for providing care to clients in the community
- Chapter 2 introduces the ethical and cultural issues of providing care to the client in the community and the community at the client
- Chapter 3 presents the Alliance Model
- Chapter 4 relates health policy and evidence-based research in the care of the community as client
- Chapter 5 introduces the notion of communication and the provision of information to the community
- Chapter 6 establishes the voice of the client and the role of the community health nurse in discovering that voice
- Chapter 7 brings in issues related to the expertise of the community health nurse (CHN) working in community-based care, which is examined from a number of perspectives
- Chapter 8 examines the topics of epidemiology and environmental health
- Chapter 9 explores the concept of inquiry, including how to assist the client in making proper and productive health choices
- Chapter 10 provides skills necessary for care management in the community
- Chapter 11 presents resource allocation for the family and community
- Chapter 12 explores community program development
- Chapter 13 examines the use of project management for successful community program change
- Chapter 14 presents how to prepare and provide emergency disaster management in the community
- Chapter 15 explores global community health issues
- Chapter 16 discusses the future of health care

Please refer to the walkthrough earlier in the front of this book for information on the pedagogical elements within the text, as well as the inside front cover for details on the student and instructor resources available.

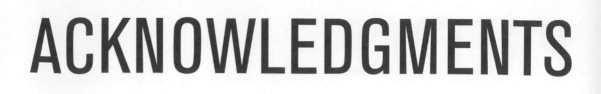

ACKNOWLEDGMENTS

The words "thank you" are insufficient to express my appreciation to all to family, colleagues, and friends who have made this venture possible. I would like to say a special thank you to:

The students who have enriched my experience of community, and serve as a source of change in the profession of nursing, and to Marilyn Klainberg, and her generosity of spirit.

The men and women who have served as mentors, guides and most significantly, healers of this damaged world. I dedicate this work to them, some living, others deceased, but all quite alive in my heart.

Barbara McCampbell Holzemer	Lee Holzemer
Sister Pauline Brick	Beth Roop Holzemer
Barbara Burke	Judy Bell Holzemer
Katherine Wehe	Foddie Keogh-Holzemer
Jane Titus	Dee Dee Lovette Spiva
John Shannon Keogh	Nancy Shaver
Carolyn Fish	Diane Holzemer
Betty Jo Blauner	Good-Bob Holzemer

—Stephen

I thank the faculty and students who have used the previous editions of this book. Their feedback has encouraged us to redesign and present this updated version. I especially wish to thank the original authors of the first edition of this book, as well as the contributors for this edition. My sincerest thanks to Dr. Stephen Holzemer who has done an incredible job in leading this venture to fruition.

On a personal level, I thank my family and friends who have put up with me during the preparation of this book. My husband Bernie, who is the love of my life, and my children and their spouses: Dennis and Dana, Danielle and Mark, Gregory and Jenny, Joshua and Shelly; and to my grandchildren, who LOVE to see their names in print: Adam, Emma, Sydney, Jacob, Sofia, Simon, Max, Samantha, Shayna, and Sari.

—Marilyn

We would also like to thank the editorial and production staff at Jones & Bartlett Learning for their publishing guidance and support: Amanda Harvey, Sara Bempkins, and Carolyn Pershouse.

—Stephen and Marilyn

CONTRIBUTORS

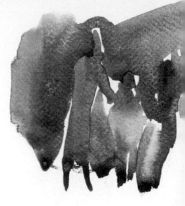

Judith Aponte, DNSc, RN, BC, CCM
Associate Professor
Hunter-Bellevue School of Nursing
Hunter College of the City University of New York
New York, NY

Helen Christina Ballestas,
PhD, RN, ANP
Assistant Professor
Adelphi University School of Nursing
Garden City, NY

Anne E. Belcher, PhD, RN
Associate Professor
Director, Office for Teaching Excellence
Johns Hopkins University School of Nursing
Baltimore, MD

Christine Coughlin, EdD, RN
Associate Professor
Adelphi University School of Nursing
Garden City, NY

Patricia Donohue-Porter, PhD, RN
Associate Professor and Director of the PhD Program
Adelphi University School of Nursing
Garden City, NY

Patricia Eckardt, PhD, MBA, RN
Adjunct Assistant Professor
Adelphi University School of Nursing
Garden City, NY

Patricia Facquet,
RN, MEdN, MSPH, CCRC
Doctoral Candidate, Walden University
Assistant Professor
Adelphi University School of Nursing
Garden City, NY

Patricia F. Garofalo, MS, RN
Clinical Faculty and Assistant Director of Simulation
New York University College of Nursing
New York, NY

Clarilee Hauser, PhD, RN
Clinical Assistant Professor
Adelphi University School of Nursing
Garden City, NY

Stephen Paul Holzemer, PhD, RN
Associate Dean and Associate Professor
Adelphi University School of Nursing
Garden City, NY

Marilyn Klainberg, EdD, RN
Associate Professor
Adelphi University School of Nursing
Garden City, NY

Andrea McCrink, EdD, WHNP, BC, RN
Director, PATH Program
Assistant Professor
Adelphi University School of Nursing
Garden City, NY

Deborah J. Murphy, MS, RN
Clinical Assistant Professor
Coordinator of Clinical & Community Affairs
Adelphi University School of Nursing
Garden City, NY

Maureen C. Roller, DNP, ANP, BC
Clinical Assistant Professor
Adelphi University School of Nursing
Garden City, NY

Kenneth C. Rondello, MD, MPH
Assistant Professor, School of Nursing
Academic Administrator, Emergency Management
Adelphi University
Garden City, NY

Danielle Smith, BSN, RN
University of Miami
Miami, FL

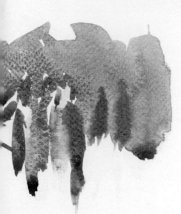

REVIEWERS

Angeline Bushy, PhD, RN, FAAN
University of Central Florida College of Nursing
Orlando, FL

Amber Dallwig, RN, MSN
University of Michigan School of Nursing
Ann Arbor, MI

**Annemarie Dowling-Castronovo,
PhD(c), RN**
Evelyn L. Spiro School of Nursing
Wagner College
Staten Island, NY

Monty Gross, PhD, RN, CNE
James Madison University
Harrisonburg, VA

Marcia Roth, MSN, MST, RN
Grand View University
Des Moines, IA

**Bonnie Jerome-D'Emilia,
PhD, MPH, RN**
The State University of New Jersey, Camden
Newark, NJ

**Jennifer L. Johnson,
RN, MSN, WHNP-BC**
University of North Carolina, Pembroke
Pembroke, NC

Kelly Ann Krumwiede, PhD, MA, RN
Minnesota State University, Mankato
Mankato, MN

Jeanne Leffers, PhD, APHN, RN
University of Massachusetts, Dartmouth
Dartmouth, MA

Kathleen Masters, DNS, RN
School of Nursing
University of Southern Mississippi
Hattiesburg, MS

Tom Mauro

Cheryl Nadeau, RN, MS, FNP-BC
New York University College of Nursing
New York, NY

Terrilynn Fox Quillen, MSN, RN
Department of Environments for Health
Indiana University School of Nursing
Indianapolis, IN

Diana Shenefield, PhD(c)
Huntington University
Huntington, IN

Deborah Williams, EdD, MSN, RN
Western Kentucky University
Bowling Green, KY

INTRODUCTION

Developing Contemporary Skills for Community Work: Concepts and Questions

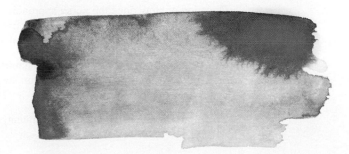

Nurses working in the community need an additional skill set—sometimes the same, but often different—than that of nurses working in acute care settings. With the exception of home care and subacute care settings in the community, the focus on prevention of illness as the goal of practice requires the nurse to approach nursing care differently. The different ways of thinking (cognitive), feeling (affective), and performing (psychomotor), when applied to the work of nursing in the community, assist the nurse in developing a new skill set.

A number of concepts, when applied broadly to practice, help the nurse working in the community to think, feel, and perform nursing differently. These concepts are reflective practice, respect, vision, relatedness, clarity, courage, compassion, inquisitiveness, validity/reliability, flexibility, justice, precision, viability, alertness, responsibility, and evidence-based future. Using these concepts is intended to make the guiding paradigm of community health nursing practice support nursing's social contract with society (American Nurses Association [ANA], 2003, 2010). These concepts are also key to implementing the Quality and Safety Education for Nurses (QSEN) undergraduate, prelicensure competencies (Cronenwett et al., 2007) that are critical within community-based care settings.

These 16 concepts are presented as a way to address six significant questions, whose answers help to reveal the scope of community health nursing practice. These questions are answered more fully throughout the chapters of the textbook. **Table I-1** summarizes these concepts and questions. **FIGURE I-1** suggests that all the following concepts have a place in the creation of an evidence-based future for community health nursing.

TABLE I-1
Concepts Helpful to Understanding the Nursing Concerns in the Community

Central Question	Concepts	Placement in the Textbook
Question 1: What are the guiding principles and a theoretical orientation for community health nursing?	Reflective practice Respect Vision Relatedness Clarity	Chapters 1–5
Question 2: What is the meaning behind the assessment and diagnosis of the voice of the client?	Courage Compassion	Chapters 6–7
Question 3: How does the nurse approach assessment and diagnosis of community-based needs?	Inquisitiveness Validity/reliability	Chapters 8–9
Question 4: How does the nurse approach assessment and diagnosis of systems of care management and resource allocation solutions?	Flexibility Justice	Chapters 10–11
Question 5: What is the meaning of community health program planning, implementation, evaluation, and termination?	Precision Viability Alertness	Chapters 12–14
Question 6: What is the future of community health nursing?	Responsibility Evidence-based future	Chapters 15–16

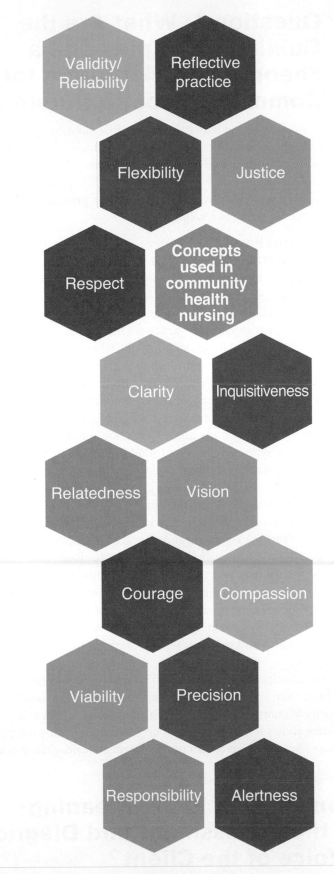

Figure I-1 Concepts helpful for creating an evidence-based future.

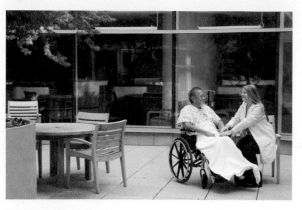
© Mark Kostich/iStockphoto.com

Question 1: What Are the Guiding Principles and a Theoretical Orientation for Community Health Nursing?

The concepts that may help answer this question are the concepts of reflective practice, respect, vision, relatedness, and clarity. These concepts allow the nurse to engage in the processes of thinking, feeling, and performing work in the community. They assist the nurse to care for others safely, or to refer the work to a provider with a better skill match for problem resolution.

Reflective Practice. Reflecting on nursing practice allows the nurse to commit to the plan of care, and make changes in the plan of care in a timely and efficient manner. The nurse accepts personal and professional responsibility for the creation of a safe and productive client–nurse relationship through reflection. The nurse reflects on current practice, with a historical understanding of former practice, to create ideas about best practice for the future.

Respect. Respect for the ethical beliefs and the cultural experience of the client is the core of a successful nurse–client relationship. Without an ethical–cultural awareness of the client by the nurse, the client remains invisible. The client may be an individual, a family, another group, or the community as a whole.

Vision. Having a vision of the potential for a well-developed client–nurse relationship allows for the client and the nurse to address specific concerns within the healthcare delivery system. Conceptual models emerge that can, for example, assist the nurse in obtaining a clearer understanding of the integration between community-based needs, the systems of care management, and resource allocation strategies to meet these needs. The Alliance for Health Model (discussed later in this book) is one model that represents the integration of community-based needs, systems of care management, and resource allocation so as to promote the vision of providing comprehensive health services to clients in the community.

Relatedness. The success of supporting healthy communities is intimately related to the progress of sound health policy and evidence-based quantitative and qualitative research. The community health nurse relates policy and research concerns to the specific needs of the community where practice is occurring. The relationship between health policy and evidence-based research promotes the development of best practices.

Clarity. Clear intradisciplinary and interdisciplinary communication is key to information management and validation of coordinated, successful health outcomes of clients. Clarity of communication between and among nurses and other healthcare providers allows for the support of best practices in care delivery, and the termination of practices that do not positively effect healthy client outcomes.

Question 2: What Is the Meaning Behind the Assessment and Diagnosis of the Voice of the Client?

The concepts that may help answer this question are the concepts of courage and compassion. These concepts describe the intimate relationship between the client and the nurse as they, for example, seek health solutions or tolerate limitations of care delivery. The language of courage and compassion eliminates the meaninglessness of noncompliance on the part of the client. The client and nurse work together to answer questions that the contemporary healthcare system may or may not address. Clients are compliant with their choices in health care.

Courage. It takes courage for clients to navigate the healthcare system as they seek health, accept the limitations imposed by illness, and define their quality of life. The lived experience, or story of the client, must be heard in every client–nurse interaction. The uniqueness of every family, group, aggregate, or community story takes courage to share.

Compassion. Compassion for clients allows nurses to sustain their commitment to the client–nurse relationship. Compassion is an action whose scope goes well beyond empathy. Compassion requires an ongoing and informed commitment to act in a way that responds to the actual and potential needs of clients. The nurse needs to summon compassion to hear the uniqueness of every family, group, aggregate, or community story.

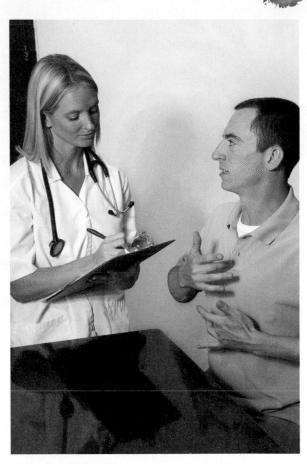

© Loretta Hostettler/iStockphoto

Question 3: How Does the Nurse Approach Assessment and Diagnosis of Community-Based Needs?

To answer this question, we turn to the concepts of inquisitiveness and validity/reliability.

Inquisitiveness. Inquisitiveness on the part of the nurse allows the nurse to develop skill in the assessment and diagnosis of community-based needs that may be met by the spectrum of health promotion, health maintenance, and health restoration services available to clients. Matching client needs with available services is possible only after successful assessment and diagnosis.

Validity/Reliability. Validity and reliability assist with translating information from epidemiology and environmental health into a practicable plan of care for the community. The use of scientific data that accurately portray what is known about the relationship between illness and the environment that supports it is the first step in problem resolution through research. Validity clarifies the concepts and concerns under study, whereas reliability refers to understanding research findings over time.

Question 4: How Does the Nurse Approach Assessment and Diagnosis of Systems of Care Management and Resource Allocation Solutions?

The concepts that may help answer this question are the concepts of flexibility and justice.

Flexibility. Creating systems of care management for families, groups, aggregates, and communities requires flexibility. Systems that are effective in one setting may

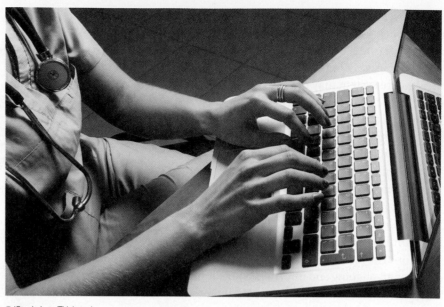

© iStockphoto/Thinkstock

fail in another setting. Systems of care management must adapt to changing community-based needs, along with the mix of resources that are made available to meet them.

Justice. Resource allocation for families, groups, aggregates, and communities should be grounded in the ethical principle of justice. Justice as fairness promotes meeting of community-based needs with available resources, in a way that is acceptable to the community. Fostering justice can be used to respond to changing needs over time.

Question 5: What Is the Meaning of Community Health Program Planning, Implementation, Evaluation, and Termination?

The concepts that may help answer this question are precision, viability, and alertness.

Precision. Community health program planning, implementation, evaluation, and termination require precision to meet the needs of the community. The evolution of programs depends on the concept of precision to keep them relevant to the community. Questions of how to prioritize limited resources are answered, in part, by precise program development.

Viability. Coordinating community health program planning, implementation, evaluation, and termination through thoughtful project management fosters program viability in the community. Engaging in the process of the strategic use of material and personnel resources keeps programs functioning at an optimal level.

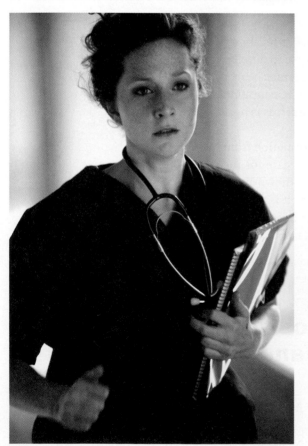

© iStockphoto/Thinkstock

Alertness. Alertness to the realities of natural and human-made disasters in the community allows for adequate care to be delivered to the community if and when they occur. Maintaining the integrity of the community requires vigilance in avoiding, as well as preparing to cope with, threats that could destroy or cripple the status of health in the community.

Question 6: What Is the Future of Community Health Nursing?

The concepts that may help answer this question are responsibility and evidence-based practice, education, and research.

Responsibility. Attention to the effects of interstate, national, and global health concerns on local communities is a growing responsibility of community health nursing (International Council of Nurses [ICN], 2011). Nurses have the responsibility to foster a professional dedication to resolve community-based needs and to keep communities safe and healthy on an ongoing basis.

Evidence-Based Future. The nurse accepts personal and professional responsibility for the creation of models of care for a changing community through evidence-based care delivery, education, and research. Dedication to the future of nursing is a professional responsibility nurses need to take seriously (Institute of Medicine [IOM], 2011).

REFERENCES

American Nurses Association (ANA). (2003). *Nursing's social policy statement* (2nd ed.). Silver Spring, MD: Author.

American Nurses Association (ANA). (2010). *Nursing's social policy statement: The essence of the profession.* Silver Spring, MD: Author.

Cronenwett, L., Sherwood, G., Barnsteiner, J., Disch, J., Johnson, J., Mitchel, P., ... Warren, J. (2007). Quality and safety education for nurses. *Nursing Outlook, 55*(3), 122–131.

Institute of Medicine (IOM). (2011). *The future of nursing: Leading change, advancing health.* Washington, DC: Author.

International Council of Nurses (ICN). (2011). *Closing the gap: Increasing access and equity.* Geneva, Switzerland: Author.

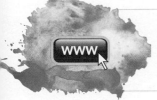

For a full suite of assignments and additional learning activities, use the access code located in the front of your book to visit the exclusive website: http://go.jblearning.com/Holzemer/. If you do not have an access code, you can obtain one at the site.

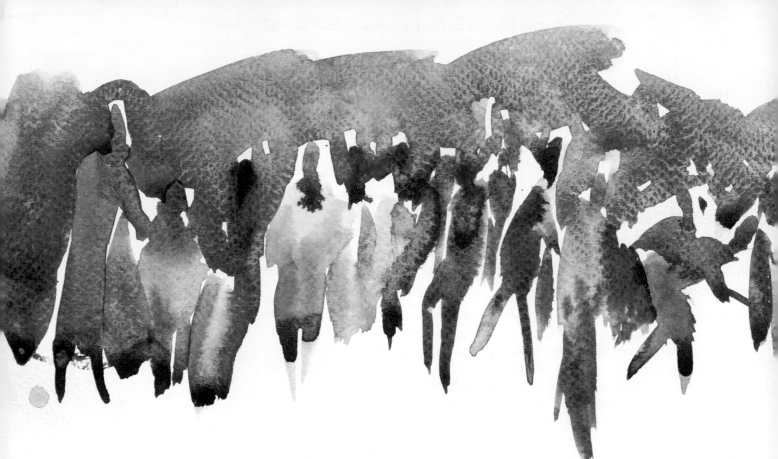

Guiding Principles and Theoretical Orientation for Community Health Nursing

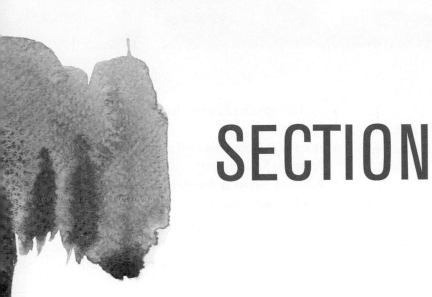

SECTION 1

CHAPTER OUTLINE

- Introduction
- Providing Care in the Community Using Reflective Practice
- Reflecting on the Essentials: Core Functions of Nursing in the Community
  - Assessment
  - Policy Development
  - Assurance
- Reflecting on a Guiding Paradigm of Community Health Nursing Practice
  - Client
  - Nursing
  - Health
  - Environment
  - Caring as Informed by Distributive or Social Justice
- The Nursing Social Contract as a Mandate to Develop and Maintain Role Competence

- Legal and Voluntary Guidelines for Providing Care in the Community
- Essentials of Education and Professional Credentialing for Community Health Nursing
- A Historical Context for Providing Care in the Community
  - Eighteenth Century
  - Colonial America
  - Nineteenth Century
  - Twentieth Century: Establishment of Community Service
- Health Care in the Twenty-First Century
- Reflecting on the Possibilities for the Future
- Summary

OBJECTIVES

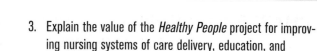

1. Define the types of nursing interventions, focused on families, groups, and communities that are useful in community health nursing practice.

2. Identify the role of the community health nurse in supporting the core functions of public health.

3. Explain the value of the *Healthy People* project for improving nursing systems of care delivery, education, and research.

4. Define the meaning of incorporating distributive or social justice in the definition of community health nursing care delivery, education, and research.

KEY TERMS

Accreditation

Assessment

Assurance

Client

Community

Community health nursing

Healthy People

Home care services

Justice

Nursing

Nursing of special interest

Policy development

Public health nursing

Public health nursing practice

Reflective practice

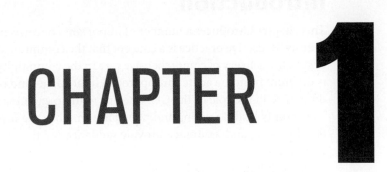

CHAPTER 1

Reflecting on Providing Care to Clients in the Community

Stephen Paul Holzemer

Marilyn Klainberg

REFLECTION

A moral being is one who is capable of reflecting on his past actions and their motives—of approving of some and disapproving of others.

—Charles Darwin (1809–1882)

Introduction

This chapter introduces a number of important concerns in providing care in the community. Reflective practice is a concept that the community health nurse (CHN) uses to ensure the delivery of comprehensive care in the community. Nursing in the community is different from the acute care approach in hospitals and other acute care settings. The difference in the role of the CHN begins with an examination of the core functions of community health nursing and public health. The core functions of assessment, policy development, and assurance provide guidance for the performance of nursing in the community.

In addition, the paradigm of providing care requires a special understanding of the concepts central to nursing practice in the community. In community health nursing practice, the concepts of client, nursing, health, environment, and caring as informed by distributive or social justice take on special meaning. As in other settings, the key to providing quality nursing care in the community is role competence. The CHN must demonstrate competence in meeting the needs of clients in a number of settings in the community. Role competence is augmented by the legal and voluntary guidelines in place to support the systems of care management. In addition, the essentials of education and credentialing in the community inform nurses about how best to prepare themselves for safe and effective nursing practice. Role competence is a concern of CHNs over the course of their entire careers.

A brief historical overview of some of the important aspects of the development of community health nursing practice is also provided here. History informs the nurse of where the profession has been, with an eye toward how to create better and more efficient systems of care for the future. The chapter ends by reflecting on nursing's future as outlined by two important documents. This reflection on the possibilities for nursing's future in community health begins by examining the Institute of Medicine (IOM, 2011) guidelines for the future of nursing and the Quality and Safety Education for Nurses (QSEN) competencies (Cronenwett et al., 2007).

Providing Care in the Community Using Reflective Practice

Reflective practice: Practice in which the nurse considers how all parts of the nursing process relate to the care of individuals, families, other groups, and the community as a whole.

Community health nursing: The provision of nursing care for collectives of people, bound in relationships that are called families, other groups, aggregates, and communities.

Providing care to clients in the community through **reflective practice**, or the way nurses provide care, has many challenges in community health nursing. Nursing in the community is unique because at any one time the nurse may be caring for clients (patients) who are young and old, are sick or well, and are making different levels of progress on their path to health and wellness. The CHN continuously reflects upon how all parts of the nursing process relate to the care of individuals, families, other groups, and the community as a whole (American Nurses Association [ANA], 2010a, 2010b), and takes steps to create best practices in care delivery, using ethical and culturally appropriate guidelines.

Definitions of **community health nursing** from the perspective of the ANA, and the American Public Health Association (APHA), Public Health Nursing Section, are helpful in identifying the focus of community health nursing. The Association of Community Health Nursing Educators (ACHNE) provides guidance to educators in the field. For the purpose of this discussion, public health nursing is a component of community health nursing, with a specialized focus on promoting wellness in communities, or among populations.

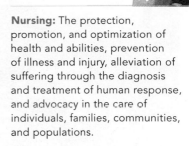

ANA Definition of Nursing

Nursing is the protection, promotion, and optimization of health and abilities, prevention of illness and injury, alleviation of suffering through the diagnosis and treatment of human response, and advocacy in the care of individuals, families, communities, and populations (ANA, 2010b).

ANA Standards and Scope of Public Health Nursing Practice

The ANA Standards and Scope of Public Health Nursing Practice are based upon the ANA definition of nursing and act as a guide to the role and "expectations of the professional role within which all public health registered nurses should practice" (ANA, 2010a, p. vii). **"Public health nursing** is the practice of promoting and protecting the health of populations using knowledge from nursing, social, and public health sciences" (APHA, Public Health Nursing Section, 1996).

APHA Definition of Public Health Nursing Practice

Public health nursing practice is affected by biological, cultural, environmental, economic, social, and political factors. As part of the healthcare system, public health nursing practice responds to these factors through working with the community to promote health and prevent disease, injury, and disability (APHA, 2010).

ACHNE Guidelines of Community Health Nursing

The **ACHNE** makes available to nurse educators suggestions and plans to implement and evaluate community/public health nursing (C/PHN) baccalaureate nursing curricula relevant for meeting the needs of the public in the twenty-first century. The C/PHN designation identifies the nurse generalist within the specialty. The *Essentials* document provides recommendations of core knowledge, values, and competencies that should be in the curriculum (ACHNE, 2009).

Nursing: The protection, promotion, and optimization of health and abilities, prevention of illness and injury, alleviation of suffering through the diagnosis and treatment of human response, and advocacy in the care of individuals, families, communities, and populations.

Public health nursing: "The practice of promoting and protecting the health of populations using knowledge from nursing, social, and public health sciences" (APHA, Public Health Nursing Section, 1996).

Public health nursing practice: A part of the healthcare system that responds to biological, cultural, environmental, economic, social, and political factors through working with the community to promote health and prevent disease, injury, and disability.

Providing nursing care to clients in the community involves meeting specific personal and professional responsibilities. The CHN, like nurses who work in acute care settings, cares for clients in a personal and professional way. The CHN, however, has the additional responsibility of caring for the client in the community setting, which adds a

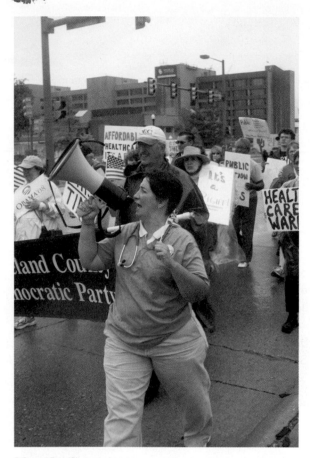

© Samuel Perry/Shutterstock.com

unique twist to the care provided. As identified by the various professional associations related to community health nursing, the CHN has the privilege and responsibility to care for the community as a whole.

Reflecting on the Essentials: Core Functions of Nursing in the Community

Three core functions are related to the work nurses perform in the community. Although considered core functions of public health, these three functions—assessment, policy development, and assurance—have meaning for the CHN in all settings. The nurse becomes fluent in these three functions so as to provide safe and effective care to the community as the client of nursing care.

Assessment

The first aspect of **assessment** that is significant for the CHN is monitoring health status. This is an ongoing activity that continuously alters the picture of health in a community. In addition, the CHN investigates the outcome of assessment. The CHN, using the nursing process, diagnoses and further explores problems and concerns in the community. Working with members of the community, the nurse better understands the significance of problems from the perspective of the community's experience of living with various challenges. The CHN, in conjunction with other professionals and laypersons, identifies the healthy and less healthy patterns of behavior in the community.

Policy Development

Policy development begins with the process of interacting with the community. The CHN actively informs the community of concerns, educates the members of the community of their choices, and empowers them to act. The CHN, after establishing a therapeutic relationship with the community, mobilizes community partnerships for change. Change efforts are molded into policies and plans to support the evolution of healthy communities. The nurse is active in moving policies into the legal system for protection of the health of the people living in the community (Milstead, 2008).

Assurance

Assurance relates to the public's perception that the providers of health care and the systems of care management are operating in their best interest. The CHN can participate in assurance by fostering linkages between people and services, and monitoring the interaction closely so that people get their needs met. On a larger scale, the CHN has a part in monitoring the competence of professionals working in the community, and participating in the enforcement of laws and regulations to support health in the community.

Reflecting on a Guiding Paradigm of Community Health Nursing Practice

The CHN approaches nursing care from a special perspective. The guiding paradigm of nursing practice—that is, the unique relationship between (and among) the concepts

Assessment: The community health nurse's practice of monitoring health status, investigating outcomes, and using the nursing process to diagnose and further explore problems and concerns in the community.

Policy development: A process in which the community health nurse interacts with the community, mobilizes community partnerships for change, and molds policies and plans to support the evolution of healthy communities.

Assurance: Efforts directed at enhancing the public's perception that the providers of health care and the systems of care management are operating in their best interest.

of nursing–health–client–environment and distributive or social justice—gives substance to the roles and responsibilities of the community health nurse (ANA, 2010a, 2010b). The relationship between these concepts is referred to as a paradigm because it attempts to grasp or represent the concepts central to nursing's development as a profession. **FIGURE 1-1** provides a representation of the concepts that traditionally define community health nursing.

Some nursing scholars suggest that a major concept has yet to be explicated in the paradigm of nursing—namely, the concept of caring as informed by distributive or social justice. If this idea has merit, it suggests that knowing caring informed by justice is as critical as knowing the concepts of nursing, health, client, and environment. **FIGURE 1-2** depicts the addition of this fifth concept in the nursing paradigm.

Nursing in the community has a somewhat different relationship with the concepts of health, client, and environment, and a unique relationship with social justice. The emphasis on understanding health relates to the prevention of illness as well as the progression of illness. This approach focuses on health promotion, the antithesis of high-technology hospital-to-home care. The emphasis on the recipient of care (client) reflects the many different collectives of individuals who make up families, other groups, aggregates, and communities. The influence of the environment on the practice of community health nursing defines the location of practice as local, regional, national, and even global in nature. Community/public health nurses partner with communities, states, nations, organizations, and groups in addition to individuals in assessment and policy development (APHA, 2010). These environments' impact on the client's health has local, regional, national, and global significance.

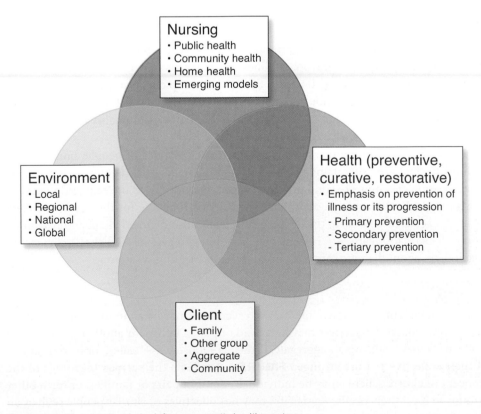

Figure 1-1 Concepts that help define community health nursing.

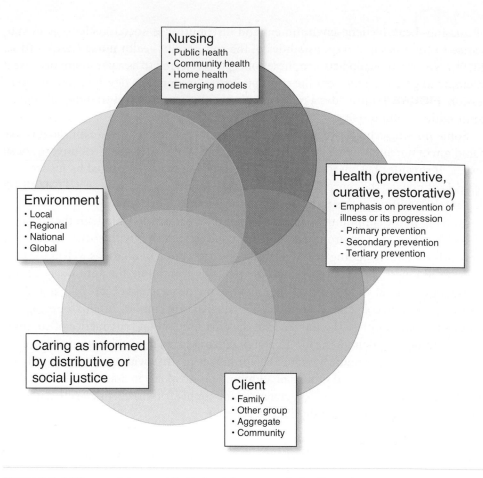

Figure 1-2 A fifth essential concept that helps define community health nursing.

As stated earlier, nursing in the community focuses on the meaning of health in terms of both prevention and progression of illness. Primary, secondary, and tertiary prevention (of illness) strategies are all part of the drive to keep clients as healthy as possible, as reflected in their health choices, and are discussed later in this text. The meaning of health also reflects the ability of the client to find meaning and quality of life in his or her state of health and wellness.

Nursing in the community involves caring for collectives of people, bound in relationships that are called families, other groups, aggregates, and communities. Many nursing strategies move beyond physical care of individuals, as the required interventions may include teaching, counseling, referral, and lobbying for the needs of collectives. An acute care nurse in the hospital may teach an individual client and his family about diabetic foot care. A CHN may identify an aggregate of 30 diabetic clients and teach them about diabetic care at a parent–teacher meeting, as a group.

Client

The client, patient, or recipient of CHN interventions may be an individual or a collective of individuals. Collectives may be a dyad or pair, a family, or another group. These collectives may make up an aggregate, if they are loosely associated, or a community, if their collective ties are stronger. **FIGURE 1-3** reflects the various meanings of the concept of **client**. Clients may be individuals, bond in pairs or families, or form other groups to meet their needs. Aggregates may be collectives of similar people such as an

Client: The individual or collective of individuals who are the focus of community health nursing.

aggregate defined by gender, race, religion, or income. If the aggregate becomes a close, well-functioning group, we refer to it as a **community**. Communities are described by geography, special interest, or special belief.

Some individuals, for various political or psychological reasons, place themselves outside of a community (the yellow circle in Figure 1-3). The behavior of some individuals is so disruptive to the community that the community or society restricts their participation in the community. Examples of clients who are not in touch or have restrictions on their interaction with their communities may include some mentally ill persons, political prisoners, and persons convicted of serious crimes.

Nursing

Nursing in the community comprises blended practice—that is, an amalgam of strategies used to provide care that is preventive, curative, restorative, and custodial/supportive. This type of care is provided within three subspecialties of community health nursing: public health nursing, nursing of special interest, and home care nursing. **FIGURE 1-4** represents the three types of community health nursing. The pyramid shape reflects the largest amount of services being offered as **home care services**. These services mirror hospital-based acute care services, which are centered on disease or system dysfunction. These curative, restorative, or custodial/supportive services are provided to individuals and families where they live.

Community: A collective of individuals that becomes a close, well-functioning group, and that may be described by geography, special interest, or special belief.

Home care services: Curative, restorative, or custodial/ supportive services that are provided to individuals and families where they live.

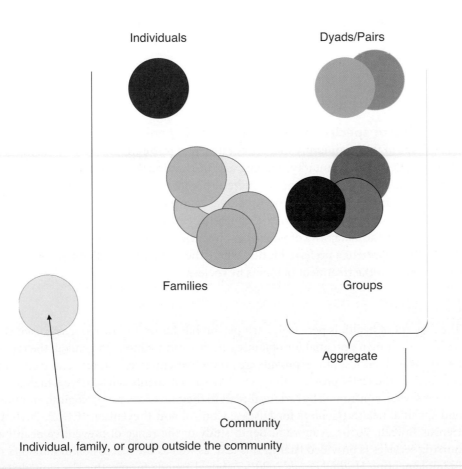

Figure 1-3 Meanings of "client."

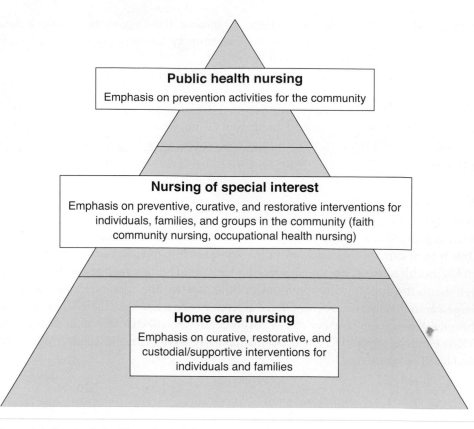

Public health nursing

Emphasis on prevention activities for the community

Nursing of special interest

Emphasis on preventive, curative, and restorative interventions for individuals, families, and groups in the community (faith community nursing, occupational health nursing)

Home care nursing

Emphasis on curative, restorative, and custodial/supportive interventions for individuals and families

Figure 1-4 Community health nursing includes various nursing specialties working in the community.

Nursing of special interest: Provision of services to individuals, families, and groups in the community that are curative and restorative in nature.

Nursing of special interest relates to services provided to individuals, families, and groups in the community that are curative and restorative in nature. Examples include parish (faith community) nursing and occupational health nursing. These types of nursing are designated as "special interest" because in one example they serve a faith community, and in the other an occupational aggregate.

FIGURE 1-5 provides a futuristic, theoretical example of how resources might be altered to provide a majority of public health services, with an emphasis on prevention. This would represent a preferred future where the prevention of illness would be more important than the treatment of illness by society.

Health

The concept of health is personal. Each person has his or her own journey; each client has his or her own potential for obtaining health and wellness. In general, the types of health-related services nurses provide are preventive, curative, restorative, and custodial/supportive. The CHN provides these services so that clients can achieve a high level of wellness when confronted by serious threats to their physical, psychological, emotional, and spiritual health (Centers for Disease Control and Prevention [CDC], 2010; U.S. Census Bureau, 2010). A more in-depth study of the range of preventive health and nursing services is provided later in this text, as well as the discussion of nursing's role in implementing *Healthy People 2020*, a national agenda for meeting the United States' healthcare needs.

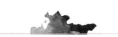

Environment

The local environment of care delivery (i.e., where care is delivered) occurs in, for example, hospitals, nursing homes, clinics, rehabilitation settings, and locations where people reside or live. The political environment of care delivery occurs on a national and global stage where important decisions are made about who will receive care, which types of services will be available, and who will provide services to society. **Table 1-1** provides a structure through which to examine the relationship between the concepts of client, nursing, health, and environment as they relate to community health nursing.

Caring as Informed by Distributive or Social Justice

Justice is an ethical concept that suggests that there is a fair way to allocate resources (Rawls, 1971). Justice requires the existence of a transparent way of meeting the needs of persons with various threats to their health in the community, and of distributing medical goods and services fairly. The CHN needs to participate in creating a just culture, in which the needs of clients are met in a way that maximizes their potential and properly reflects the ethical principles of the profession (Lackman, 2009; Mayer & Cronin, 2008).

Justice: An ethical concept that suggests that there is a fair way to allocate resources.

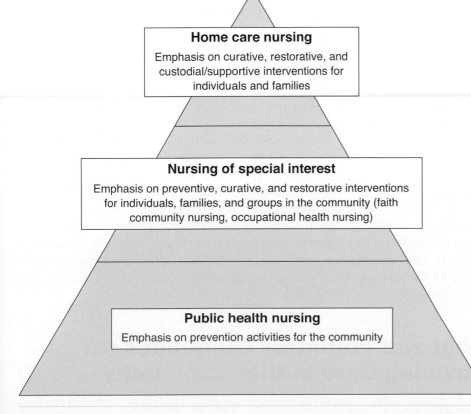

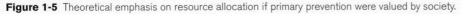

Figure 1-5 Theoretical emphasis on resource allocation if primary prevention were valued by society.

TABLE 1-1

Relationship Among the Concepts of Health–Nursing–Client–Environment in the Community

Focus of Health Outcomes	Characteristic of Nursing Model of Care Delivery	Client Focus of Care Delivery	Environment Settings of Care Delivery
Preventive outcomes	Public health nursing	Aggregates and communities	Local, regional, national, and global settings
Curative outcomes	Acute care nursing	Individual and family	Hospitals and skilled nursing settings
Curative outcomes	Home care (acute and subacute) nursing	Individual and family	Home and assisted living settings
Restorative	Rehabilitation nursing	Individual, family, group, and aggregates	Short-term rehabilitation, home, and assisted living settings
Custodial/supportive	Rehabilitation nursing	Individual, group, and aggregates	Long-term care settings

The Nursing Social Contract as a Mandate to Develop and Maintain Role Competence

Nurses serve at the pleasure of society. Society gives nurses "permission to act" because the profession of nursing has established guidelines to promote the provision of safe and effective nursing care. Nurses, taking this social mandate to heart, are responsible for monitoring their personal skill in providing safe, preventive, curative, restorative, and end-of-life care to people of all ages (ANA, 2011a, 2011b). Nurses in the community have the unique challenge of providing care where people live and congregate outside of acute care settings. Central to the idea of providing safe and effective care in the community is the meaning of professional role competence.

Nurses working in the community have the responsibility for monitoring their own competence to meet the needs of the public. A more detailed discussion of how nurses develop and maintain role competence in community health nursing is offered later in this text. Role competence is possible, in part, through adherence to the guidelines required for the systems of care delivery in the community, and the educational and credentialing expectations that guide nursing practice in the community.

Legal and Voluntary Guidelines for Providing Care in the Community

The provision of health care in the community is regulated by federal, state, and city laws and regulations. Of particular concern are agencies that seek reimbursement from Medicare and Medicaid for services rendered. Agencies are licensed by each state to provide

> ### ANA's Official Position on Professional Role Competence
>
> The public has a right to expect registered nurses to demonstrate professional competence throughout their careers. ANA believes the registered nurse is individually responsible and accountable for maintaining professional competence. The ANA further believes that it is the nursing profession's responsibility to shape and guide any process for assuring nurse competence. Regulatory agencies define minimal standards for regulation of practice to protect the public. The employer is responsible and accountable to provide an environment conducive to competent practice. Assurance of competence is the shared responsibility of the profession, individual nurses, professional organizations, credentialing and certification entities, regulatory agencies, employers, and other key stakeholders (ANA, 2011a).

services according to specific criteria. The Department of Health and Human Services (DHHS) is a federal agency that oversees government healthcare programs such as Social Security, Medicare, and Medicaid. The Health Resources and Services Administration (HRSA) and the Office of Prepaid Health Care Operations and Oversight (OPHOO) are both parts of DHHS. The Health Care Financing Agency (HCFA) is the federal agency responsible for the oversight of Medicaid and Medicare. The federal agency HRSA is part of the U.S. Public Health Service, within DHHS, responsible for developing primary healthcare services and resources, for the health of mothers, infants, and children, and those persons with special needs (National Center for Health Statistics, 2010).

Accreditation is a voluntary process by which a healthcare organization is evaluated by an objective body of its peers on particular standards. The process utilizes established standards so that a specific level of quality is provided. Accreditation bodies monitoring quality in the community include the Community Health Accreditation Program (CHAP), The Joint Commission (an agency often associated with accreditation in acute care settings), and the National Committee for Quality Assurance (NCQA). These organizations, and others, are involved in the accreditation process on national and international levels.

Accreditation: A voluntary process by which a healthcare organization is evaluated by an objective body of its peers on particular standards.

Essentials of Education and Professional Credentialing for Community Health Nursing

Nurses working in the community are expected to be educated, for the most part, with a baccalaureate of science (BS) degree in nursing. These nurses often maintain a caseload of clients, and work fully as a member of the healthcare team in the community. Pre-baccalaureate-educated registered nurses, with associate degree preparation, usually provide more supportive services to BS-prepared nurses and nurses with advanced practice credentials.

Nurses seek graduate education in community health nursing (MS, MSN degree) to assume leadership roles in a variety of institutions. Some nurses working in the community seek master's-level preparation in public health (MPH degree) to complement

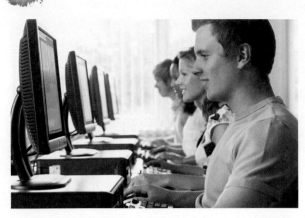

© Monkey Business Images/Shutterstock.com

their employment goals. Doctoral preparation may include completing a doctor of philosophy (PhD degree) to conduct research, a doctor of public health (DrPH degree), or a doctor of nursing practice (DNP degree) for participation in advanced clinical practice in public health and nursing (Buerhaus, Straigler, & Auerbach, 2009).

In addition to formal education, nurses can participate in the process of certification to demonstrate expert clinical practice. The American Nurses Association Credentialing Center and other specialty nursing organizations provide credentialing services for this purpose. The CHN should consider seeking certification in areas that support his or her career goals. For example, nurses in the community may become certified in a specialty such as diabetes care or psychiatric nursing because it fits their role in the community. Certification in community health nursing as a specialty is also available; it demonstrates competence in general or advanced practice.

The guidelines required for the systems of care delivery in the community, and the educational and credentialing expectations that guide nursing practice in the community, were not developed in a vacuum. The long and rich history of nursing in the community is a key aspect of how community health nursing is practiced today.

A Historical Context for Providing Care in the Community

Although a thorough historical overview of how nurses have provided care in the community is beyond the scope of this text, the history of nursing in the community must be respected. The identification of key historical aspects is important to provide evidence of the evolution of healthcare services, so that the community health nurse can better understand those systems that are currently in place. History allows the nurse to review past patterns of care delivery with attention to how they can be improved (Donahue, 2011).

Caring for the sick is as old as humankind. From the beginning of civilization, people have made attempts to relieve the myriad of afflictions that brought pain, agony, suffering, and death to society. Early on, care was mostly palliative because there were no answers to the many questions posed in diagnostic medicine and nursing. The little care that could be provided took place in the home or community. It was much later on that the notion of providing care in hospitals or other places outside of the home developed. After the emergence of hospitals and other care facilities, various economic variables served to promote today's return to providing an increasing amount of care in the home and other community settings (Fungiello, 2005).

The earliest people viewed illness and death as part of the natural phenomena of life, and later as the work of the supernatural beings who were angry or displeased with them. They believed that the sickness and suffering experienced by individuals was caused by wrathful gods and evil demons. Both death and recovery were often looked upon as magical in nature. These beliefs and practices gave rise, in part, to the custom of priests and religious orders serving as healers and formal caregivers.

As awareness of the relationship between hygiene and sickness evolved, efforts turned toward the development of sanitariums and other facilities to provide care. Epidemics (plagues) were a major source of illness, and when these scourges broke out, there was virtually no way to stop them other than to let them run their natural course. Today, the eruption of new and or mutated communicable disease continues to threaten human life (Hays, 2009).

It was not until the eighteenth century that any formal health interventions toward community health were noted. Although the study of community health problems dates back to ancient Greece and Rome, the first indication of government interest in the recording or investigation of disease or issues relating to sanitation occurred during the eighteenth century.

Eighteenth Century

The eighteenth century was notable for the beginning of the sanitary revolution that began to take hold in Europe, especially in England and then ultimately in colonial America. During this time, surveys, geographical mapping of diseases, and sanitation investigations and commissions were commonly undertaken by regional governments. As cities grew during this era, slums grew along with them, as did the concomitant problems associated with the inner-city environment, such as high morbidity and mortality rates.

In England, as a result of the Industrial Revolution, people began to flock to cities for work. This wave of immigration created slums and quickly spread infectious diseases. The most significant healthcare discovery during that time was the 1796 discovery of inoculation by Edward Jenner (1749–1823). At that time, the vast majority of the English population was afflicted with smallpox to some degree. Jenner realized that those persons who worked with cattle had milder and fewer cases of smallpox, and this observation led him to an understanding of the idea of immunity, a concept previously unknown in science. At the same time, immigration of colonists to America and the rush to large cities in America as part of industrialization in that country ensured that communicable disease also became an American healthcare problem.

Copper engraving (c. 1656) of Doctor Schnabel, a plague doctor in seventeenth-century Rome, with a satirical macaronic poem ("Vos Creditis, als eine Fabel, / quod scribitur vom Doctor Schnabel") in octosyllabic rhyming couplets.

Die Karikatur und Satire in der Medizin: Medico-Kunsthistorische Studie von Professor Dr. Eugen Holländer, 2nd ed. (Stuttgart: Ferdinand Enke, 1921), Fig. 79 (p. 171).

Colonial America

Crossing the Atlantic Ocean did not improve the quality of available health care. In early America, hospitals comprised either almshouses for the poor and indigent or pesthouses for those persons with contagious diseases. Most care of the ill and most births took place at home, with care being provided by physicians or lay midwives. Institutions, by comparison, were often created to keep the impoverished away from the general public rather than to serve their needs.

The medical profession, still without the benefit of antiseptics and antibiotics, could do little to help those afflicted with disease. Treatment remained crude, as did methods for sanitation and hygiene. Physicians in America had no formal education; instead, skill and training in health care were acquired in an apprentice system. Hospital nurses were responsible for nothing more than general cleaning, scrubbing floors and pots, and doing the laundry. Many nurses were illiterate, disinterested, and totally untrained persons working in hospitals.

Infectious disease remained the major healthcare problem, especially smallpox, which was estimated to affect one in five people, including President George Washington. Later, it was yellow fever that brought terror to the colonies. The first hospital in America was located in Philadelphia, and was established at the urging of Benjamin Franklin. It was his belief that the general public had a responsibility to the poor, sickly, and needy immigrant populations. Franklin wrote a petition seeking permission to build what was to become Pennsylvanian Hospital (1751). Later, New York Hospital was built under a charter granted by King George III in 1770 and opened in 1790. Its stated pur-

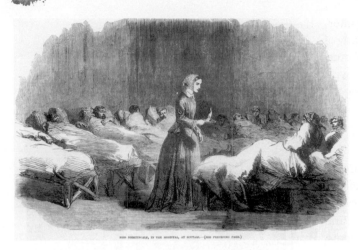

© Photos.com/Thinkstock

pose was to prevent the spread of infectious diseases that were brought into the port city by new immigrants and sailors.

Nineteenth Century

In the nineteenth century, communicable diseases such as typhoid and typhus ravaged Europe, killing more people than any of the wars fought on the continent. So desperate were the conditions that England passed the first sanitary legislation in 1837. Nevertheless, child mortality rates in industrial cities were still 50% before children reached the age of five.

Sir Edwin Chadwick (1800–1890), an English social reformer, was instrumental in amending the Poor Law in 1834. As an outcome of his efforts, issues such as child welfare, care for the mentally ill, care of the elderly, standards for factory workers, and education were addressed. In 1842, Chadwick's publication, *The Sanitary Conditions of the Labouring Population*, increased the public's awareness of public health to such an extent that the Public Health Act of 1848 was passed, which established a Board of Health.

An important discovery in England was made during this time by John Snow, a physician, anesthetist, and epidemiologist. During the major cholera epidemic of 1854 in London, Snow proved that water was the source of contamination and spread of cholera. These discoveries helped to bring about an increase in civic understanding and moral commitment to the betterment of people's lives through economic, social, and environmental reform. This shift in the way people felt about their civic and moral responsibilities helped healthcare providers move from the sole care of individuals to the care of populations.

Florence Nightingale and the Beginning of Modern Nursing

In freeing herself from the constraints of Victorian society, Florence Nightingale (1820–1910) changed the profession of nursing forever. Actually, before Nightingale, there was no profession of nursing. Nightingale came from the upper class at a time when it was considered unseemly for a well-bred lady to be involved in the unsightly and unsanitary care of the sick. She was always attracted to philanthropic works, planning programs for the care and welfare of the needy.

With the outbreak of Crimean War between Russia and England in 1854 came newspaper reports of the appalling health conditions of the wounded English solders. More lives were lost to contaminated wounds, infections, and an epidemic of cholera than were lost fighting the actual battles. Members of the upper strata of London society were stunned and horrified by the accounts they read. The stories of the plight of their young men were more than they could bear, and they let their political leaders know of their displeasure. Nightingale was asked to help, and she and 14 nurses arrived at the military hospital to find that there were no beds, blankets, soap, or wash basins for the sick and wounded soldiers.

The death rate among the wounded was almost 50%. Nightingale and her meager staff cleaned the barracks, washed clothes, cooked, and fed those patients too weak to feed themselves. At first they were resented by the medical and administrative staff, but in short order, upon seeing the extraordinary changes that were made, Nightingale won their admiration. She also wrote to her family's wealthy friends and government officials to acquire much needed supplies and equipment. Reading the stories of her phenomenal work, the English responded overwhelmingly to her appeal, and contributions for provisions poured forth.

Upon returning to London, Nightingale was asked to turn her efforts to the needs of England. In 1859, she published a 77-page text entitled *Notes on Nursing: What It Is and What It Is Not.* This text, which addressed issues of prevention and general good health, was an immediate best seller. In her classic work, Nightingale stressed the need for hygiene, good food, sunlight, sanitation, sewerage, and attractive and comfortable surroundings for healing.

According to Nightingale, nurses were to be sober, educated, well trained, cleanly dressed, and, above all, kind and caring to their charges. Nightingale always stressed the importance of prevention as well as prompt and efficient care. Perhaps the most famous quote attributed to her is the description of nursing that identifies two major components of nursing: health nursing and sick nursing. Health nursing was "to keep or put the constitution of a healthy person in such a state as to have no disease," and sick nursing was "to help the person suffering from disease to live and regain a state of wellness" (Dolan, 1968; Klainberg & Dirschel, 2010).

Nightingale's work filtered across the Atlantic Ocean and became the basis for the modern nursing movement in the United States—a movement also driven by the horrors of war and the healthcare needs created by war. Military nursing today remains an important factor in caring for society. During this time, Florence Nightingale encouraged nurses to be assigned to work in the community with physicians in a local dispensary, a practice that has been referred to as the forerunner of community health nursing.

The Civil War

The Civil War created the impetus for the improvement of health care in the United States. The catastrophic number of wounded and mutilated soldiers that resulted from the Civil War created the need to provide health care for the troops wounded in battle. More than 2,000 untrained nurses participated in the Civil War, but that number was not nearly enough. If wounded soldiers survived their immediate injuries, they were then susceptible to various infections and diseases.

Seeing the inhumanity of the Civil War and outraged by its atrocities, Clara Barton, trained as a teacher and often referred to as the "American Florence Nightingale," became a national heroine as her reputation spread throughout the country. Founder of the American Red Cross, Barton began her one-woman crusade against the horrors of war after she witnessed many of them. Like Nightingale, Barton delivered lanterns to surgeons so that they could continue to treat and operate throughout the night. She brought food, clean bandages, and blankets, but mostly—like Nightingale—she brought caring, kindness, and the knowledge that she could help save the lives of the young men in battle. Untrained but not unskilled, Barton proved to the military leaders of the day that her presence, and those she brought with her, would be a help and not a hindrance to the war effort.

Immigration to the United States

New York City has always been a major disembarkation point for immigrants who were seeking to start new lives in the United States. In this sense, its experience is reflective of that of other cities that have served as ports of disembarkation, such as New Orleans and Miami. New York City has also been a place where economically deprived people have lived in large numbers, bringing their own unique set of healthcare needs to be tended. Historically, their presence has posed a dilemma, as the city has often had insufficient resolve or resources to address these needs, which have differed with every new wave of immigrants.

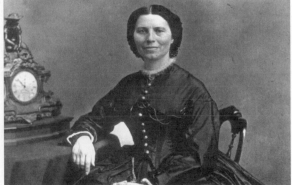

© National Library of Medicine

The late 1800s saw a shift in U.S.-bound immigration patterns. Originally, most immigrants came from England, Ireland, and Germany, largely in reaction to the economic and political conditions found in Europe at that time. That influx was followed by a wave of immigrants from southern and eastern parts of Europe. Jewish and Italian immigrants moved into the slums previously occupied by their German and Irish predecessors. Little attention or consideration was given to light, air, or sanitation in the densely populated tenements, creating a slum environment filled with discontent and unrest. It was the extremes of poverty, illiteracy, ignorance, misery, wretchedness, disease, filth, crime, corruption, depravity, and human degradation that allowed the political structure of the cities to become so corrupt, and planted the seeds for the social reform movement of the 19th century.

Nursing in Early American Communities

In the United States, trained nurses visiting at the homes of the sick first appeared in 1813. The Ladies Benevolent Society was the first to organize women in Charleston, South Carolina, to visit the sick poor. In 1819, the Hebrew Female Benevolent Society of Philadelphia organized a visiting nurses' organization comprising volunteer nurses who visited the sick. In 1839, the nurses' society of Philadelphia assigned female home visitors to care for the sick at home; in 1877, the first educated nurses were sent to care for the sick poor at home; and in 1885, Lillian Wald was closely associated with the establishment of the Visiting Nurses Association.

Perhaps an even more important and profound development during this era was the beginning of the social reform movement and the spirit of advocacy that the settlement workers brought to the consciousness of wealthy Americans. Most of these settlement workers themselves came from the privileged class, but they informed and ultimately interested their peers in the problems and plight of the poor. Social reformers were inspired with a sense of unrelenting mission to bring about change; although they worked on several of large cities' problems at the same time, the common thread among all of these endeavors was the belief that the most important task was education.

Lillian Wald, Mary Brewster, and Lavinia Dock

Born in 1867, Lillian Wald, influenced by family relatives who were physicians, came to New York and entered the New York Hospital School of Nursing (Kalisch & Kalisch, 1978). Wald trained for the standard three years, graduating in 1891. She then went to work at the Juvenile Asylum for a year, but left this position after becoming unhappy and frustrated by her lack of medical knowledge. This frustration brought her to the Woman's Medical College in New York. During her time there, she and another nurse, Mary Brewster, were asked to go to the Lower East Side of New York to lecture to immigrant mothers about how to care for their sick children and family members.

Together, Wald and Brewster began a district nursing service in New York City. They moved into the neighborhood that they were planning to serve because they felt it would help people in the community view them as friends and be more willing to confide their problems. Years later, in 1895, Wald and Brewster opened the Nurses' Settlement at 265 Henry Street, working with other nurses including Lavinia Dock. It was Wald who first used the term "public health nurse." She put a preface on Florence Nightingale's term "health nursing" to signify that these nurses would be concerned directly with the needs of the people in general.

By 1900, as many as 20 district nursing organizations with more than 200 nurses were operational; most were found in large cities, although some did exist in small communities. Nursing also expanded

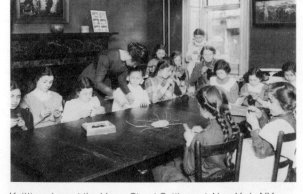

Knitting class at the Henry Street Settlement, New York, NY (1910).

Courtesy of the Library of Congress. Photographed by Lewis Wickes Hines.

into school and occupational settings. School nursing rapidly became an integral and indispensable part of the health care of the young, while occupational health nursing served those in the workplace.

Twentieth Century: Establishment of Community Service

Nursing can and should be viewed as one of the earliest forms of community service. It is related to the strong, perhaps instinctive, desire to preserve and protect the members of one's own group. As civilization grew, this notion was extended to include other groups, tribes, clans, townspeople, and ultimately strangers. It could be argued that the earliest form of nursing was that which took place in the community.

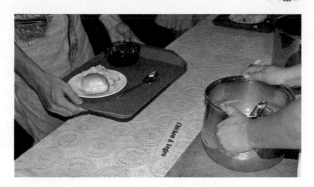

© Bob Denelzen/ShutterStock.com

It was during the beginning of the twentieth century, in a time characterized by the enormous and persistent demands of immigration and infectious disease, that American nursing had the foresight, intuition, and historical experience to move into community-based care. Always aware that social context was important to the health care of its population, nurses fed the hungry in neighborhood soup kitchens and tended to the needs of schoolchildren with immunizations, growth scales, and hygiene classes. When the sick could not get to the physician's office, the community health nurse came to the client.

With the dawn of the new century, perhaps the greatest reforms in nursing occurred in relation to public health. The knowledge and information nurses needed to provide care in the community far outstripped anything they had learned in nursing school. It was out of necessity that the specialty of the public health nurse emerged as an essential service. Originally the term "public health nursing" was used more often than "community health nursing," although for a while they were thought to be interchangeable. Community health nursing is the result of the ever growing and changing needs of a rapidly changing society. Community health nursing, influenced by reforms in public health, education, and societal needs, is a direct reflection of the growth and change in the modern world.

Today, the ANA uses the term "community nursing" to encompass the care provided by those nurses who work in public health, schools, industry, and other community-based clinics, services, and organizations. The twentieth century saw many gains in the general health of the public, and the twenty-first century began with a focus, in part, on the high cost of health care. Today, a major reevaluation of how healthcare dollars are spent is under way. Concerns about healthcare costs pose threats to government programs such as Medicare, hospital stays are becoming shorter, and there is a possibility that caps on spending will be placed on health care for special interest groups such as the elderly. New problems in healthcare financing are emerging, in part because some people are unable to pay for care due to inadequacies in insurance coverage or lack of any coverage at all.

Health Care in the Twenty-First Century

A priority of twenty-first-century health care relates to healthcare insurance issues and the individuals, families, and communities who are either uninsured or underinsured. An attempt to provide insurance for all has become a hot-button political

Healthy People: A U.S. federal government initiative that has generated lists of objectives and desired outcomes of health care for the decades 2000, 2010, and 2020.

issue and, at this book's writing, continued to be addressed by the members of the U.S. Congress and the president of the United States. Many factors impinge on the healthcare insurance (and general cost) debate, including the increased cost of basic healthcare services, decreasing government contributions to payment of healthcare services, inconsistent patterns of "length of stay" in healthcare institutions, aging of the U.S. population, and aging of both lay and professional caregivers (Anderson, Rice, & Kominski, 2007).

The United States has, to some extent, implemented a coordinated national response to the many ethical, legal and financial complexities of providing healthcare services. With a focus on health promotion and disease prevention, the *Healthy People* initiative has generated lists of objectives and desired outcomes of health care for the decades 2000, 2010, and now 2020 (Sultz & Young, 2011). The development of objectives is intended to identify important health concerns and specifically address ways to measure progress every 10 years. The resulting objectives focus on interventions that are designed to reduce or eliminate illness, disability, and premature death among individuals and communities. Some identify broader concerns such as the elimination of health disparities, dealing with either social determinates of health, or improving public health services and access to care (National Center for Health Statistics, 2009, 2010).

As previously mentioned, the Patient Protection and Affordable Care Act (Affordable Care Act) became law (P.L. 111-148) in March 2010. The Affordable Care Act (ACA) is complex legislation with a multi-year phase-in process. It is essentially a measure to make health care available to all but a few exempt groups dramatically changing issues that relate to individual responsibility to participate in access, restructuring cost systems to pay for care (including insurance coverage), and redefinition of Medicaid coverage (Kaiser Family Foundation, 2011, April 15). Exempt groups, like incarcerated persons, and Native Americans will receive care from different government programs.

The law, having been challenged as to its constitutionality, was supported, for the most part, by the Supreme Court in June 2012. The court supported the need for individuals to participate in securing health care, but did not fully support the expansion of Medicaid, a joint state–federal venture to provide care primarily for people living in poverty (Kaiser Family Foundation, 2012; *New York Times*, 2012).

In the first two decades of the twenty-first century, increasing attention has been given to healthcare reform. Legislation is dramatically changing the landscape of who can have access to care and how they will obtain it. The Patient Protection and Affordable Care Act of 2010 and the Health Care and Education Affordability Act of 2010 call for major changes in healthcare delivery over the next 20 years (Henry J. Kaiser Family Foundation, 2011). **Table 1-2** identifies some reasons why people are for or against the many reform changes.

It is difficult to be "against" the sweeping changes of healthcare reform; after all, many more people will get the care they need to improve their health. A question does surface, however, about how the United States will be able to afford the sweeping reforms. How will the federal and state pool of resources need to be altered to pay for healthcare reform? Is the American public willing to shift money from military spending, education, or public health prevention to provide more acute illness care to the public? What will be the consequences of shifting resources from one set of priorities to another in an effort to realize healthcare reform?

TABLE 1-2
Rationale for Supporting Healthcare Reform

1. Americans will have access to quality, affordable health care.
2. The ability for all consumers to purchase affordable health care.
3. Extend much needed relief to small businesses.
4. Expand Medicare to help seniors and people with disabilities afford their prescription drugs.
5. Prohibit denials of coverage based on preexisting conditions.
6. Limit out-of-pocket costs so that Americans have greater security and peace of mind.
7. Require insurers to include children on their parents' healthcare plan until age 26.
8. Increase access for Medicaid to low-income Americans.
9. Provide sliding-scale subsidies to make insurance premiums affordable.
10. Hold insurance companies accountable for how healthcare dollars are spent.
11. Prevent insurance company abuses.
12. Increase and improve preventive care services.

Source: Adapted from Stand Up for Health Care. (2010). *12 reasons to support health care.* Retrieved from http://www.standupforhealthcare.org/learn-more/quick-facts/12-reasons-to-support-health-care

Reflecting on the Possibilities for the Future

Today, healthcare delivery is experiencing turbulent changes in its legal, political, and application settings. Two documents have emerged that may help stabilize the healthcare environment, as participants in this environment reexamine critical issues related to access to care, healthcare financing, and nursing's role in current and future systems of care. The IOM guidelines for the future of nursing (IOM, 2011) and the QSEN competencies (Cronenwett et al., 2007) challenge the CHN to actively participate in the creation of a future for the nursing profession in increasingly complex care delivery systems. The IOM and QSEN documents, discussed in more detail later in this text, provide a common sense of direction for nursing's involvement in keeping the public healthy for generations to come.

Summary

This chapter introduced a number of important concerns in providing care in the community. Reflective practice was introduced as a concept that the CHN uses to ensure the delivery of comprehensive care in the community. Nursing in the community is different from the acute care approach to care used in hospitals and other acute care settings, with the major difference in care being related to the core functions that guide nursing practice in the community.

The functions of assessment, policy development, and assurance link the work of nurses in the community with that of other healthcare providers. The needs of the public require continuous assessment. The public must engage in policy development to secure the health services they need. Communities can proceed to get their needs met when they feel assured that services and personnel will be available to the community.

The paradigm of providing care in the community requires a special understanding of the concepts central to community health nursing practice. In community health nursing practice, the concepts of client, nursing, health, environment, and distributive justice take on special meaning. As in other settings, the key to providing quality nursing care in the community is role competence.

The CHN needs to participate fully in the process of community engagement, so as to demonstrate competence as a provider of nursing care to the community. This chapter linked the idea of role competence with legal and voluntary guidelines for providing care from a regulatory perspective, and the essentials for professional education and credentialing that support community health nursing practice.

A brief historical overview of some key aspects of the development of community health nursing practice was presented in this chapter as well. Of particular importance is the link between the history of yesterday and the history that is being made today, in the context of healthcare reform. The process of deciding who will receive the care that they request or require, and who will provide it, is central to the ongoing development of community health nursing as a discipline in the service of the public's health.

The chapter ended with a beginning reflection upon the possibilities for nursing's future in community health by introducing the IOM guidelines for the future of nursing and the QSEN competencies, developed to improve community health and all other types of nursing care.

REFERENCES

American Nurses Association (ANA). (2010a). *Nursing: Scope and standards of practice* (3rd ed.). Silver Spring, MD: Author.

American Nurses Association (ANA). (2010b). *Nursing's social policy statement: The essence of the profession.* Silver Spring, MD: Author.

American Nurses Association (ANA). (2011a). *ANA's official position on professional role competence.* Retrieved from http://www.nursingworld.org/MainMenuCategories/ThePracticeofProfessional Nursing/NursingEducation.aspx

American Nurses Association (ANA). (2011b). *Definition of nursing.* Retrieved from http://www .nursingworld.org/MainMenuCategories/ThePracticeofProfessionalNursing.aspx

American Public Health Association (APHA). (2010). *Definition of public health nursing practice.* Retrieved from http://www.apha.org/membergroups/sections/aphasections/phn/about/ defbackground.htm

American Public Health Association (APHA), Public Health Nursing Section. (1996). *The definition and role of public health nursing.* Washington, DC: Author.

Anderson, R. M., Rice, T. H., & Kominski, G. F. (Eds.). (2007). *Changing the U.S. health care system: Key issues in health services policy and management* (3rd ed.). San Francisco, CA: John Wiley & Sons.

Association of Community Health Nursing Educators (ACHNE). (2009). *Essentials of baccalaureate nursing education for entry level community/public health nursing.* Wheat Ridge, CO: Author.

Buerhaus, P. I., Staiger, D. O., & Auerbach, D. I. (2009). *The future of the nursing workforce in the United States: Data, trends, and implications.* Sudbury, MA: Jones and Bartlett.

Centers for Disease Control and Prevention (CDC). (2010, June 25). Summary of notifiable diseases—United States, 2008. *Morbidity and Mortality Weekly Report, 57*(54).

Cronenwett, L., Sherwood, G., Barnsteiner, J., Disch, J., Johnson, J., Mitchel, P., ... Warren, J. (2007). Quality and safety education for nurses. *Nursing Outlook, 55*(3), 122–131.

Dolan, J. A. (1968). *History of nursing*. Philadelphia, PA: W. B. Saunders.

Donahue, M. P. (2011). *Nursing the finest art: An illustrated history* (3rd ed.). Maryland Heights, MO, MO: Mosby Elsevier.

Fungiello, P. J. (2005). *Chronic politics: Health care security from FDR to George W. Bush*. St. Louis, MO: Mosby.

Hays, J. N. (2009). *The burdens of disease: Epidemics and human response in western history*. New Brunswick, NJ: Rutgers University Press.

Henry J. Kaiser Family Foundation. (2011). *Health reform source*. Retrieved from http://health reform.kff.org/timeline

Henry J. Kaiser Family Foundation. (2011, April 15). Summary of the new health reform law. *Focus on Health Reform (Pub. #8061)*. Menlo Park, CA: Author.

Henry J. Kaiser Family Foundation. (2012, January). A guide to the Supreme Court's review of the 2010 health care reform law. *Focus on Health Reform (Pub. #8270)*. Menlo Park, CA: Author.

Institute of Medicine (IOM). (2011). *The future of nursing: Leading change, advancing health*. Washington, DC: Author.

Kalisch, P. A., & Kalisch, B. J. (1978). *The advance of American nursing*. Boston: Little, Brown.

Klainberg, M., & Dirschel, K. (2010). *Today's nursing leader: Managing, succeeding, excelling*. Sudbury, MA: Jones and Bartlett.

Lackman, V. D. (2009). Practical use of the nursing code of ethics: Part II. *MEDSURG Nursing, 18*(3), 191–194.

Mayer, C. M., & Cronin, D. (2008). Organizational accountability in a just culture. *Urologic Nursing, 28*(6), 427–430.

Milstead, J. A. (2008). *Health policy and politics: A nurse's guide* (3rd ed.). Sudbury, MA: Jones and Bartlett.

National Center for Health Statistics (NCHS). (2009). *Health, United States, 2009: With a special feature on medical technology*. Hyattsville, MD: U.S. Government Printing Office. Retrieved from http://www.cdc.gov/nchs/hus.htm

National Center for Health Statistics (NCHS). (2010). *Health, United States, 2010: With a special feature on death and dying*. Hyattsville, MD: U.S. Government Printing Office.

New York Times. (2012, July 17). Health care reform and the Supreme Court (Affordable Care Act). Retrieved from http://topics.nytimes.com/top/reference/timestopics/organizations/s/supreme _court/affordable_care_act/index.html

Rawls, J. (1971). *A theory of justice*. Cambridge, MD: Harvard University Press.

Sultz, H. A., & Young, K. M. (2011). *Health care USA: Understanding its organization and delivery* (7th ed.). Sudbury, MA: Jones & Bartlett Learning.

U.S. Census Bureau. (2010). *Statistical abstract of the United States: 2010* (129th ed.). Washington, DC: Author. Retrieved from http://www.census.gov/statab/overview.html

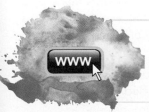

For a full suite of assignments and additional learning activities, use the access code located in the front of your book to visit the exclusive website: http://go.jblearning.com/Holzemer/. If you do not have an access code, you can obtain one at the site.

LEARNING ACTIVITIES   `WWW`

1. Which of the following is the best example of a public health nursing intervention?

    A. Applying wet-to-dry dressings in the home, three times a week

    B. Developing a program for an aggregate that demonstrates a changing need for services in the community

    C. Answering an emergency crisis phone line for abused women

    D. Attending risk-reduction meetings for recovering alcoholic adolescents in a shelter

2. Which of the following nursing interventions is most important to implement, from a public health perspective?

    A. Installing handrails for senior adults in a nursing home

    B. Instructing neighbors in a community to create a "Safety Watch"

    C. Monitoring toxic emissions from a clean water plant

    D. Implementing statewide screening for scoliosis

3. Which term is used by the American Nurses Association to encompass the work done by nurses in areas such as industry, schools, and community-based clinics?

    A. Public health nursing

    B. Community nursing

    C. Community-based health care

    D. Community-focused nursing

4. John Snow was famous for his discoveries in 1854 in London related to a disease outbreak associated with which of the following pathogens?

    A. *Escherichia coli*

    B. Yellow fever

    C. Cholera

    D. Bubonic plague

5. The discoveries of John Snow helped to bring about an increase in which of the following health-related ideas?

    A. A civic understanding and moral commitment to the betterment of people's lives through economic, social, and environmental reform

    B. A commitment of the government to reduce taxes on health care

    C. The need for health insurance for all citizens of London

    D. The understanding that there needed to be more control by the police in enforcing health laws

6. The focus of *Healthy People 2020* is related to which of the following ideas?

    A. Economic provision of low-cost health care for all citizens

    B. Development of objectives and outcomes intended to identify and address important health concerns in society

    C. Healthcare reform that will require health insurance for all

    D. Development and implementation of required healthcare services for citizens of every state in the United States

7. Which of the following statements made by a nurse reflects the idea that a major change is necessary in the delivery of nursing care in the community?

    A. "The amount of home care services needs to be increased."

    B. "Special interest groups need to provide services that are missing in the community."

    C. "There is too much regulation in the care that is provided to people in the community."

    D. "Nurses need to help people learn the value of preventive services."

8. Which of the following is an example of nursing services sponsored by a special interest group?

   A. State monitoring of safe drinking water
   B. A diabetic foot-care program offered in a large, regional nursing home
   C. A variety of health screening events taking place in a collection of houses of worship
   D. Bereavement counseling provided after the death of domestic pets

9. A nurse is discussing the core functions of public health. Which of the following activities relates to assessment?

   A. Meet with members of the community to explain services
   B. Evaluate the competencies of the home care staff
   C. Review laws on communicable disease prevention
   D. Monitor proper seatbelt use in children

10. A nurse is discussing the core functions of public health. Which of the following relates to assurance?

   A. Families feel safe in their communities.
   B. Groups have a place to meet for their planned activities.
   C. People believe that the care is safe and available.
   D. Individuals decrease their use of emergency departments for routine care.

ADDITIONAL QUESTIONS FOR STUDY

1. Visit the website of *Healthy People* and compare the goals of *Healthy People 2020* with those of *Healthy People 2000*. Write a brief paper describing what you see as the differences, if any, between these goals. What would you like to see incorporated into *Healthy People 2030*?

2. Identify a health-related problem in the community and examine the core functions of public health. For each aspect, explain how the core function relates to the problem.

3. Define the terms associated with the community health nursing paradigm. Compare your definitions with those of your classmates, and expand your definitions based on their ideas.

CHAPTER OUTLINE

- ▸ Introduction
- ▸ The Relationship Between Respect and an Ethical and Cultural Context for Care in the Community
- ▸ An Ethical Context for Care in the Community
  - Ethics Defined
  - Code of Ethics
  - Selected Ethical Principles
  - Ethical Issues in the Community
  - Community Engagement and Social Action in Health Care

- Ethics, Values, and Moral Reasoning Related to Community Health Nursing
- Ethical Decisions of the Community Health Nurse
- ▸ A Cultural Context for Care in the Community
  - The Influence of Health Beliefs and Culture on Health Care
  - Cultural Variations in Social Interaction
  - Cultural Sensitivity of the Community Health Nurse
- ▸ Summary

OBJECTIVES

`www`

1. Explain how the concept of respect relates to both an ethical and cultural context for providing care in the community.

2. Identify the ethical principles that guide community health nursing care delivery, education, and research.

3. Discuss how personal values influence the types of community-based services that are made available to the public.

4. Prioritize the list of major community health problems that need resolution in the learner's local community.

KEY TERMS

`www`

Advance medical
directives

Autonomy

Beneficence

Code of ethics

Confidentiality

Curandero

Distributive justice

"Do not resuscitate"
(DNR) order

Egalitarian justice

Environmental press

Ethical pluralism

Ethics

Health Insurance
Portability and
Accountability Act
(HIPAA)

Informed consent

Ladder of participation

Scope of practice

Third-party payment

Utilitarian justice

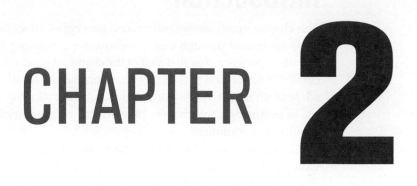

CHAPTER **2**

Respect for an Ethical and Cultural Context for Care in the Community

Marilyn Klainberg

Introduction

This chapter examines two interrelated concepts—ethics and cultural beliefs. These concepts are related through their fundamental grounding in the client's personal beliefs and life experience. The first part of the chapter defines ethics and discusses ethical concerns that are central to the practice of community health nursing. These issues include advance directives, quality of life, the cost and rationing of health care, the increasing use of technology, and the way in which the community health nurse (CHN) works in an ethical environment.

The second part of the chapter examines culture and the influence of culture on providing and receiving nursing care in the community. In the United States, clients seeking nursing care in the community come from a variety of cultural backgrounds. For some of these individuals, understanding the importance of culture is the key to developing a therapeutic and lasting nurse–client relationship.

The Relationship Between Respect and an Ethical and Cultural Context for Care in the Community

Demonstrating respect for the health-related choices of clients (as individuals, families, aggregates, and communities) is the responsibility of nurses working in the community. Respect becomes authentic when it encompasses the ethical and cultural context or setting where care is delivered. This chapter examines both the ethical and cultural context for providing care in the community, and considers how the CHN can participate in care with respect for the decision-making process employed by various clients. Ethical and cultural concerns arise when working with all individuals, families, other groups, and communities as a whole. The CHN needs to be aware that respect for the client, in whatever configuration, is central to the success of providing care from a sound ethical and culturally sensitive perspective.

An Ethical Context for Care in the Community

Like other healthcare providers, the CHN faces innumerable moral decisions and ethical dilemmas each day. Working in a community setting may entail working in community-based agencies, public health institutions, clients' homes, or other places where clients reside. The CHN, therefore, operates within a framework of ethical and moral decision making that is often unique. Each community has its own culture, values, and morals that may be distinct and influence the decision-making process. Ethical and moral decisions are based on a standard of behavior developed within a culture or society. Nurses are guided by a professional code of ethics as they develop various nurse–client relationships (American Nurses Association [ANA], 2001; Fowler, 2010).

An ethical approach to the provision of health care is a mandate of nursing. Nurses' code of ethics interprets moral principles upon which nursing actions are measured. These principles include respect for a person's autonomy and the ideas of beneficence, nonmaleficence, veracity, confidentiality, and justice. Since 1953, guidance on ethical action has also been provided on an international level by the International Council of Nurses (ICN). The international code of ethics addresses the need for nurses to respect human rights as they provide care to their clients. The ICN code has been made available in a variety of languages, and is available on the organization's website (http://www.icn.ch).

Ethics Defined

The definition of **ethics** is complex. Although ethics are intensely personal, they also reflect the society in which one lives. Ethics is often referred to as a system of moral principles, or the rules or guidelines of a particular group, culture, or society. It is the branch of philosophy that deals with values and moral principles related to human conduct. Whether one's actions are considered right or wrong or good or bad is often determined by one's culture (Dayer-Berenson, 2011; Skott, 2003).

The impact of a culture on ethical decision making was identified by Kurt Lewin as environmental press. **Environmental press** refers to the pressure brought upon individuals by a culture or society that produces specific behaviors. Environmental pressures may either facilitate or inhibit a person in behaving in certain ways (Lewin, 1936). A person's behavior, according to Lewin's theory, is a function of the relationship between the person and the environment. This theory is illustrated by the following example.

Since the late 1980s, as a result of economics and improved technology, providers of healthcare services in the United States have begun to debate the issue of rationing health care for severely disabled and elderly persons. Until this time, it had been the goal of health care providers to dispense equal care to all. Recently, however, cost factors and issues of quality of life related to health care have raised fundamental questions about the aims and goals of health care. Despite this dialogue concerning cost containment, basic values related to health care presently remain the same. It is, however, a significant matter, and with changes occurring in society and how health care is provided, it is an issue that continues to be deliberated (Ray, 2010).

Code of Ethics

Many professional groups have a code of ethics or principles that acts as a beacon, guiding group members toward the way in which the profession is conducted. A **code of ethics** comprises the rules by which a profession is guided. The American Nurses Association has developed a code of ethics that expresses the duties, values, and ethical responsibilities of the professional nurse. Nurses accept a moral and legal obligation to abide by this code when they accept the role of the nurse in all client-care settings. **Table 2-1** summarizes the key aspects of the ANA code (ANA, 2001; Fowler, 2010).

Selected Ethical Principles

Autonomy

The term **autonomy** means independence or self-determination. Autonomy is the right of individuals and society to decide for themselves how to mandate their own lives. The notion of autonomy implies respect for each person as unique and maintains each person's right to determine his or her own destiny. Autonomy is an important part of American bioethics and means that adults have the right to make their own healthcare decisions. When the community determines how persons should choose, even if the client's choice is considered "bad" by the larger society, the society is imposing its will over the rights of an individual.

Although this imposition may seem to be in conflict with human rights, a society imposes its decisions when it believes that those decisions will ensure the betterment and safety of the larger community or are in the best interest of the individual. Examples include mandated laws related to the use of seatbelts and the deterrence of smoking in

Ethics: A system of moral principles, or the rules or guidelines of a particular group, culture, or society.

Environmental press: The pressure brought upon individuals by a culture or society that produces specific behaviors.

Code of ethics: The rules by which a profession is guided.

Autonomy: Independence or self-determination.

TABLE 2-1
Code of Ethics of the American Nurses Association

1.	The nurse, in all professional relationships, practices with compassion and respect for the inherent dignity, worth, and uniqueness of every individual, unrestricted by considerations of social or economic status, personal attributes, or the nature of health problems.
2.	The nurse's primary commitment is to the patient, whether an individual, family, group, or community.
3.	The nurse promotes, advocates for, and strives to protect the health, safety, and rights of the patient.
4.	The nurse is responsible and accountable for individual nursing practice and determines the appropriate delegation of tasks consistent with the nurse's obligation to provide optimum patient care.
5.	The nurse owes the same duties to self as to others, including the responsibility to preserve integrity and safety, to maintain competence, and to continue personal and professional growth.
6.	The nurse participates in establishing, maintaining, and improving healthcare environments and conditions of employment conducive to the provision of quality health care and consistent with the values of the profession through individual and collective action.
7.	The nurse participates in the advancement of the profession through contributions to practice, education, administration, and knowledge development.
8.	The nurse collaborates with other health professionals and the public in promoting community, national, and international efforts to meet health needs.
9.	The profession of nursing, as represented by associations and their members, is responsible for articulating nursing values, for maintaining the integrity of the profession and its practice, and for shaping social policy.

Source: © 2001 Code of Ethics for Nurses with Interpretive Statements. By American Nurses Association. Reprinted with permission. All Rights Reserved.

Advance medical directives: Legal orders that permit clients to choose in advance the type of healthcare treatment they want.

"Do not resuscitate" (DNR) order: A medical order to abstain from cardiopulmonary resuscitation if the client's heart stops beating.

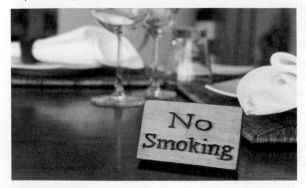

public places. These issues of prevention and safety are controversial: On the one hand, they are aimed at increasing wellness; on the other hand, they create are an ethical dilemma in that they interfere with the autonomy of the individual. Autonomy means that people have the right to make their own healthcare decisions, whether good or bad, without interference from the society in which they live.

The degree of participation and a striving toward autonomy by the individual or the community as a whole often indicate how well the community or an individual has succeeded in self-care or wellness. The degree of autonomy often predicts the degree of success that will be achieved in regard to a health goal. Because the extent to which individuals have control over their own lives affects their well-being, empowering clients to take charge of healthcare decisions is a primary health promotion strategy.

Advance medical directives such as a **"do not resuscitate" (DNR) order** are examples of how clients can have a voice in their care. A DNR is a medical order to abstain from cardiopulmonary resuscitation (CPR) if the client's heart stops beating. Other advance directives permit clients to choose in advance the type of treatment they want if they become too ill to indicate the care they want. Likewise, the right to receive or refuse treatment is a major ethical issue. The growth in the number of clients with long-term care needs or hospice care needs at home (either by family members or home health attendants) raises ethical questions of a different nature.

In caring for a client at home, the principle of autonomy related to medical issues remains clear; however, unlike in institutional settings, issues related to client care issues at home are often complex. Outside of the institution, there are other persons whose rights and interests are affected by the client's choices, and these considerations must be included when decisions are made. In these situations, autonomy may give way to accommodation, as part of an effort to include the needs of the family in the decision-making process. For example, if the main caregiver is unable to provide all the care necessary and desired by the client, the community health nurse may need to assist the family to accommodate and meet the needs of all parties concerned.

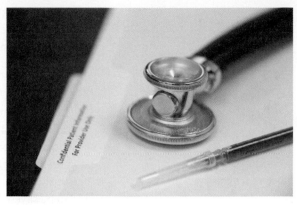

© SNEHIT/Shutterstock.com

Beneficence

Beneficence is a healthcare principle that mandates that the healthcare provider "do good for the client." Adhering to this principle may become a complicated issue when the healthcare provider also attempts to do that which the client wishes. If there is conflict between what is considered good by the profession and what the client wants, the nurse must abide by the client's wishes as long as it is within the professional scope of practice.

Nurses have the responsibility to inform and teach clients about their healthcare needs but should not attempt to impose their own or society's wishes upon the individual. For many religious groups, as a result of their beliefs and restrictions, this is an important issue. Hospitals in affiliation with such populations are developing outpatient as well as in-hospital settings to meet the needs of specific groups; for example, bloodless clinics have been established to care for Jehovah's Witnesses so that they may receive health care in a setting that is appropriate and supportive of their religious beliefs. Bloodless medical and surgical programs provide options for other individuals who do not wish to have a blood transfusion because of religious beliefs, personal choice, or other medical restrictions such as allergies, fever, or fear of infection.

Beneficence: A healthcare principle that mandates that the healthcare provider "do good for the client."

Confidentiality: The obligation to uphold a client's privacy, maintain certain information in confidence, and respect the client's autonomy.

Confidentiality

An important component of all healthcare professions, but especially nursing within a community, is **confidentiality**. An obligation to uphold a client's privacy and maintain certain information in confidence has long been part of nurses' code of ethics. Health information that an individual considers private must be kept confidential. The issue of privacy envelops the values of individual autonomy. Privacy also encompasses the right of the individual to be left alone and free from unwanted publicity. Confidentiality is merely the tool for privacy protection (Goodman, 2010; Sheldon, 2009).

In health care, the meaning of confidentiality goes beyond keeping information imparted to the healthcare provider secret—it reaches to the core of the relationship between the client and the community nurse. It is an obligation of the nurse to preserve the confidentiality of the client. The code of ethics for nurses developed by the ANA embodies the concept of a client's right of privacy by stating that the nurse has an obligation to protect the client's privacy and confidentiality. Without such protection, the client may not be completely honest with the nurse, which might inhibit other aspects of the client's care as well as the well-being of the community.

In rare situations, the nurse may need to break this confidentiality, such as in a situation in which the failure to disclose information could cause serious harm to the client, the family, or others; in this case, disclosure may be legally binding upon the healthcare provider in some states. For example, if a mentally ill client threatens the life of another person, or if a client with acquired immunodeficiency syndrome (AIDS) confides that he or she is knowingly spreading the disease through unprotected sexual activity, the nurse may be required to break confidence with the client. In some states, healthcare providers (usually the physician) have a "duty to warn"; in other states, however, disclosure of information remains prohibited by law.

Justice

The most common perspectives of justice are distributive, egalitarian, and utilitarian. An important notion of **utilitarian justice** is that benefits should be first given to those who need them the most; thus, if there is a choice or a decision related to the provision of care, the best or most efficient choice should be made. An example of utilitarian justice is a situation, such as an accident, in which there are limited resources and one victim can be saved and another cannot; in these circumstances, care would be provided to the victim with the best chance of survival.

The concept of justice in providing care to a community is based on the notion that people are treated fairly (Mayer & Cronin, 2008; Rawls, 1971). The basis of this concept of justice is **egalitarian justice**. The notion of egalitarian justice or equal justice is that each person has equal access to the health services he or she needs. The idea of fair and equal treatment is dependent, however, on issues that may be difficult to determine or may even be immeasurable. Equal access to care may be affected by many factors; for example, where one lives (e.g., an urban versus rural location) may influence the actual delivery or access availability of services to a client or a community, thereby influencing the equity of care. In some situations, justice as fairness requires allocation of resources that does not reflect equality. People in need may need more resources than others, and it would be just to recognize that reality.

Economics certainly has an effect on how health care is provided for a population or an individual client. If communities or nations have limited economic resources, the health care they provide, although equal among their members, may be less than the services provided to residents in other communities or nations. Although nurses should provide care as needed to all clients regardless of financial status, inequities may occur based on financial realities.

In a healthcare system that uses **distributive justice**, healthcare services are distributed in the fairest way possible to all according to need. Although the principle of justice is the promotion of equity, using equity alone to measure justice is not sufficient. The needs of the community or an individual and availability of resources must be established to determine a just distribution of care (Lachman, 2009; Mayer & Cronin, 2008).

Ethical Issues in the Community

The need to explore ethical issues in relation to community health is not new, but has certainly grown in importance in recent years. The healthcare system in the United States is undergoing an enormous transformation caused in part by factors such as the high cost of health care, improved technology, increased awareness by a concerned and informed population, the aging of the population, the high cost of health insurance, and the lack of health insurance for some individuals.

Advance Directives

Rapid advancements made in healthcare technology, in addition to a changing economic climate, have had an enormous influence on the home care system. Formerly limited to hospitals, highly technological care—such as that requiring intravenous therapy or respirators—may now be provided to clients at home. Some clients may be sent home on respirators or with intravenous lines with little or no support system in

Utilitarian justice: A system of justice based on the principle that benefits are first given to those who need them the most.

Egalitarian justice: A system of justice based on the principle that people are treated fairly; also known as equal justice.

Distributive justice: A system of justice based on the principle that benefits are distributed in the fairest way possible to all according to need.

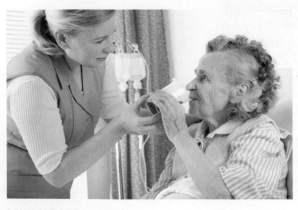

© Alexander Raths/Shutterstock.com

place other than home care visits by the community health nurse; however, these visits are also limited by insurance coverage. Thus, advance directives, such as DNR orders and the healthcare proxy, which are standard in hospitals, are now available to clients at home. Other advance directives include a living will and a durable power of attorney for health care. As noted earlier, advance directives are documents of empowerment that extend the autonomy of clients beyond the point at which they lose their capacity to choose their own care. Because this has become an issue of concern in the care of clients in the community, nurses must provide information to clients about advance directives that are available for use at home.

The living will and healthcare proxy appoint a surrogate decision maker to act on the client's behalf. DNR orders, by comparison, are related only to resuscitation. At-home DNR orders tell emergency staff or attending personnel not to transfer the client to a hospital for CPR. Signing a healthcare proxy allows clients to appoint someone they trust to make decisions about care in case they lose their ability to make decisions. Clients select someone they know as their healthcare agent; they can give that individual as little or as much authority as desired regarding the client's health care or healthcare treatments.

As an advance medical directive is a legal document, clients need to discuss carefully with their healthcare agent what they would or would not want the agent to do if a decision had to be made. This could include not providing CPR, artificial nutrition, hydration, transplant, and so on. The community health nurse provides information to a community about the availability of the healthcare proxy and other advance directives to clients in the hospital as well as to individual clients at home. An example of a pocket-size healthcare proxy is shown in **FIGURE 2-1**, and a standard advance directive/

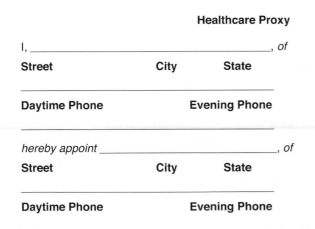

Healthcare Proxy

I, _____, of

Street   **City**   **State**

_____

Daytime Phone   **Evening Phone**

_____

hereby appoint _____, *of*

Street   **City**   **State**

_____

Daytime Phone   **Evening Phone**

_____

as my healthcare agent to make all healthcare decisions for me if I become unable

to decide for myself, including decisions about artificial nutrition and hydration.

_____

Signature (Proxy Initiator)   Date

This proxy was signed in my presence. The signer is known to me and appears

to be of sound mind and to act of his/her own free will.

_____

Witness   Date

_____

Witness   Date

Figure 2-1 Pocket-size healthcare proxy.

(1) I, _____,

(please print your first, middle, and last names)

hereby appoint _____,

(please print your proxy's first, middle, and last names)

of _____

(please print your proxy's home address and telephone number)

as my healthcare agent to make any and all healthcare decisions for me, except to the extent that I state otherwise. This proxy shall take effect when and if I become unable to make my own healthcare decisions.

(2) Optional instructions: I direct my proxy to make healthcare decisions in accord with my wishes and limitations as stated below, or as he or she otherwise knows. (Attach additional pages if necessary.)

_____

_____

Unless you state your wishes about artificial nutrition and hydration [feeding tubes], your agent will not be allowed to make decisions about artificial nutrition and hydration. See instructions on the back for samples of language you could use.

(3) Name of substitute or fill-in proxy if the person I appoint above is unable, unwilling, or unavailable to act as my healthcare agent.

_____

(please print your substitute proxy's first, middle, and last names)

_____

(please print your substitute proxy's home address and telephone number)

(4) Unless I revoke it, this proxy shall remain in effect indefinitely, or until the date or condition stated below. This proxy shall expire (specific date or conditions, if desired):

_____

_____

(5) Signature _____ Address _____ Date _____

(6) Statement by witnesses (the person who is appointed agent or alternate agent cannot sign as witness, and must be 18 or older) *I declare that the person who signed this document is personally known to me and appears to be of sound mind and acting of his or her own free will. He or she signed (or asked another to sign for him or her) this document in my presence.*

Witness 1 _____ Address _____

Witness 2 _____ Address _____

Figure 2-2 Standard advance directive/healthcare proxy.

healthcare proxy is shown in **FIGURE 2-2**. The CHN should find copies of these documents used by their employing institution so that the most up-to-date forms are used.

The Economics of Health Care in the Community

The influence of the insurance industry on the healthcare system exemplifies the impact of business on healthcare services, including home health care. The emergence of managed care reflected the sway of these changes, and is yet another indicator of a need for change in the way health care is financed. At this moment, the need for changes in the healthcare system or healthcare reform is a hot political issue.

Economics certainly has an effect on how health care is provided for a population or an individual client. If communities or nations have limited economic resources, the health care they provide, although distributed equally among their members, may be less than the services provided to other communities or nations. Ethicists are concerned with many issues related to the right to equal care and the equivalent provision of health care.

Prior to the availability of health insurance, patients paid physicians directly for health care—an example of a direct fee-for-service financing model. The introduction of a third-party payment system (health insurance) significantly altered how a client receives healthcare services and, therefore, influenced and changed every aspect of health care. **Third-party payment** refers to a system in which the healthcare provider is paid by insurance companies for services rendered; that is, the fees for care are paid by the insurance provider rather than solely by the patient. Until recently, this meant the client would seek out the services of a physician, and the insurer would pay a percentage of the cost of those services. The insurance company had guidelines as to what would or would not be covered by its policy and the amount it would pay for a specific service.

Third-party payment: A system in which a healthcare provider is paid by insurance companies for services rendered; that is, the fees for care are paid by the insurance provider rather than solely by the patient.

The client and the physician had the most control over the selection of service. The physician could then order almost unlimited laboratory work, and the client could select any physician. This approach also meant patients could obtain direct access to specialists without prior consultation with a family doctor. Over time, this flexibility grew to be very costly in terms of dollars and provided fragmented patient care and, at times, expensive or unnecessary care for the client. The concept of managed care was introduced in response to this trend. Managed care attempted to control cost and prevent fragmented care by having the caregiver act as the gatekeeper for services provided to the client.

In the United States, the high cost of health care is largely due to a system of care that has traditionally focused on crisis intervention as opposed to prevention. In addition, an aging population has created demands and put pressure on the healthcare system to change from the existing insurance-based system and to provide a new healthcare delivery system, with an emphasis on prevention, health promotion, and wellness. Adding to this challenge are increasing costs for traditional hospital care, which have led to shorter hospital stays and an increased need for care following hospitalization, given that patients are sicker while being treated on an inpatient basis. As the system continues to evolve and change, health care—particularly care of the client in the community and at home—has been and continues to be significantly influenced by these changes.

To deal with the high cost of care, some countries have decided to withhold high-tech care from elderly clients because the cost to society is too great. Ceilings on surgical procedures exist in many countries simply because the economic burden upon the community is too great; thus, clients older than a certain age may not be entitled to certain medical procedures. This approach raises the ethical dilemma of for whom and at what age it is reasonable to receive healthcare services. Financial issues are presently a concern in the United States, as the guidelines for health care are based on cost factors that are changing how health care is provided. The alternative to limited health care based on economics is a society that provides care in spite of its cost or because there are no limits.

Today, a U.S. physician and institution can collect insurance compensation regardless of whether there is a logical basis for an intervention. For example, if a 90-year-old woman with end-stage Alzheimer's disease is scheduled for a hysterectomy for fibroids, the surgeon is paid by the insurer despite the questionable logic of performing such a procedure. Clients can be exploited in this way when the benefit of treatment is not clear. Unfortunately, when resources are used ineffectively, other people who need care may not receive the care they need. Problems with allocating limited resources becomes a dilemma for the community health nurse manager, who often must decide which community or person receives the limited healthcare services that are available.

Technology and the Cost of Care

Changes in demographics and shifts in populations affect a healthcare system. In the United States, for example, the increase in the country's aging population is altering the delivery of care. Limited resources to meet the needs of the elderly in hospitals are creating a need to expand services at home, which in turn is increasing the burden on the community healthcare provider. Utilizing limited funds to provide programs to promote wellness and healthcare services has placed an economic strain on the healthcare system.

Improved technology, the high cost of health care, and deep financial cuts have further diminished the pool of healthcare services for many, particularly those with no or limited health insurance. Allocation of limited services to the community and individuals at home places a strain on the community health nurse. Ethical dilemmas concerning community health issues have grown as the general needs of society have changed and transformed how healthcare needs are met.

Like falling dominoes in a row, the effects on one component of health care affect another healthcare element; for example, shorter hospital stays make increased home care

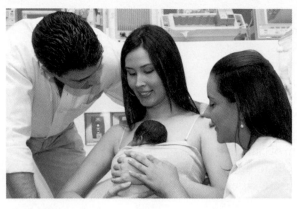

© Reflekta/Shutterstock.com

necessary, which has had a major effect on home healthcare services. People are discharged from hospitals earlier than ever before following childbirth, surgery, and other medical treatments. Such early discharge often limits the time available for pre-discharge healthcare education and may restrict the development of a thorough discharge assessment and plan for many clients at home.

Economics certainly has an effect on how health care is provided, whether for a population or for an individual client. When communities or nations have limited economic resources, the amount of health care they provide, although equal among their members, may fall short of the amount of services provided to other communities or nations. Although ideally nurses will provide care as needed to all clients regardless of financial status, some inequities may arise based on financial realities.

Technological advances in health care and innovative research in recent years have increased longevity, but economic constraints make it difficult to provide safe environments for many aging or debilitated clients at home. Care of the client at home, using sophisticated equipment such as a respirator, is often offered with limited support to the family or the client. The burden of care sometimes proves too great for families, and it is the family and the community health nurse who must deal with the resulting dilemmas, often facing closed doors for the financial support from an overburdened insurance structure. Self-help or voluntary help programs are sometimes available to add support.

Community Engagement and Social Action in Health Care

Social concerns of a society may help to create a basis for meeting community needs. Health concerns of a society are often reflected in the development and implementation of health education and prevention programs. The need for a preventive approach, rather than a strictly curative effort, has grown and changed the role of the nurse. Examples of this trend include health promotion and educational programs within a community to offer immunization against the flu, to provide injection drug users with clean needles, and to instruct members about the use of condoms to prevent the spread of sexually transmitted diseases and avoid pregnancy among adolescents. Additionally, healthcare concerns involving substance abuse, spousal abuse, child abuse, and AIDS are situations addressed by the CHN, whether the CHN serves as a community health educator, as a group leader, or in the expanded role of the school nurse.

Volunteer hospice workers who become friendly visitors to the dying and hospice professionals provide care at minimal cost; support groups for caregivers and respite programs are examples of communities negotiating these situations together in a positive manner. Although such services do not replace services lost to clients, they represent positive ways in which a community can begin to address its own healthcare needs. Many self-help groups exist for individuals with serious diseases such as Parkinson's disease, multiple sclerosis, cancer, and many others. These groups may initially be organized by or utilize the expertise of the CHN. Most local libraries have information about finding local self-help and volunteer groups in the community.

For any community program to be successful, there needs to be acceptance of that program by the community and an understanding of the needs fulfilled by the program. It is costly and of questionable benefit to a community to simply provide a healthcare program without the understanding by the community of need for the program. Arnstein, a social planner in the late 1960s, developed a method of measuring community participation called the **ladder of participation**, which measures the participation of

Ladder of participation:
Arnstein's method for measuring the participation of a community in eight steps, ranging from nonparticipation to citizen control.

a community in eight steps, ranging from nonparticipation to citizen control (Shetland Islands Council, 2011). The first step is manipulation and the second step is therapy, both of which are considered areas of nonparticipation by a community. During these first two steps, the CHN can educate the community or client or provide services to the community.

Steps 3, 4, and 5 are considered degrees of tokenism by the community. Step 3 is the informing step, step 4 is consultation, and step 5 is identified as placation. During these steps, clients may heed information and attempt to have a voice, but they are not considered in the community healthcare planning. The CHN must include clients during the planning stages of programs and provide for client input during this phase.

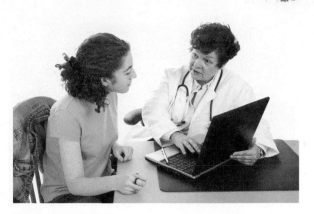

© Lisa F. Young/Shutterstock.com

Steps 6, 7, and 8 of the ladder are considered various stages of empowerment. Step 6 is partnership, step 7 is delegation of power, and step 8 is citizen control. During these stages, citizens engage in a partnership with healthcare providers, but it is not until step 8 that communities fully participate in an equal partnership with health professionals, with clients taking charge of their own health and community members making a commitment to carry out a healthcare plan.

The ladder of participation illustrates how a community embraces an issue (e.g., a healthcare issue), takes charge of its own health decisions, and improves its own health promotion activities. The CHN has an important role in providing information by educating the community. How the members of a community decide to implement or participate in the community's health is influenced by a variety of issues (ANA, 2010).

Ethics, Values, and Moral Reasoning Related to Community Health Nursing

Today, the CHN, as part of the healthcare team, must often deal with situations unlike those encountered in the past. Even as technology has developed and enhanced our lives, it has also brought many moral dilemmas. Community health nurses must be concerned with the growing responsibility to confront these ethical and moral decisions in today's complex society.

Moral Reasoning and Health Care

Moral attitudes and behaviors are developed through a combination of many factors. The environment in which one is raised, the family, the culture, and the society all play important roles in the development of one's morals. Kohlberg's work suggests that moral development goes through various stages of development that are characterized by different ways of understanding right or wrong (Crain, 1985). According to Kohlberg, individuals pass through these stages in an orderly fashion, moving from a lower stage of moral development to a higher stage. Moreover, all individuals in all cultures go through these stages, albeit to varying degrees. Kohlberg also claims that each successive stage is at a morally and cognitively higher level than the previous stage. Furthermore, his work indicates that at each higher stage of moral development, individuals are able to deal with moral and ethical problems of greater complexity. The choices one makes, then, depend on one's moral and ethical development.

Gilligan's work on moral development elicits differences in the moral understandings between men and women (Gilligan, 1982). Gilligan suggests that men and women interpret moral problems from distinct orientations; that is, men's moral development is based on the ethic of rights and justice, whereas women's moral development is based on the ethic of care and responsibility.

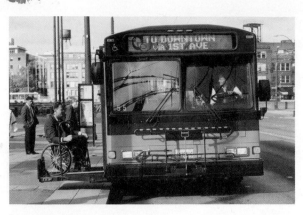

© John A. Rizzo/Photodisc/Thinkstock

Both Kohlberg's and Gilligan's theories are useful to the CHN in working with aggregate populations or individuals to create a positive and informed environment in which to help the client make health-care decisions.

Moral action should support the needs of society. Health care, until recently, claimed to be grounded in this idea. However, as the health-care system previously functioned in a curative domain, there was little interest in prevention. Thus a question arose about whether this perspective was truly in the collective interest of society. The notion of collective interest may not have changed, but how we provide care to the society has certainly been challenged.

Individual Good Versus Societal Good

Sometimes, the CHN in working with communities must consider the needs of an individual or an aggregate over the needs of the community. The health needs of one member or an aggregate population of a community may vary in terms of time, cultural differences, physical needs, technological levels, and economics from the health needs of the community as a whole. At times, this diversity may indicate a need for an individual approach to meeting some immediate or long-term goals. Accommodating the needs of individuals may place an economic burden on the larger community, which may benefit only a few. Examples might include a community that provides sidewalk cuts to meet the demands of wheelchair users and a community that provides kneeling buses to meet the needs of persons who are otherwise unable to access public transportation. As identified previously, the planning process for such a program must consider how the community will participate in the program.

Legal Issues

Providing health care to the community presents legal issues that concern the community nurse. All healthcare workers are responsible for practicing within a framework of laws. These laws reflect the mandates of local, state, and federal legislation. Community health nurses practice under three types of laws: constitutional law, legislative law, and common law. These legal guidelines shape how community health workers practice, as well as govern the private and community healthcare agencies under which nurses provide service. Therefore, nurses have legal standards, in addition to ethical standards, under which they practice.

Scope of practice: The legal limits of nursing practice within the community being served, as defined by state law and the Nurse Practice Act.

Informed consent: A process in which a research subject is educated about the terms, procedures, and potential risks and benefits before agreeing to become involved in research.

The community nurse must know and follow closely the state laws and the Nurse Practice Act, which designates the **scope of practice** under which the nurse operates. The CHN may be a generalist, a clinical nurse specialist, a midwife, an occupational health nurse, a school nurse, or a nurse practitioner. It is important that the nurse operate in the appropriate scope of practice, according to the role designated by each state. To do so, the CHN must know the legal limits of nursing practice within the community being served. Furthermore, scope of practice differentiates between the nurse's role in the care of the client and that of other healthcare professionals.

What may be good for society may sometimes come at the cost of endangering an individual—for example, when human subjects participate in research. Because many CHNs are nurse researchers, they must be cognizant of the risks involved with human subjects in the research process. Ideally, by informing the client of the risks, a collaboration develops between the researcher and the subject. At the core of the research process is the informed consent procedure, which attempts to balance the risks to human subjects against the potential benefits to society (Burns & Grove, 2005).

Community health nurses involved in research, like any other researcher working with human subjects, need to obtain **informed consent** from clients. Research involving human subjects should not be carried out unless the importance of the research is in proportion to the risk to the subject (Burns & Grove, 2005). It is a most important moral principle of informed consent that the client understand the terms, procedures, and potential risks and benefits before agreeing to become involved in research.

Quality of Life Versus Quantity of Life

Issues such as equity in allocation of resources to individuals or society, the client's right to choose his or her quality of life, euthanasia for home-bound clients, and decisions on how one should live with an illness or potential illness are examples of ethical dilemmas regarding quality of life versus quantity of life with which community health nurses are concerned. Choices regarding clients' right to the quality of life they desire versus greater longevity are often driven by economics related to the healthcare system. Clients with large economic resources or with celebrity often stand a better chance of being a recipient of improved services. This has recently become a concern, particularly in situations related to organ transplantation.

A burden falls upon the resources of society when a client's behavior contributes to an illness or injury. Treating the client who drives without a seatbelt and is injured in a motor vehicle accident imposes an economic burden on society. This is so even if the client can afford to pay for his or her medical expenses or has health insurance to pay for care. The actual care provided to one client requires time and energy to support that care despite the cost, and the time it takes to provide care reduces the time that can be devoted to another client. Is it not the responsibility of citizens to comply with laws to decrease this burden? Does this interfere with a person's rights?

Similarly, obese clients who choose not to take measures to lose weight may be in danger of ill health because of this choice. Obese clients are at higher risk for hypertension, adult-onset diabetes, and heart disease. The need for treatment of health problems that are directly or indirectly caused by such clients' decisions places an economic burden on the healthcare system, just like the burden imposed by the driver who refuses to wear a seatbelt and experiences a traumatic injury. Being able to pay for care does not burden the system less, yet the wealthy obese person or the wealthy smoker or alcoholic has a better chance of receiving care or services than the person with fewer economic resources.

Organ transplant allocation becomes an ethical dilemma for some. Organ procurement, along with the issue of limited organ availability and selection of who gets an organ, is a difficult decision in many cases. The sale of organs is illegal in the United States, but not internationally. Should the person who can afford to purchase an organ have preference over one who cannot? At this moment in the United States, individuals must directly give permission before donating an organ or indicate on a document (such as an advance directive or on their driving license) that they will permit their organs to be donated, but cannot decide to whom the organ goes in most cases. Patients must be officially brain dead before most organs can be taken, although kidney and liver donations may be allocated to a designated individual for living donation.

The client's right to self-determination poses another ethical dilemma that may affect the healthcare system. Individuals have the right to make their own decisions. However, if a client chooses not to follow a healthcare provider's healthcare plan at any level of prevention when that plan is based upon research, should the client be considered to be noncompliant or to be using his or her own judgment or values to make an independent decision? Clients may choose not to follow the suggestions or plan of the healthcare provider. Indeed, clients have a right to choose their own care and decide most issues related to their own health, as long as that choice does no harm to others. However, the cost to the healthcare system may be great and in some situations may do harm inadvertently to others.

Personal and Social Responsibility

In the United States, an individual's right to liberty is protected by the U.S. Constitution and can be affected by disclosure by a health professional. Consider a situation in which a client with an active case of tuberculosis refuses treatment, yet continues living in close proximity to young children. Such a case confronts the nurse with ethical, safety, and legal dilemmas. The nurse must choose between issues related to confidentiality and safety issues—that is, the nurse must weigh the safety of one client against the confidentiality of another. The nurse faces an ethical dilemma when client confidentiality clashes with the obligation to obey laws directed by society. This situation requires that the nurse obey the law by reporting the situation to the health department and breaking the seal of patient confidentiality with the client to whom he or she is committed by the code of the profession. The CHN may face these kinds of conflicting ethical choices on a regular basis (ANA, 2001; Butts & Rich, 2005).

The Health Insurance Portability and Accountability Act

Health Insurance Portability and Accountability Act (HIPAA): Federal legislation enacted in 1996 that identifies requirements for protection of confidentiality of information related to medical records and services. It protects information related to a person's health care, authorizes release of healthcare information by patients, and clarifies ownership of their health records.

The **Health Insurance Portability and Accountability Act (HIPAA)** was enacted in 1996 and signed into law by President Bill Clinton. It identifies requirements for protection of confidentiality of information related to medical records and services. The original intent was to stop healthcare fraud and enforce healthcare confidentiality and to create health insurance portability and management. Furthermore, HIPAA protects information related to a person's health care, authorizes release of healthcare information by patients, and clarifies ownership of their health records. The privacy requirements limit the release of patient information without the patient's consent or knowledge, thereby preventing access to a person's healthcare information without that individual's consent. The increased use of electronic records makes HIPAA regulations particularly important for the privacy and security of patient records that reside on shared computer systems (Sheldon, 2009).

Ethical Decisions of the Community Health Nurse

Using the ethical decision-making process, the nurse assists the client in developing a plan of care. **Table 2-2** compares the nursing process and the ethical decision-making process. Both processes are used to move a client problem from assessment through evaluation, so as to best meet the client's needs. Ethical decision making does not occur

TABLE 2-2
Comparison of the Nursing Process and the Ethical Decision-Making Process

Nursing Process	Ethical Decision-Making Process
1. Assessment	1. Assessment—gathering of relevant information
2. Diagnosis and analysis	2. Clarification of ethical component and social and legal implications
3. Plan	3. Identifying possible outcomes
4. Implementation	4. Implementation
5. Evaluation	5. Evaluation

in a vacuum; rather, the CHN works with other providers to solve ethical dilemmas. Agencies in the community, such as acute care facilities, may establish ethics committees to help resolve ethical problems. A critical part of both approaches is the incorporation of cultural beliefs so that the client can participate fully in the healthcare process.

A Cultural Context for Care in the Community

The Influence of Health Beliefs and Culture on Health Care

The impact and influence of cultural and ethical beliefs on the provision of health care in a society are great. Differences in customs and values influence healthcare beliefs and practices among different cultures; regardless of how healthcare professionals evaluate a client's state of health, clients are inclined to measure their own sense of well-being based on their beliefs and values (Raholm, 2008). The way people assess health is highly individual and often has strong ties to culture. In some cases, a client's cultural beliefs or behaviors may conflict with the standards of the healthcare providers in a community. Nonetheless, the responsibility for acquiring health care and maintaining one's personal health is largely placed upon the individual (Andrews & Boyle, 2008).

Placing the burden of responsibility upon the individual for maintaining his or her own health suggests that there is a common standard of acceptable health in the United States. Therefore, self-care becomes an additional responsibility of one's health mainte-nance. In the United States, many consider health care to be a right, but it is also con-sidered to be a responsibility by many clients and providers.

The CHN may experience a sense of conflict when working with clients who, based on certain societal expectations, have not done all they could to maintain their health. Furthermore, the CHN's response to a client's health needs or demands is inevitably influenced by the nurse's own cultural heritage and health beliefs. Healthcare provid-ers must be sensitive to the enormous impact of culture both on clients' health and on providers' attitudes toward clients.

Culture is learned from a person's environment, and cultural learning is often lik-ened to the way in which humans learn to speak (Spector, 2008). Accordingly, cultural norms are mostly implied and are often unexpressed by individuals. Most members of a family or cultural group have no need to discuss rules among themselves related to their culturally connected behaviors. Culture influences the foods we eat, how our children are reared, how we react to pain, how we cope with stress, how we respond to health care, and how we deal with issues related to death. Cultural influences and organized support systems often set guidelines for living and provide foundations for client behaviors (Andrews & Boyle, 2008; Ray, 2010). In short, culture provides the underpinnings for a person's social development.

Health beliefs or mores are not limited to cultural beliefs. They of-ten incorporate what clients have learned to expect from their social environment (environmental press). Perceptions of health that clients have also reflect the environment in which they live as well as the culture into which they have been socialized. Although ethnic differ-ences are often key to the care of the client, health beliefs frequently organize and manipulate how individuals interpret their own health and how they seek access to health care. Therefore, clients may believe

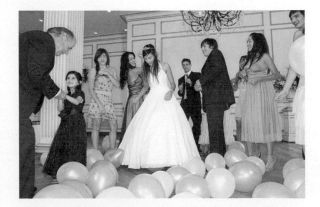

© AISPIX by Image Source/Shutterstock.com

that certain conditions are the norm for their age or condition and see no reason to seek out health assistance.

Cultural diversity is found in geographic environments in which a variety of culturally different persons or groups live together. Each group brings its own expectations of health into the larger society. These expectations are, in turn, influenced by a variety of forces, including changes in technology, advancements made in health care, and the influence or pressures from the environment of the greater society. All of these forces shape individuals' interpretation of their rights as members of a society and may create ethical dilemmas within a society (National Center for Cultural Competence, 2006; Purnell, 2009).

The United States for many years was likened to a melting pot, but it is actually more like a salad bowl—that is, it is a mix of people with many groups maintaining their own cultural, ethical, and religious identities and histories, making up one country (**FIGURE 2-3**). Thus, when considering an ethical approach to health care (particularly in the community), one must account for the impact of culture and the values of the members of a community. A more contemporary approach to consider when exploring ethics and community practice is to move away from the traditional approach, which focuses on the individual, and to address the targets of health care at an aggregate, community, or societal level.

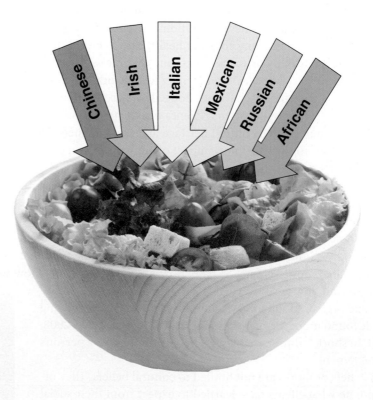

Figure 2-3 American culture as a salad with unique ingredients, not a "melting pot."
Photo © Hemera/Thinkstock

Cultural Variations in Social Interaction

Culture influences how the CHN approaches clients in relation to time and space. **Ethical pluralism** (also known as moral diversity) maintains the position that culturally diverse societies display multiple moral standards, which may lead to conflicting moral realities (Purnell, 2009). However, divergence in values and differences in moral standards across cultural boundaries are valued and considered to be resources that have historically led to the evolution of moral thinking (Dayer-Berenson, 2011, pp. 56–57).

In the United States, persons from the dominant culture tend to be very time dependent and, therefore, very concerned with the importance of time—that is, most Americans set appointments and are disturbed if the person with whom they have an appointment is late. Time is cut up into segments, with work scheduled between the hours of 9 A.M. and 5 P.M., and entertainment similarly kept to a prescribed schedule. Television shows are divided into 30- or 60-minute segments; theater or film begins at a specific time. Because Western culture tends to connote time with productivity, time is regarded as an important commodity. Accordingly, most Americans try to never waste time and to be on time for appointments.

What has just been said about mainstream American culture is not true of all the diverse cultures within the United States, however. Some cultures view time as never ending, and they get to where they are going when they get there. If something does not get finished today, it is believed that it will get done tomorrow. Persons from such cultures have a different approach to keeping appointments and a different understanding of what it means to be "on time." For persons from Ghana, for example, punctuality is of little importance. It is more important to continue a social interaction than to be on time for another event.

The physical distance people maintain when interacting also differs from culture to culture. In the United States, people from the dominant culture remain approximately 2 feet away from persons with whom they are conversing. In contrast to this practice, persons from many other cultures stand either closer to or farther away from the person with whom they are speaking. Other cultural practices, such as those related to human touch, can also play an important part in how the CHN should approach a client from the nondominant culture. Additionally, eye contact has a significant meaning in most cultures. Many persons native to the Australian culture, for example, may combine direct eye contact with intermittent looking away, which they interpret as showing interest. Although direct eye contact may not be sustained by Native Australians, Argentines tend to maintain intense eye contact during conversation. In short, cultural variation is the rule in the area of social interaction.

The degree to which physical touching is permitted is also dictated by cultural values and mores. While some degree of touching between persons of different sexes is generally acceptable to the dominant culture in the United States, Orthodox Jewish men are not permitted to be touched by women other than their wives. If hands-on care is to be delivered to an Orthodox Jewish male, the CHN delivering the care should also be a man whenever possible. If the CHN is a woman, she should instruct the wife or another man as to how to provide direct care to these male clients at home. The female nurse may oversee procedures to ensure that they are done correctly. South Korean clients also consider physical touching by members of the opposite sex inappropriate.

In Singapore and Vietnam, the head is considered sacred; thus, it is considered an affront to reach over someone's head and an offense to pat or touch a child on the head (Geissler, 1994). Strangers touching children is frankly frowned upon by many Hispanic parents (Andrews & Boyle, 2008), as Mexican parents believe that such behavior can cause illness. For example, caida de la mollera is a serious illness with a high mortality among infants and children 1 to 3 years of age. Its cause is often related to diarrhea or vomiting; as a result of dehydration, the anterior fontanelle becomes depressed below the contour

Ethical pluralism: The position that culturally diverse societies display multiple moral standards, which may lead to conflicting moral realities; also known as moral diversity.

Curandero: A folk healer within Hispanic cultures.

of the skull. Some poorly educated or rural Hispanic parents believe that this condition is caused by a nonfamily member touching the head of the infant. As it is common for the CHN to measure infants' skulls, this procedure is easily mistaken for the cause of the problem (Spector, 2008). If caida de la mollera afflicts a child, a **curandero** (folk healer) may be called to rid the child of the mal ojo (evil eye) attributable to the stranger. In an attempt to heal the child, the curandero may hold the infant upside down to help the fontanelle resume its correct placement; sadly, this practice may result in retinal hemorrhages. To prevent such tragedies, the parents must be encouraged to hydrate the infant. If they wish to use the curandero, such services can be provided in addition to hydration.

In fact, regardless of their level of education and assimilation into a more cosmopolitan health system, many Mexican Americans and other Hispanics may use the curandero for a variety of ailments and problems. Often these problems may be psychosocial. It is important for the CHN to understand the role and functions of the folk healers and work collaboratively with them. Without acceptance by the folk healer, Hispanic clients may not comply with the recommendations of the CHN or other provider.

Folk beliefs regarding illnesses and their cures can be found in all cultures. Nurses who wish to be optimally effective within the communities they serve should develop familiarity with and appreciation of folk beliefs and other cultural differences, thereby empowering themselves to help their clients toward wellness.

Cultural Sensitivity of the Community Health Nurse

In an effort to reflect cultural sensitivity, the CHN can assist clients in adapting to the care environment in the community. The CHN should explain all schedules and expectations, and ask clients if they understand and can comply with the plan of care. Asking clients about their preferences in care needs to include a clear explanation when client requests cannot be met. Open-ended questions and statements will elicit the most useful information for the CHN to use and incorporate into the plan of care.

Anticipatory guidance is a tool that is useful in supporting the client as he or she adapts to the requirements of the healthcare system. As always, obtaining input from family members and significant others is a critical aspect of providing care. Taking the time to validate the ongoing willingness of the client to participate in his or her care is central to the overall success of moving the client to a higher level of health and wellness. Excellent resources are available from the Health Resources and Services Administration (HRSA) for the CHN to use in examining culture, language, and health literacy. Assessing the response of the community health agency in terms of its cultural sensitivity to client needs allows the CHN to ensure that all providers are working from a culturally sound perspective. This perspective is central to providing anticipatory guidance when meeting the needs of the public (National Center for Cultural Competence, 2006).

Summary

This chapter examined two interrelated concepts—ethics and cultural beliefs. These concepts are related because of their fundamental grounding in the client's personal beliefs and life experience. The first part of the chapter defined ethics and discussed ethical concerns that are central to the practice of community health nursing. These issues include advance directives, quality of life considerations, the cost and rationing of health care, increased use of technology, and the ethical environment in which the CHN practices.

The second part of the chapter examined culture—specifically, the influence of culture on providing and receiving nursing care in the community. In the United States, clients seeking nursing care in the community come from a variety of cultural backgrounds, and the CHN must be aware of and respectful toward all clients' cultural grounding.

When working with some individuals from nondominant cultures, understanding the importance of culture is the key to developing a therapeutic and lasting nurse–client relationship. A strong ethical foundation and cultural appreciation of how to best meet the needs of the community are central to professional nursing practice.

REFERENCES

American Nurses Association (ANA). (2001). *Code of ethics for nurses with interpretive statements.* Silver Spring, MD: Author.

American Nurses Association (ANA). (2010). *Scope and standards of practice: Nursing* (2nd ed.). Silver Spring, MD: Author.

Andrews, M. M., & Boyle, J. S. (2008). *Transcultural concepts in nursing care* (5th ed.). Philadelphia, PA: Lippincott, Williams & Wilkins.

Burns, N., & Grove, S. (2005). *Study guide for the practice of nursing research: Conduct, critique, and utilization* (5th ed.). Philadelphia, PA: Elsevier Saunders.

Butts, J., & Rich, K. (2005). *Nursing ethics: Across the curriculum and into practice.* Sudbury, MA: Jones and Bartlett.

Crain, W. C. (1985). Kohlberg's stages of moral development. In *Theories of development* (pp. 118–136). Upper Saddle River, NJ: Prentice Hall.

Dayer-Berenson, L. (2011). *Cultural competencies for nurses.* Sudbury, MA: Jones & Bartlett Learning.

Fowler, M. D. (2010). *Guide to the code of ethics for nurses: Interpretation and application.* Silver Spring, MD: American Nurses Association.

Geissler, E. M. (1994). *Mosby's pocket guide to cultural assessment.* St. Louis, MO: Mosby.

Gilligan, C. (1982). *In a different voice: Psychological theory and women's development.* Cambridge, MA: Harvard University Press.

Goodman, K. W. (2010). Ethics, information technology, and public health: New challenges for the clinician–patient relationship. *Law, Medicine & Ethics, 38*(1), 58–63.

Lachman, V. D. (2009). Practical use of the code of ethics: Part II. *MEDSURG Nursing, 18*(3), 191–194.

Lewin, K. (1936). *Principles of topological psychology.* New York, NY: McGraw-Hill.

Mayer, C. M., & Cronin, D. (2008). Organizational accountability in a just culture. *Urologic Nursing, 28*(6), 427–430.

National Center for Cultural Competence. (2006). *A guide for using the cultural and linguistic competence policy assessment instrument.* Washington, DC: Author.

Purnell, L. D. (2009). *Guide to culturally competent health care* (2nd ed.). Philadelphia, PA: F. A. Davis.

Raholm, M-B. (2008). Uncovering the ethics of suffering using a narrative approach. *Nursing Ethics, 15*(1), 62–72.

Rawls, J. (1971). *A theory of justice.* Cambridge, MA: Harvard University Press.

Ray, M. A. (2010). *Transcultural caring dynamics in nursing and health care.* Philadelphia, PA: F. A. Davis.

Sheldon, L. K. (2009). *Communication for nurses: Talking with patients* (2nd ed.). Sudbury, MA: Jones and Bartlett.

Shetland Islands Council. (2011). *The ladder of participation.* Retrieved from http://www.shetland.gov.uk/consultation/guidelines/theladderofparticipation.htm

Skott, C. (2003). Storied ethics: Conversations in nursing care. *Nursing Ethics, 10*(4), 368–376.

Spector, R. E. (2008). *Cultural diversity in health and illness* (7th ed.). Upper Saddle River, NJ: Pearson Education.

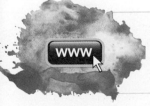

For a full suite of assignments and additional learning activities, use the access code located in the front of your book to visit the exclusive website: http://go.jblearning.com/Holzemer/. If you do not have an access code, you can obtain one at the site.

LEARNING ACTIVITIES

1. The Code of Ethics, which set the standards for ethical nursing behavior, was developed by which of the following organizations?

    A. U.S. Department of Health and Human Services

    B. National League for Nursing

    C. American Nurses Association

    D. The Joint Commission

2. The obligation of the healthcare professional to "do good" is represented by which of the following principles?

    A. Beneficence

    B. Justice

    C. Nonmaleficence

    D. Confidentiality

3. After the nurse carefully explains the implications of identifying a "healthcare proxy" and the meaning of instituting a "do not resuscitate" medical order, Ms. Jones, a 96-year-old patient with congestive heart failure, who is mentally competent, refuses to participate in any further discussion of the topics. Which of the following statements, made by a nurse, is probably correct?

    A. "Ms. Jones is making a mistake she will regret."

    B. "The staff should call Ms. Jones's family and encourage her to change her mind."

    C. "This is Ms. Jones's decision and needs to be respected."

    D. "Ms. Jones's physician will have to serve as healthcare proxy in this situation."

4. Which statement made by a nurse to a client refers to the concept of autonomy?

    A. "It is a person's right to independence or self-determination."

    B. "It refers to the right of a society, not the right of an individual."

    C. "It relates to individuals' freedom to do whatever they want concerning their health."

    D. "It is the individual's responsibility to do the right thing to improve his or her own destiny."

5. What is the goal of the Health Insurance Portability and Accountability Act (HIPAA) ?

    A. The act protects the integrity of Medicaid and Medicare information shared with other agencies.

    B. The act protects the client against disclosure of identifiable health information.

    C. The act restricts sharing of health information with unregulated insurance companies.

    D. The act is primarily intended to control electronic health records.

ADDITIONAL QUESTIONS FOR STUDY

1. Our values are influenced by many things. Develop a brief overview of what you believe has affected your personal values related to health care, and then create a list of what you believe has or will affect your professional values.

2. Pretend that you have won $1 million in the lottery. List the first three items on which you would spend your money (e.g., pay off loans, share with family, take a trip or vacation, retire). Share with your classmates how, as a group, you would spend the money. Keep track of each item and determine whether they are repeated by others. This is an indication of what you value.

3. Identify three nursing or healthcare problems you would like to solve with part of your winnings from the lottery (see Question 2). Share the information with classmates as suggested in Question 2.

CHAPTER OUTLINE

- ▶ Introduction
- ▶ Philosophy of Nursing Care
- ▶ Structure of the Alliance for Health Model
  - The Voice of the Client
  - The Expertise of the Provider (Nurse and Interdisciplinary Team)
  - Community-Based Needs
  - Systems of Care Management
  - Resource Allocation

- ▶ The Alliance for Health Model as a Complement to Evidence-Based Nursing
  - Evidence from Research
  - Evidence from Clinical Practice
  - Evidence from the Client's Perspective
- ▶ Use of the Alliance for Health Model: Two Different Problems in the Community
  - A Problem Emerging with Community-Based Needs
  - A Problem Emerging with Resource Allocation
- ▶ Summary

OBJECTIVES

WWW

1. Consider the importance of the nurse and client sharing responsibility for using the Alliance for Health Model, to solve community-based problems.

2. Identify the role of the nurse in evaluating the effectiveness of completing a community assessment, using the Alliance for Health Model, in each of the model's five components.

3. Explain why the community health provider team is essential for completing and responding to the findings of a community assessment.

4. Consider how the Alliance for Health Model could be adapted to improve the process of community assessment.

KEY TERMS

WWW

Advocacy group

Aesthetics

Alliance for Health Model

Demographics

Interdisciplinary plan of care (IPC)

Morbidity

Mortality

Special interest group

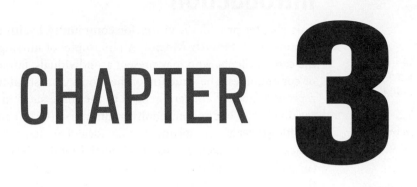

CHAPTER 3

The Vision for the Alliance for Health Model

Stephen Paul Holzemer

Alliance for Health Model: A philosophy of nursing care—a template—to assist the nurse in focusing on the relationship between nursing and the community, so as to resolve problems within the scope of nursing practice. It consists of five essential components that represent areas of concern central to the three steps in the joint-venture process of seeking health by the community health nurse and the client.

Introduction

This chapter provides a vision for community health assessment—specifically, the **Alliance for Health Model**. A philosophy of nursing care is provided that guides the care of clients, who may present as individuals, families, other groups, aggregates, or communities. The structure of the model consists of five essential components that represent areas of concern central to the three steps in the joint-venture process of seeking health by the community health nurse (CHN) and the client. The Alliance for Health Model is a complement to the idea of evidence-based nursing in care delivery, education, and ongoing research. Using this model, the CHN collects evidence of health (or the lack of health) from established research, from the expertise of professionals "in the field," and from the lived experiences of the client.

Philosophy of Nursing Care

Community health assessment is an ongoing process. Community health nurses and other healthcare providers in the community engage in ongoing assessment of the community in an effort to ensure the accuracy of their perceptions of the health of the community. This process guides their interventions with the community so that their interventions remain appropriate. The Alliance for Health Model is a tool to be used in community assessment, albeit from the most general perspective. Obtaining an overall, general perspective allows the CHN to better understand the actual and potential needs of families, groups, aggregates, and the community as a whole.

The Alliance for Health Model represents a philosophy of nursing care in the community—one that is defined as a joint venture between the nurse and the client on their journey toward health. The model provides the professional nurse with a schema for applying the nursing process to actual and potential health problems experienced by families, other groups, aggregates, and communities. **FIGURE 3-1** depicts the evolution of the Alliance for Health Model as occurring in three steps:

1. The voice of the client articulates needs, and is responded to by the nurse (or other provider) with the professional expertise to hear the client.
2. The nurse and the client identify community-based needs and validate the utility of the systems of care management in place (or needing development) to meet community-based needs.
3. The nurse and the community secure the resources needed to resolve threats to the health of the community.

The Alliance for Health Model reflects a larger set of cultural and ethical values and beliefs about health and illness, which is created by the larger collective of various healthcare providers and the communities they serve. This model should evolve with current and changing health-related concerns, like those identified through the national response to health known as *Healthy People 2020* (U.S. Department of Health and Human Services [DHHS], 2010). The usefulness of the Alliance for Health Model unfolds from the relationship between the specialty of community health nursing and the needs experienced by families, other groups, aggregates, and communities—that is, the clients of the community health nurse. The key to success when using the model rests in the therapeutic relationship that develops between nursing and the community.

The Alliance Model for Health is intended to serve as a template to inform the CHN and other healthcare providers about the various forces that interact to create a composite picture of health and illness in the community. The client and the nurse navigate the healthcare delivery system together to address the client's health needs. **FIGURE 3-2** illustrates the basic structure of the Alliance for Health Model; **FIGURE 3-3** examines the various components of the model in further detail.

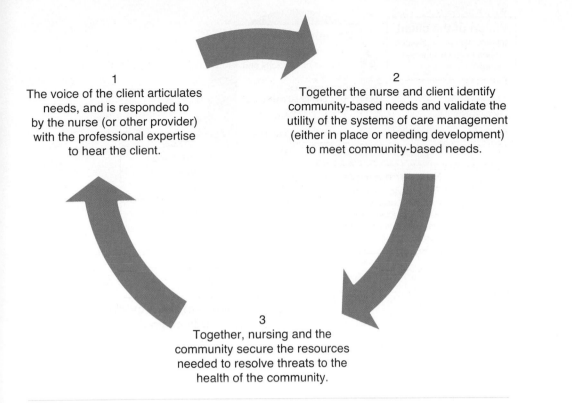

1
The voice of the client articulates
needs, and is responded to
by the nurse (or other provider)
with the professional expertise
to hear the client.

2
Together the nurse and client identify
community-based needs and validate the
utility of the systems of care management
(either in place or needing development)
to meet community-based needs.

3
Together, nursing and the
community secure the resources
needed to resolve threats to the
health of the community.

Figure 3-1 The evolution of the Alliance for Health Model.

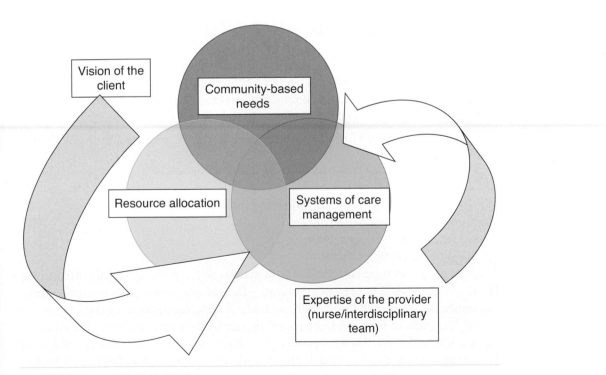

Vision of the
client

Community-based
needs

Resource allocation

Systems of care
management

Expertise of the provider
(nurse/interdisciplinary
team)

Figure 3-2 Alliance for Health Model structure.

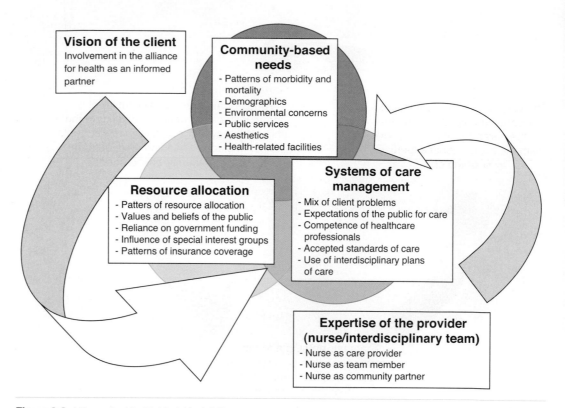

Figure 3-3 Alliance for Health Model in detail.

Structure of the Alliance for Health Model

The Alliance for Health Model is a template to assist the nurse in focusing on the relationship between nursing and the community, so as to resolve problems within the scope of nursing practice. Such a model resides within a larger model of multidisciplinary and interdisciplinary expertise geared toward meeting national and global health-related concerns.

The Alliance for Health Model includes five components:

1. The voice of the client
2. The expertise of the provider (nurse and interdisciplinary team)
3. Community-based needs
4. Systems of care management
5. Resource allocation concerns

The separateness of these components is, in many ways, artificial. In fact, the Alliance for Health Model should be seen as a dynamic whole of interacting parts or components, not unlike the concept of health itself, with many variables influencing the meaning of health. The parts of the model find meaning only in their relationship to the other aspects of the model. The whole, or picture of health, is altogether different and not limited by the linear aspects of the model. The evolutionary nature of this "picture of health" transcends the ability to capture or diagram it in a meaningful way.

The Voice of the Client

The voice of the community client articulates, in part, the pressing community-based needs, the preferred systems of care management, and the engagement in resource allocation decisions. The client should be engaged in the Alliance for Health Model as an informed partner; that is, the client needs to be fully informed about the benefits and limitations of the healthcare options at hand. Nurses need to make time to hear the voices of clients who are at times silenced, such as those with mental illness, those with undocumented immigration status, those who speak a non-English language, and those who have a history of not choosing to participate in the available standard of healthcare services (American Nurses Association [ANA], 2001; Dayer-Berenson, 2011; Fowler, 2010).

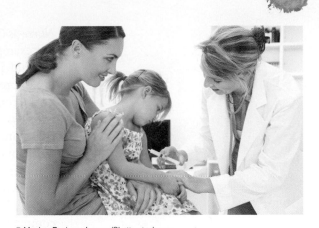

© Monkey Business Images/Shutterstock.com

It is important to recognize that the measurement of health-related outcomes depends on the response of individuals to health-related interventions. The conceptual leap of viewing families, groups, and large aggregates as the clients of nursing care allows for the construction of a more holistic view of nursing care, but complicates the measurement of outcomes. Most assessment tools used today focus on the care delivered to individuals (Allender, Rector, & Warner, 2010; Solberg, 2007; DHHS, 2010).

Families, groups, and larger aggregates, when receiving nursing care, may respond with improved or stabilized health status. The techniques needed to measure aggregate wellness, however, are not always available to nurses or other care providers. For example, a family intervention to assist all members in coping with an unexpected death is intended to improve the functioning of the family unit. The nurse might expect to see improvements in communication as the family copes with the death experience, but a tool to measure improvements in family coping may not be readily available to the community health nurse. Some of the limited areas where the measurement of aggregate health status has been successfully carried out are immunization rates, communicable disease surveillance, and monitoring of prenatal care.

One of the inherent problems with clients negotiating for healthcare services is that they may not necessarily know which services they need. Clients may have unmet or unrecognized healthcare needs because they are unfamiliar with the services that are available. Healthcare services may also be incongruent with their ethical and cultural beliefs and, therefore, not acceptable to the clients (Dayer-Berenson, 2011). It is the responsibility of the healthcare provider to keep the consumer aware of acceptable options in health care, and to create linkages between providers and consumers of health care.

The Expertise of the Provider (Nurse and Interdisciplinary Team)

The role of the nurse in the community is a prescribed function. That is, this role is generated from the permission society gives to the nursing profession to assist others in their quest for health and wellness, coping with illness and disease, and dealing with the limitations of care and recovery. Nursing has developed a rich reservoir of guidelines that enable the nurse to act from a position of ethical, legal, and cultural competence (ANA, 2010a, 2010b).

Nurses rarely act in the community as sole agents. Rather, the nurse is typically part of an intradisciplinary (within nursing) and interdisciplinary (with other providers) team whose members, acting in concert, assist clients in meeting their healthcare needs. Thus the nurse fulfills three primary roles in the community: care provider, team member, and community partner.

- *Nurse as Care Provider.* Nurses provide a wide range of services in the community. For example, they provide advanced acute care interventions in the home as well as health planning services for a whole geographic area. Nurses engage in multiple illness prevention, health maintenance, and health restoration activities as needed by the community.
- *Nurse as Team Member.* Although some nurses work in isolation, the power of community health nursing comes from an articulated intradisciplinary and interdisciplinary plan of care for clients needing services.
- *Nurse as Community Partner.* In the community, nurses work toward establishing partnership status with clients, so as to create success in meeting community-based needs. Nurses must be present in the community—and actually be a part of the community—to be effective in providing nursing care.

Intervention from many health-related disciplines is needed to improve the health of the community. Nursing, as one discipline, is a significant—but not isolated—contributor to the betterment of the public's health. Nurses need to improve their ability to work with other team members continuously so that comprehensive care can be provided to all clients. The skill of healthcare team members in providing comprehensive care should focus on care that is available, accessible, affordable, appropriate, adequate, and acceptable (ANA, 2010a, 2010b). In the community, nurses' skills and knowledge, as well as the skills of other members of the interdisciplinary team, vary from novice to expert. The team is likely to consist of both newly licensed and experienced members who are striving to work collaboratively to solve problems and meet the needs of clients (Buerhaus, Staiger, & Auerbach, 2009).

Community-Based Needs

The needs of all communities change on an ongoing basis. Continuous assessment of community-based needs is necessary for constructing a useful picture of which needs represent priorities for action. A clear image of community-based needs informs the client and the nurse which systems of care management are necessary to use or develop, and how to direct or redirect resources to make these systems of care management useful. The dynamic nature of community health nursing includes an ever-changing scope of problems and solutions, ranging from emerging pandemics such as the H1N1 influenza to changing demographics of current problems such as HIV/AIDS (National Center for Health Statistics, 2009; DHHS, 2010).

There are six areas of concern related to community-based needs: patterns of morbidity and mortality, demographics, environmental concerns, public services, aesthetics, and health-related facilities.

Patterns of Morbidity and Mortality

Morbidity: Illness.

Mortality: Death.

The patterns of **morbidity** (illness) and **mortality** (death) are central concerns with community-based needs and significant variables in community health assessment. Knowledge of the causes of death and disability assists in the development of preventive health services as well as in the provision of early treatment and rehabilitation services. Patterns of morbidity and mortality inevitably change in communities. Epidemics, changes in immunization rates in children, and variations in how disease affects certain groups can all affect patterns of morbidity and mortality, with such changes occurring as communities develop, grow, or deteriorate.

Demographics

Information about clients is coded based on characteristics such as age, employment, religious affiliation, and level of education. A community is known by both the visible characteristics of the people (e.g., age, race, gender, and location of housing) and their invisible characteristics (e.g., level of education, income, and religion). Thus **demographics** represents a way of describing a community statistically. Demographics can describe only those aspects of the community that can be measured. Some parts of the community demographics, such as the homelessness rate, may prove challenging to measure because it is difficult to obtain an accurate count of the number of people living in isolation.

In the United States, the complexity of measuring national demographics, usually through census counts performed every 10 years, results in problems with reporting findings. Some data take years to analyze and present to the public. The community may change while the old picture of a community (findings from the census) is being developed and provided to the public. The massive task of measuring characteristics of the United States makes more frequent measurement unlikely. As a consequence, changes in the population that surface immediately after a census measurement may not be captured until the next census is conducted (U.S. Census Bureau, 2010).

International demographics are difficult to use because different countries use different variables to measure health statistics. Some countries do not record any health-related information, which makes any comparison impossible. Also, exact definitions of what constitutes certain illnesses or syndromes vary from nation to nation.

Environmental Concerns

Environmental concerns relate to the quality of air, water, food, and variables such as the physical and emotional working conditions in which people find themselves. Safety is the key to environmental health regardless of where people live, eat, play, work, and pray (if appropriate). Recreational, employment, and house of worship facilities need to be as safe as where people live (shelter).

The environment is the context in which life is supported on earth. Concern about the global environment is necessary to protect the fragile ecosystem, which serves as a major determinant of health. It is important to advocate for a healthy environment, whether one is concerned about the loss of the atmospheric ozone layer and the resulting increase in harmful, carcinogenic rays from the sun, or the presence of a local chemical dump site that threatens the drinking water of a community. People need to know about the health effects of the environments in which they live, work, play, and pray, and they need to act in a way that conserves resources for future generations.

Public Services

Public services include fire, police, sanitation, and public education services; public utilities (gas, electric, water); and recreation and sports facilities. Every community provides protection from crime and disasters to its residents as well as activities that promote socialization and entertainment. A sign of a healthy community is the availability of adequate public services such that the community members are safe to enjoy life. Large communities or those in certain hubs of the country may offers more public services than other communities. In times of financial constraints, some communities limit access to public services that are not seen as essential.

Aesthetics

Aesthetics includes exposure to and participation in the fine arts, music, and spirituality, closely associated with one's cultural experience. The personal joy of seeking beauty in one's home and surrounding environment is augmented by the availability of parks, museums, and houses of worship. Communities express the joys and pains of

Demographics: A way of describing a community statistically based on the community members' visible characteristics (e.g., age, race, gender, and location of housing) and invisible characteristics (e.g., level of education, income, and religion).

Aesthetics: Exposure to and participation in the fine arts, music, and spirituality, closely associated with one's cultural experience.

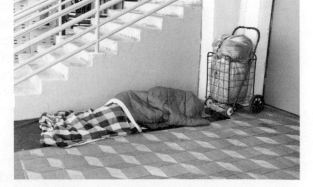
© Joe Belanger/Shutterstock.com

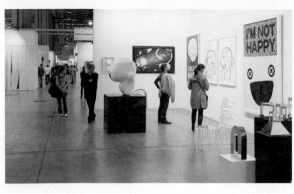

© Adriano Castelli/Shutterstock.com

living through the creation of art and beauty. People may define art and beauty as a personal valuing of pottery, paintings, or music. The personal meaning of aesthetics in a multiracial, multiethnic society such as the United States is important to consider, as people may have widely divergent views of what is artistic and beautiful.

A healthy community is one in which people can express what they find to be artistic and beautiful while tolerating the expressions of other groups different from themselves. The appreciation of diversity is key to the aesthetic component of a healthy community. Some of the ways in which communities appreciate aesthetics are by building museums, funding public sculpture, remembering holy days and festivals, and holding ethnic celebrations.

Health-Related Facilities

Although all health-related facilities are located in the community, they vary in terms of what they do and who they serve. Health-related facilities include ambulatory care clinics, hospitals, community-based organizations (CBOs), subacute and custodial care facilities, public health departments, and home care and hospice organizations. These various health-related facilities are built by communities to meet the needs of the public. Contemporary trends are to decentralize healthcare services when possible and to increase the use of CBOs. Rehabilitative services, for example, are moving into communities so that clients can receive services close to where they live.

Individuals and groups can also provide care out of private offices. In addition, health maintenance organizations (HMOs) and preferred provider organizations (PPOs) support health care by linking a number of facilities or practitioners together to provide health care with the intent of lowering costs.

Systems of Care Management

Systems of care management exist to meet community-based needs within the possibilities and realities of resource allocation. These systems need careful creation, use, and at times termination, so as to maximize the resources available for meeting community-based needs. Understanding systems of care management involves a study of the mix of client problems, expectations of the public for care, competence of healthcare professionals, accepted standards of care, and use of interdisciplinary plans of care. These five variables influence the development of the systems of care management in a number of ways.

Mix of Client Problems

The mix of client problems varies widely according to location, success in resolving existing problems, and identification of new problems as they emerge. It may necessitate an ever-fluctuating level of intensity of needed services. Some individual clients in the community may need total support, whereas others may need only minimal intervention to maintain independence in living. Nurses in the community must make daily assessments of their case loads to decide which clients need a visit, which clients need a supportive phone call, and which clients need a different level of care, perhaps involving referral and coordination.

When the client mix includes families and groups of people as in a support group, care providers have a more diverse case load and confront a wider range of human problems. For example, the community health nurse caring for a family experiencing domestic disputes will likely be managing a complex plan of care. Clients with domestic dispute problems need special intervention services and psychosocial counseling.

The family unit needs a very different type of care from interventions focused on individuals. In domestic violence, the whole family needs care and support. Groups of people meeting for a common reason, such as a 12-step Alcoholics Anonymous group, have common needs, but the group requires a variety of interventions so that all members can participate. Sometimes nursing groups of people is done for economy of time (giving similar instructions to many people at the same time), and sometimes it is done because people are better able to participate in their healing in the midst of group support. Some cancer support groups are founded on the idea that people with similar problems are best able to help other cancer survivors cope with life.

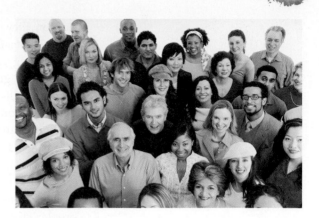

© Digital Vision/Thinkstock

Expectations of the Public for Care

The expectations of the public for health care are as complex as the various communities that exist. The desire for healthcare services by the public is a major aspect of how care is ultimately managed. For example, prior to the advent of dialysis, people had fewer expectations about long-term care of clients with renal disease than they do today. Similarly, recent trends that support consumerism and make nutritional counseling and weight-loss information a high priority encourage the public to expect this type of information from their care providers.

Advertising often attempts to inform clients what they should expect from healthcare providers. Competing advertisements often present the idea that a special service is actually the normal service, thereby suggesting that organizations without the special service are actually offering substandard care. Some deluxe maternity services are advertised as a service that a new family should expect, implying that hospitals without such a service are not providing the basic care that the new family needs. In this sense, advertisements may be misleading.

Some people avoid the healthcare system because they fear providers, do not trust that the care they receive is adequate, or have had a poor experience with care in the past. The major problem with this situation is that the client avoids the care system until the illness or problem has progressed so far that little or nothing can be done to correct it.

The challenge for healthcare providers is to assist the public to expect a *reasonable* level of care, given that *unlimited* care is no longer realistic. Even the reliance on the safety net of healthcare services for people who are uninsured or underinsured, living in poverty, or with disabilities is now being called into question. In addition, American society has not yet defined "futile care"; as a consequence, many people continue to receive care that will not help them become healthier or improve their quality of life (Public Health Leadership Society, 2002; DHHS, 2010).

Some clients are kept on high-technology life support equipment long after such care has ceased to be useful, at the expense of others who might benefit from that level of care. Such misdirected care exacts an unknown toll on families, groups, and communities that must pay for the care on both monetary and emotional levels. The focus on curative care, as discussed earlier in this book, creates a scenario in which people always want more care after a health problem emerges, instead of preventing the problem in the first place.

Competence of Healthcare Professionals

The competence of healthcare professionals is both a personal responsibility and a public mandate (ANA, 2010a; Holmes, 2006). The competence of professionals affects how care is managed. Nurses need competence in theoretical as well as technical aspects of care. Care providers need to be skilled in issues related to financial reimbursement, for example, to be fully able to manage care effectively from an economic perspective. In addition, they need specific skills in negotiation, supervision, and collective bargaining, to name but a few areas. Nurses working to guard the public's health must be skilled in epidemiology, project management, and politics.

Likewise, given the high level of acuity in home care services, nurses need the latest technical skills in areas such as intravenous home infusion therapy, use of respirators, administration of peritoneal dialysis, and managing complex medication regimens to be able to manage care in a safe way. Each member of the interdisciplinary team brings various levels of skill in the physical, emotional, spiritual, and cultural care of clients; together the team is able to provide comprehensive care to the community. The smooth functioning of the interdisciplinary team suggests that the team as a whole, though not necessarily each team member, has the skills and knowledge necessary to manage complex client situations.

Accepted Standards of Care

Effective examination of accepted standards of care requires the input of both professionals and the people whom they serve. Each healthcare discipline performs its work using accepted standards of care. The ANA sets general standards of care for the nursing profession, for example, and the ANA and specialty organizations, such as the Association of Nurses in AIDS Care, collaborate to set standards for specialized and advanced practice (Finkelman & Kenner, 2009). Legally, the state Nurse Practice Act specifies the parameters of accepted nursing care for its jurisdiction. Consortia, such as the Public Health Leadership Society, may establish principles for ethical practice from an interdisciplinary perspective (Public Health Leadership Society, 2002).

Nurses are required to uphold standards for community-based care that are adapted for home care, school health, public health, and private practice. Nurses working in the community have the opportunity to share their concerns about care with their peers and professional associations so that the standards of care reflect contemporary practice. Organizations such as the National League for Nursing and the Public Health Nursing section of the American Public Health Association are involved in solving problems in community-based practice through discussions among their respective memberships.

Use of Interdisciplinary Plans of Care

Interdisciplinary plan of care (IPC): An action plan created and used by the various disciplines involved in the process of providing care that set minimal expectations for client outcomes or responses to care interventions.

Interdisciplinary plans of care (IPCs), also known as action plans, are created and used by the various disciplines involved in the process of providing care. They influence care management by setting minimal expectations for client outcomes or responses to care interventions. These care plans are intended to capture the more general or typical response to interventions to accelerate discharge from a more acute level of care to a lesser level of care. For example, an individual client might be discharged from the hospital to home, or the home care nurse might discharge a client from a dependent care level of service to a level of greater self-care and independence.

Standardized IPCs are not useful for every client. People may respond to care in unique or unexpected ways and, therefore, may need a tailored, personal plan of care. It is important to remember that all clients, working together with the nurse, need to continuously evaluate the actual plan of care for its fit with any predetermined IPC. Each provider has the legal responsibility to plan and provide care that meets the special needs of clients.

Interdisciplinary plans of care are conceptually less useful for families, groups, and communities. Standards of care for collectives are difficult to set because of the complexities inherent in more complex, multiple-person clients. Ongoing research is needed to document an interdisciplinary approach to the care of families, groups, and communities.

Resource Allocation

Resource allocation is a complex construct, with aspects related to local, regional, national, and global availability and use of personal and material resources. Resource allocation comprises more than just cash flow from various private and public sources; it involves the material, time, and energy necessary to construct systems of care management that meet the needs of the community on physical, emotional, and cultural levels. Resource allocation is explored by examining the patterns of resource allocation, values and beliefs of the population, reliance on government funding, influence of special interest groups, and patterns of insurance coverage.

Patterns of Resource Allocation

Patterns of resource allocation include who receives resources in the present and who received them in the past. The pattern of resource allocation is an important variable when one considers who needs resources today as well as tomorrow. Every community has a pattern of how it allocates resources. Retirement communities allocate resources differently than aggregates of young families, for example. One role for nursing and other members of the interdisciplinary team is to keep a community informed about unmet needs of other parts of the community. For example, a community that does not value rehabilitative services may need to be educated about the importance of these services before it decides whether it wants or requires them.

Values and Beliefs of the Population

The values and beliefs of the population relate to concerns about who should and who should not receive resources. These considerations dictate which types of health-related services members of the population want developed. For example, a closed and isolated Amish community has different requirements for health services than a large metropolitan Hispanic community. Some populations with traditional religious beliefs could be expected to have different requisites for family planning services than groups who value various artificial birth control methods.

Populations are diverse and inevitably encompass a variety of cultural values and beliefs. The community health nurse needs to uncover and learn about these various beliefs without supporting negative stereotypes. For example, nurses can learn about beliefs different from their own by reading about other cultures as well as living and working with other groups of people. Diversity is found both between cultural groups and within the groups themselves. Most groups have members who are conservative as well as those who are liberal in how they interpret the values and beliefs held by the overall group.

Reliance on Government Funding

Reliance on government funding occurs on local, state, and national levels. Communities that receive various levels of government funding for health-related programs allocate their resources differently than communities that pay out-of-pocket for all healthcare services. In the United States, public hospitals subsidize approximately 70% of inpatient care and 50% of outpatient or ambulatory care (National Center for Health Statistics, 2009). Changes in government funding could greatly affect the services offered in certain communities that subsidize healthcare costs with public support. Each state varies in how it provides funds or services to the people who cannot pay for them. Local communities provide services after applying taxes on property and goods that are sold. The United States is different from other countries in this respect, because it does not have an integrated national–state–local level of health services guaranteed to

Special interest group: A group that uses its influence to get the services that its members want.

Advocacy group: A type of special interest group that exists to assist less empowered groups to have a voice and get their needs met.

its citizens. As a consequence, the U.S. healthcare system provides services that are not always integrated (Finkelman & Kenner, 2009).

Influence of Special Interest Groups

The influence of **special interest groups** can affect resource allocation in both overt and covert ways. Special interest groups are those that use their influence to get the services that they want. For example, a certain political group may want more acute care cardiac services while limiting reproductive services for women. One concern with special interest groups is that they may advocate for services for one group at the expense of another group's needs.

Healthcare planning can become inconsistent and chaotic when special interests are catered to without regard for the needs of the whole community. Clients from different age groups or with different diagnoses should not have to compete for care resources. Should resources in short supply go to the clients in the neonatal intensive care unit or those in the intermediate geriatric care unit? Does society want to focus on caring for people with AIDS or Alzheimer's disease? There are no easy answers to these questions.

Advocates for the homeless, prisoners, and physically and mentally challenged persons indicate that their needs are often not taken into account when healthcare choices are made by the public. **Advocacy groups**—another type of special interest group—exist to assist less empowered groups to have a voice and get their needs met. The community health nurse advocates for different types of clients at different times in their experience of health and illness. Nurses advocate for other nurses by lobbying politicians to protect professional practice legislation.

Patterns of Insurance Coverage

The influence of third-party payment for health care as it relates to who has access to healthcare services is a complex issue. Increasingly large segments of the U.S. population are now uninsured or underinsured. Insurance coverage is not just a problem for people who do not work; many of the "working poor" cannot afford health insurance either. Patterns of insurance coverage are directly influenced by employment patterns. For example, many people who work are not offered healthcare benefits or are paid per diem wages that do not include healthcare or other benefits. Some workers in the United States are undocumented nonresidents who are impossible to cover with insurance. Insurance coverage is a primary concern of emerging discussions of healthcare reform (DHHS, 2010).

The Alliance for Health Model as a Complement to Evidence-Based Nursing

The use of the Alliance for Health Model complements the evolution of evidence-based nursing in care delivery, education, and ongoing research. This model is unique in requiring the examination of the therapeutic relationship between the nurse and the client, as well as the requisite to address the realities of resource allocation. The nurse and the client—that is, the profession and the public—must do their healing work within the constraints and possibilities of allocating human and material resources. The Alliance for Health Model has a history of utility in relating these core concepts with this healing work in education and care delivery in the community (Holzemer, 1997, 2010; Holzemer, Scaramuzzino, & Kiernan, 2001).

Evidence from Research

Evidence from scholarship is central to the work of moving with clients on their journey to health and wellness. Qualitative and quantitative ways of knowing are enriched by the various, respective modes of inquiry. Studies conducted in the community can use large samples to describe, correlate, and predict phenomena of interest in quantitative research. In this sense, the community represents a living laboratory where qualitative questions find meaningful answers in how people live.

Evidence from Clinical Practice

The realities of using and improving best practices in nursing care begin at the bedside, regardless of the location of care delivery. The expertise of the nurses "in the community" provides new and innovative approaches to care that are pre-research in nature. Point-of-service experience indicates where improvements in care may be generated prior to the formal inquiry involved in quantitative and qualitative research.

Evidence from the Client's Experience

Clients live their joys and sorrows in a unique way; the result is their story—their experience. It is critical for nurses and other healthcare providers to listen closely to their clients and incorporate their experience into the plan of care. Respect for the health-related experience of the client is not part of their story, but rather the central component of their story. When the story comes from a family, group, aggregate, or other community, it is likely to be complex, and sometimes confusing.

Attention to the client's story is vital, yet it poses a challenge in community health nursing. The evidence from the client's experience is not simply a summation of the evidence from individual members in a family, group, aggregate, or other community. Instead, the story of a family in distress comprises the collective ability of the family to function in a healthy way; the story of a community includes the needs of the people and environmental influences that reflect the health and illness of the whole. The client's experience in the community is demonstrated by the community's dynamic and changing behaviors, and it takes vigilance on the part of the nurse to interpret these behaviors correctly.

The concept of vulnerability, specifically related to clients without a voice, is a particular challenge to the community health nurse. Clients who are not heard due to the overwhelming needs of special interest groups, for example, make listening to the client very difficult. The influence exerted by clients of special interest, who may control the systems of care management and resource allocation in the community, make meeting the needs of all clients problematic.

Use of the Alliance for Health Model: Two Different Problems in the Community

Two case studies are used here as examples of how the various parts of the Alliance for Health Model are related. A problem may begin with any of the primary aspects of the model. In the first example, the problem begins in the area of community-based needs; in the second example, a concern is noted with resource allocation. It is important to understand that the problems in one area influence all other areas of the model. Of interest, a problem emerging in one area may be solved by devoting attention to a related or nested concern in another part of the model.

A Problem Emerging with Community-Based Needs

Community-Based Needs. Community A is a rural community, with a population of 5,000. The public health nurse is working with an epidemiologist to review recent mortality data from the local hospital, nursing home, and emergent care center. The pair notes a rapid rise in the incidence of an influenza-like illness, especially among young women. Phone calls to the local school of nursing and a child care center validate high absentee rates among the women attending or using these facilities. The local news station reports 46 cases of the yet-to-be-named condition, with three unconfirmed deaths. The local community moves into a crisis state (**FIGURE 3-4**).

Vision of the Client. The community as a whole (vision of the client) becomes afraid of contagion and avoids care. An increased rate of voluntary discharges from the local hospital occur, against nursing advice. Some families curtail outside activities, and local support and activity groups cancel meetings. Segments of the community with financial means leave the area on "unplanned vacations." Other segments of the population, whose members were not previously participants in receiving healthcare resources, seem immobilized from acting and isolate themselves.

Expertise of the Provider. Nurses and other healthcare providers, as part of the community, also fear contagion. Unlike their lay counterparts, they secure antibiotics before a causative agent can be isolated. Although considered an unsound medical practice, the providers of care take drugs to prevent what

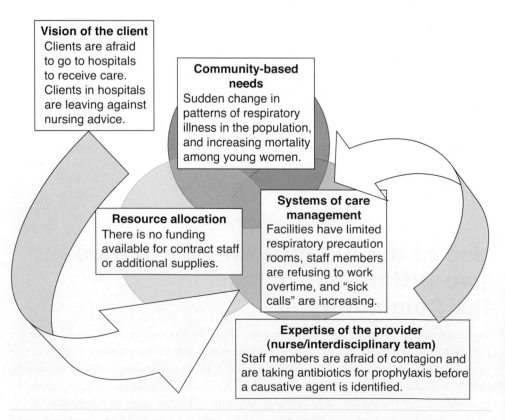

Figure 3-4 Alliance for Health Model: A problem emerging with community-based needs.

"might occur to them." They are not responding to the situation like educated professionals.

Systems of Care Management. The systems to provide care in the local hospital are experiencing problems. The facility was not constructed and is not supplied to cope with a sudden influx of patients with respiratory illness. Families are upset and angry because visiting hours have been curtailed. Even with minimal space and equipment constraints, problems are intensifying because of the number of staff who are not showing up for work. The number of "sick calls" is increasing.

A Problem Emerging with Resource Allocation

Resource Allocation. A funding plan to keep a private children's hospital fails, leading to the closure of the 75-bed institution (**FIGURE 3-5**). The private, for-profit hospital was part of a regional pediatric care system, and was losing money due to low reimbursement rates for experimental procedures. The hospital is a major source of employment for the geographic area. There are two other hospitals in the area, but the closest pediatric facility is now 150 miles away.

Community-Based Needs. Community B is an urban community, with a population of 67,000 people. The public is aware that ongoing political unrest has prevented the passing of the local budget. The "general feel" in the community is that all of the problems will be resolved during the last budgetary session.

Vision of the Client. The community as a whole (vision of the client) is very upset because there is no place for their sick children to receive care conveniently.

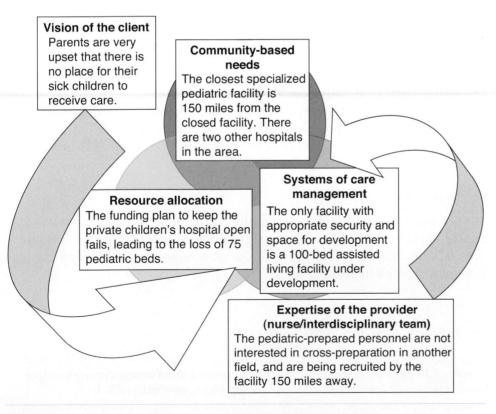

Figure 3-5 Alliance for Health Model: A problem emerging with resource allocation.

Expertise of the Provider. The pediatric-prepared personnel are not interested in cross-preparation in another field, and are being recruited by the facility located 150 miles away.

Systems of Care Management. The only facility with appropriate security and space for development is a 100-bed assisted living facility under development.

Summary

The Alliance for Health Model represents a philosophy of nursing care in the community, defined as a joint venture between the nurse and the client on their journey toward health. The model provides the professional nurse with a schema for applying the nursing process to actual and potential health problems experienced by families, other groups, aggregates, and communities. There are three steps in the joint venture process of seeking health by the nurse and the client:

1. The voice of the client articulates needs, and is responded to by the nurse (or other provider) with the professional expertise to hear the client.
2. The nurse and the client identify community-based needs and validate the utility of the systems of care management (either in place or needing development) to meet community-based needs.
3. The nurse and the community secure the resources needed to resolve health-related threats to the community.

The Alliance for Health Model should be seen as a dynamic whole of interacting parts or components, which find meaning in their relationship to the other aspects of the model. It includes five components:

1. The voice of the client
2. The expertise of the provider (nurse and interdisciplinary team)
3. Community-based needs
4. Systems of care management
5. Resource allocation concerns

The Alliance for Health Model complements the idea of evidence-based nursing in care delivery, education, and research. Using this model, the nurse collects evidence of health (or the lack of health) from established research, accesses the expertise of professionals "in the field," and appreciates the lived experience of the client. The Alliance for Health Model can serve as a useful tool to better capture the relationship between the CHN and the client on their search for health.

Acknowledgments

The development and utility of the Alliance for Health Model is due in great part to Joan Arnold, PhD, RN. Dr. Arnold, a community health nurse scientist, continues to advance the science of community health nursing education–research–care delivery to improve the health of people in need.

REFERENCES

Allender, J. A., Rector, C., & Warner, K. D. (2010). *Community health nursing: Promoting and protecting the public's health* (7th ed.). New York, NY: Lippincott Williams & Wilkins.

American Nurses Association (ANA). (2001). *Code of ethics for nurses with interpretive statements.* Silver Spring, MD: Author.

American Nurses Association (ANA). (2010a). *Nursing: Scope and standards of practice* (3rd ed.). Silver Spring, MD: Author.

American Nurses Association. (2010b). *Nursing's social policy statement: The essence of the profession.* Silver Spring, MD: Author.

Buerhaus, P. I., Staiger, D. O., & Auerbach, D. I. (2009). *The future of the nursing workforce in the United States: Data, trends, and implications.* Sudbury, MA: Jones & Bartlett.

Dayer-Berenson, L. (2011). *Cultural competencies for nurses: Impact on health and illness.* Sudbury, MA: Jones and Bartlett.

Finkelman, A., & Kenner, C. (2009). *Teaching IOM: Implications of the Institute of Medicine reports for nursing education* (2nd ed.). Silver Spring, MD: American Nurses Association.

Fowler, M. D. (Ed.). (2010). *Guide to the code of ethics for nurses: Interpretation and application.* Silver Spring, MD: American Nurses Association.

Holmes, C. A. (2006). The slow death of psychiatric nursing: What next? *Journal of Psychiatric and Mental Health Nursing, 13,* 401–415.

Holzemer, S. P. (1997). The Alliance for Health Model: Helping students to understand community health assessment and care delivery. In B. Marckx & E. Tagliareni (Eds.), *Teaching in the community: Preparing nurses for the 21st century.* New York, NY: National League for Nursing Press.

Holzemer, S. P. (2010). Creating a culture of care for the maturing nurse. In M. Klainberg & K. M. Dirschel, *Today's nursing leader: Managing, succeeding, excelling* (pp. 277–290). Sudbury, MA: Jones and Bartlett.

Holzemer, S. P., Scaramuzzino, M., & Kiernan, J. (2001). Community-based primary care for children. In C. G. Hernandez, J. K. Singleton, & D. Z. Aronzon (Eds.), *Primary care pediatrics.* Philadelphia, PA: Lippincott.

National Center for Health Statistics (NCHS). (2009). *Health, United States, 2009: With special feature on medical technology.* Hyattsville, MD: U.S. Government Printing Office. Retrieved from http://www.cdc.gov/nchs/hus.htm

Public Health Leadership Society. (2002). *Principles of the ethical practice of public health* (Version 2.2). Retrieved from http://www.phls.org

Solberg, L. I. (2007). Improving medical practice: A conceptual framework. *Annals of Family Medicine, 5*(3), 251–256.

U.S. Census Bureau. (2010). *Statistical abstract of the United States: 2010* (129th ed.). Washington, DC: Author. Retrieved from http://www.census.gov/statab/overview.html

U.S. Department of Health and Human Services (DHHS). (2010, July). *Healthy people 2020: The road ahead.* Retrieved from http://www.healthypeople.gov/hp2020

ADDITIONAL RESOURCES

Centers for Disease Control and Prevention (CDC). (2010, June 25). Summary of notifiable diseases—United States, 2008. *Morbidity and Mortality Weekly Report, 57*(54).

Milstead, J. A. (2013). *Health policy and politics: A nurse's guide* (4th ed.). Burlington, MA: Jones & Bartlett.

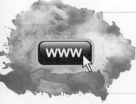

For a full suite of assignments and additional learning activities, use the access code located in the front of your book to visit the exclusive website: http://go.jblearning.com/Holzemer/. If you do not have an access code, you can obtain one at the site.

LEARNING ACTIVITIES

www

Read the following questions slowly and choose the best answer. Questions that have more than one correct answer are identified with the statement "Choose all that apply."

Using the Alliance for Health Model in **FIGURE 3-6**, match the various sets of data with the five key aspects of the model. The key aspects may be used more than once.

For Questions 1–6, match the following examples with the key aspect of the Alliance for Health Model (A–E) each represents.

A. Community-based needs
B. Systems of care management
C. Resource allocation concerns
D. Vision of the client
E. Expertise of the provider

1. Insurance coverage.

2. Creation of special hospital units for respiratory infections.

3. Experience of being a client in the hospital.

4. Availability of sanitation services.

5. A nurse does not make a referral to a physical therapist when such a referral is indicated.

6. A client and family decide to institute a "do not resuscitate" directive.

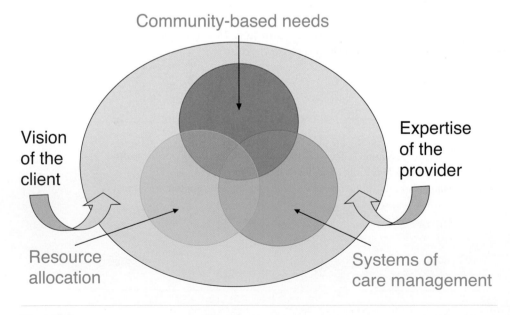

Figure 3-6

7. A nurse is interested in obtaining evidence of the client's perspective of care while developing an evidence-based protocol. Which of the following statements, made by a nurse, reflect an attempt to capture the client's perspective of care? Choose all that apply.

   A. "Contact the Health Department to obtain the latest morbidity data."

   B. "Reviewing the patient satisfaction data will provide useful information."

   C. "A new protocol will allow the staff to make follow-up calls to clients."

   D. "Ask the nurse managers to submit their thoughts on best practices."

   E. "Interview the financial staff to identify the lowest-cost interventions."

8. A nurse who is working in "high-tech" home care feels that he is not prepared to provide comprehensive care to clients receiving chemotherapy in the home. From which resource would the nurse *initially* seek help to resolve the problem?

   A. The board of nursing in the state where the nurse works

   B. The specialty organization related to the type of care that is provided

   C. The school of nursing from which the nurse graduated

   D. The education department of the employing agency

9. A community health nurse would anticipate using an interdisciplinary plan of care with which of the following clients?

   A. A 12-year-old boy with an arm fracture and of normal weight

   B. An 87-year-old man with unstable angina and dementia

   C. A 45-year-old woman with chest trauma and poor health history

   D. A newborn with failure to thrive after a home delivery

10. A community health nurse working in a large, politically conservative community would expect limitations in which of the following healthcare services?

    A. Coronary care services for men

    B. Supportive care services for older people

    C. Women's reproductive health services

    D. Services for infants and children

ADDITIONAL QUESTIONS FOR STUDY

The Alliance for Health Model will be greatly influenced by the unfolding of the Patient Protection and Affordable Care Act (Affordable Care Act), which became law in 2010. Although the exact way the law will take effect state by state may be different, the concerns of the five components of the model will be, in some ways, redefined.

Go to the website Health Care and You (http://www.healthcareandyou.org), or another similar site, and review the various components of the Affordable Care Act. Discuss with your classmates the impact of the Affordable Care Act on the following:

1. The voice of the client

2. The expertise of the provider (nurse and interdisciplinary team)

3. Community-based needs

4. Systems of care management

5. Resource allocation concerns (components of the Alliance for Health Model)

APPENDIX 3-A

Alliance for Health Model Community Assessment Tool

Name of team (group) members; identify the team leader. (Your instructor may assign any number of people to make up a community assessment team.)

1. _____ (Team Leader)

2. _____

3. _____

4. _____

5. _____

6. _____

Please identify the dates and times of data collection, as well as the sources of information used in all parts of this assessment. Omit the names of the people you interview for the purposes of privacy and confidentiality. Place your original assessment notes where indicated.

Description of the Community

Use Census Tract or other statistical resources to determine the boundaries of the community. In this description, include pictures, newspaper articles, and direct quotes from residents for the community you select. Write a summary statement in the space provided. Place pictures and other supplemental material in the "Supplemental Data" section. Do not take pictures of residents that can reveal their identity. Distant group shots without identifying information are acceptable.

Areas of Assessment

Focus on Community-Based Needs

1. **Patterns of Morbidity and Mortality:** What are the leading causes of death and disability? Why do people seek health care? Are there unusual patterns of illness and death in the community?
2. **Demographics:** What are the characteristics of the community related to age, gender, education level, income and types of housing available? Have the demographics changed over the last 5 to 10 years?

3. **Environmental Concerns:** What does the community look like? Which types of environmental problems could cause accidents or disease? Are there any areas in the community where the movement of people is restricted due to pollution or other barriers?
4. **Public Services:** Which types of public services exist related to fire, police, education, sanitation, recreation, and sports? Has an emergency disaster plan been developed for this community? How do people evaluate the quality of these services?
5. **Aesthetics:** Which types of art, music, cultural, and religious institutions are reflected or available in the community?
6. **Health-Related Facilities:** Describe the various health-related facilities available to the community under study. What is the response rate of the emergency medical services? How do the health-related facilities relate to the characteristics and needs of the community?

Care Management Techniques

1. How do the patterns of morbidity and mortality of the community relate to the use of resources (e.g., is the local hospital so burdened with trauma cases that other clients do not receive timely emergency care)?
2. Do people in the community want care that is not being provided? Do people perceive inequality in who obtains care?
3. How do healthcare providers define the type of care that is provided to the community? How is the care evaluated?
4. How are standards of care set, followed, and evaluated?
5. Is there evidence of an interdisciplinary plan of care for the community? Which disciplines are involved in providing interdisciplinary care?

Influences on Resource Allocation Decisions

1. What are the influences on allocation of resources?
2. What are the values and beliefs of the community, as they relate to health and illness? How do you know this?
3. In what ways does the community depend on government funding for its healthcare services? Are there alternative sources of funding?
4. Which special interest groups exist in the community? How do they influence healthcare services?
5. What are the patterns of healthcare insurance coverage?
6. What is the process for involving the consumer in healthcare decisions for the community?
7. How are care providers oriented for their work? Is there continuing education available or required?

Application: Diagnostic Statement(s) About the Community

Write diagnostic statements that are developed from the assessment *after the entire assessment is completed*. They should be listed in the priority of how your team thinks they should be addressed. Identify whether they represent actual or potential problems. Write the group's rationale for the order in which the diagnoses are listed.

Evaluation of the Community Assessment Project

1. What were the benefits and limitations of completing this project?
2. Which aspects of the project would you change to improve your learning?

Assessment Notes

Identify the dates and times of data collection, as well as the sources of information used in all parts of this assessment. Each team member may collect notes separately, and the information for the whole group should be placed in this section.

Supplemental Data

Place pictures, newspaper articles, fliers, and other supplemental material here. (Do not take pictures of residents that can reveal their identity. Distant group shots without identifying information are acceptable.)

CHAPTER OUTLINE

▸ Introduction
▸ The Relationship Between Health Policy and Evidence-Based Research
▸ Health Policy
  • Forms of Policy
  • Health Policy Encoded into Law
  • Ethical and Philosophical Concerns
  • The Policy Process
  • Politics and Power
  • How a Bill Becomes Law

• Assessing the Policy Environment and Getting Involved
▸ Evidence-Based Research
  • Definitions
  • Scientific Research
  • Types of Studies
  • Clinical Research and Evidence-Based Practice: An Example
▸ Summary

OBJECTIVES

1. Define the relationship between health policy and evidence-based research (and practice).

2. Discuss the challenges in securing evidence from research, the experience of expert practitioners, and clients (the community) to improve community health nursing care delivery, education, and research.

3. Explain the complex nature of developing health policy that accurately reflects the needs of the public.

4. Identify problems in the learner's local community that would benefit from research from both a quantitative and qualitative perspective.

KEY TERMS

Advocacy

Clinical research

Control (in research)

Evidence-based practice (EBP)

Experimental studies

Health policy

Inclusion/exclusion criteria

Lobbying

Lobbyist

Nonexperimental studies

Policy

Policy process

Political power

Politics

Power

Procedure

Public policy

Qualitative studies

Quantitative studies

Quasi-experimental studies

Randomization

Research

Scientific research

CHAPTER 4

Relating Health Policy and Evidence-Based Research in the Community

Clarilee Hauser

Introduction

This chapter discusses the relationship between health policy and evidence-based research (EBR). Health policy and EBR are related because of their close fit. For example, research informs the community health nurse (CHN) about better ways to provide care, and this information is then translated into health policy to improve care delivery systems and implement programs that have been shown to be effective.

This chapter begins with a review of how health policy is defined and how the policy process works. Because health policy on the state and national levels involves law, a description of how an idea about health becomes a bill, and how a bill becomes a law is provided. In addition, the process by which a CHN assesses the policy environment and ways that nurses can become involved in the process are explained. An example of a fictitious bill on providing support to women choosing the Lamaze process of childbirth preparation is reviewed. In the example, the idea to improve birthing services for women came from the most recent information representing best practice, or evidence-based practice (EBP). Evidence-based practice, like EBR, includes information gleaned from client preferences, expert clinical practice, and quality research.

Evidence-based research is the second major concept discussed in this chapter. The various aspects of scientific research are identified, along with the types of studies that nurses may use in community health nursing; these may be research models from a qualitative or quantitative perspective. The example of Lamaze training is re-introduced as an idea that could be studied in EBR. A specific technique of transforming a concept into a clinical topic for problem solving, known as the PICO (**P**atient/problem–**I**ntervention–**C**omparison/control–**O**utcome/effects) process, is reviewed. Findings from such a study could be used to set health policy, making the final connection between the concepts of research and health policy.

The Relationship Betwen Health Policy and Evidence-Based Research

Community health nursing practice encompasses the core functions of public health delineated by the Institute of Medicine in 1988—namely, assessment, policy development, and assurance. Although all nurses are very familiar with assessment, policy development and assurance may be new to nursing students. This chapter examines health policy and the way it affects the profession of nursing, public health services, and the health of the public. It has been claimed that the voice of nursing has historically been absent from policy decisions and, therefore, has had little impact upon the promotion of social action (Porter-O'Grady, 1994; Porter-O'Grady & Malloch, 2011). Today, given the spirited debate about the future of health care in the United States, it is now imperative that nursing discovers its voice. To that end, this chapter explores ways that individual nurses can become involved in the policy process.

To be successful, health policy and health programs must be based on sound scientific research. Scientific research is the foundation upon which EBP is built. To bridge the gap between research and EBP, the nurse must be familiar with the research process and be able to distinguish between sound and flawed research. In this chapter, the research process and the critique of research studies are presented with an eye toward the understanding that best practices (EBP) are based on strong scientific evidence. This evidence is essential to the formation of health policies supporting services that are cost-effective, beneficial, accessible, and acceptable to the public. **FIGURE 4-1** visually depicts the relationship between health policy and evidence-based research.

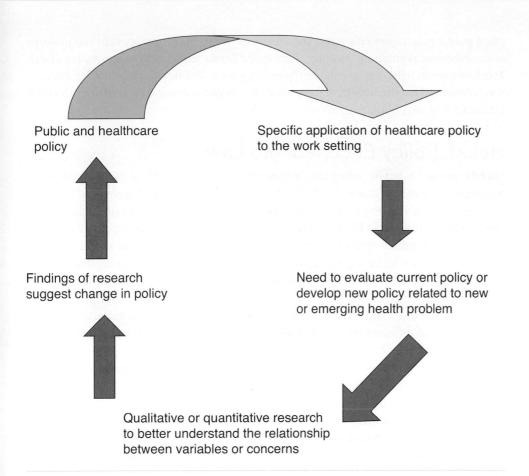

Public and healthcare policy

Specific application of healthcare policy to the work setting

Findings of research suggest change in policy

Need to evaluate current policy or develop new policy related to new or emerging health problem

Qualitative or quantitative research to better understand the relationship between variables or concerns

Figure 4-1 The relationship between health policy and evidence-based research.

Health Policy

Forms of Policy

Policy has been described as a "purposeful, overall plan of action or inaction developed to deal with a problem or a matter of concern in either the public or private sector" (Sudduth, 2008, p. 173). What does that statement mean? Think about your introduction to clinical practice. One of the first tasks you had to accomplish was to read the policies and procedures manual. The policy portion told you how you were expected to act. It outlined the institution's position on the use of drugs and alcohol; smoking on the premises; discrimination, sexual harassment, and creation of a hostile work environment; and many other policies intended to guide your behavior.

Policy making is intended to anticipate areas that may cause confusion and that are open to interpretation; policies clearly state the expected behavior in an effort to prevent problems from arising. These statements identify what "should" happen, not what actually happens (Blakemore & Griggs, 2007). **Procedures** are then developed to explain the actual mechanics of how to do something. Simply stated, policy is a statement of "what," whereas a procedure is a statement of "how" to do a task.

Public policy is policy formed through a governmental body for the benefit of the public (Bourne, 2010). It takes the form of regulations and is backed by the force of law. Policy is usually referred to as existing on the corporate level, whereas public policy is policy enacted at the governmental level. If you were to violate a corporate policy, you would risk reprimand and perhaps the loss of employment. By comparison, if you vio-

Policy: A "purposeful, overall plan of action or inaction developed to deal with a problem or a matter of concern in either the public or private sector" (Sudduth, 2008, p. 173).

Procedure: A statement that explains the actual mechanics of how to do something.

Public policy: Policy formed through a governmental body for the benefit of the public.

late a public policy, you risk arrest and/or prosecution. Public policy is broad in scope and establishes regulations ranging from speed limits to building codes to tax codes. Much of human behavior is regulated by public policy. Public policy is "public" because it is formulated for the benefit of the public, and because much of it comes from and is influenced by the public.

Health Policy Encoded into Law

Health policy: Public policy that is concerned with the health of the public and the healthcare system that maintains it.

Health policy is public policy that is concerned with the health of the public and the healthcare system that maintains it (Hanley & Falk, 2007). It is a statement of what we, as a society, believe is important about our health and the health of our communities. On its website, the World Health Organization (WHO) defines health policy as follows:

> Health policy refers to decisions, plans, and actions that are undertaken to achieve specific health care goals within a society. An explicit health policy can achieve several things: it defines a vision for the future which in turn helps to establish targets and points of reference for the short and medium term. It outlines priorities and the expected roles of different groups; and it builds consensus and informs people. (WHO, 2010)

In the United States, health policy is established at the local, state, and federal levels of government. For instance, at the local level, a school board might determine how much and which type of information about practicing safer sex is to be included in health classes at the local high school. At the state level, each state has its own Nurse Practice Act that defines the scope of nursing practice within the state, and a Board of Nursing that issues licenses, as part of the regulation of nursing practice. Much of the policy process regarding the health of the public is accomplished at the state level. Examples of health policy formulated at the national level include the various health-related bills that are a part of every political administration's legislative agenda. **Table 4-1** summarizes some of the most significant health policies developed at the national level. Five of the most significant pieces of federal legislation that have affected health care in the United States are briefly discussed in this section.

The Social Security Act of 1935

In part as a response to the ravages of the Great Depression, President Franklin D. Roosevelt signed the Social Security Act in 1935. This legislation provided for the "general welfare" by delivering federally subsidized old-age benefits and by empowering the states to provide for elderly and blind persons and dependent and crippled children. It also provided for public health, especially maternal and child health and welfare and unemployment insurance. While many of the programs were contributory in nature, some were financed by taxation. This legislation was significant because it represented the first time Americans had some government-sponsored protection from illness and old age (Gerber & McGuire, 1995).

The Social Security Act Amendments of 1965

Two programs were created under the aegis of the Social Security Act Amendments of 1965. Medicare provided federally funded health insurance for people 65 years and older and for disabled individuals, with the funds being derived from taxes on employee wages that were matched by the employer. Medicaid provided federal grants to states to provide healthcare benefits for low-income families and individuals. The signing of this act by President Lyndon B. Johnson was seen as an attempt to achieve some sort of universal health insurance coverage, a concept that was promoted by President Harry S. Truman.

TABLE 4-1
Examples of Significant Federal Health Policy Legislation

1921: The Sheppard-Towner Act, also known as the Sheppard-Towner Maternity and Infancy Protection Act of 1921, was enacted to provide education on maternity and childbirth using federal funding. It also provided incentives for states to develop women's healthcare clinics.

1963: The Maternal Child Health and Mental Retardation Planning Amendments provided grants to states to develop programs addressing mental health issues and improved programs and services for low-income, high-risk women and children.

1965: The Heart Disease, Cancer, and Stroke Amendments provided for regional medical centers to concentrate on specific programs. This legislation was intended to promote cooperation and coordination of healthcare services.

1966: The Comprehensive Health Planning and Public Health Service Amendments Act was designed to aid communities and states in coordinating services. It was an attempt to improve effectiveness and efficiency in health care.

1968: The Health Manpower Act extended funding to institutions for the training of physicians, nurses, and allied health personnel to meet the healthcare needs of the United States.

1970: The Occupational Safety and Health Act was enacted to ensure that employers provide a safe working environment.

1973: The Health Maintenance Organization Act established grants for the development of federally certified HMOs and required all employers who offered health insurance to their employees to also offer an HMO option.

1983: The Social Security Amendments introduced the concept of diagnosis-related groups (DRGs) and retrospective payments in an effort to control medical costs.

1985: The Consolidated Omnibus Budget Reconciliation Act extended hospice services and authorized coverage for health promotion to Medicare recipients.

1988: The Medicare Catastrophic Coverage Act extended Medicare to include home health and posthospital coverage.

1988: The Family Support Act strengthened welfare while stressing education and training for employment.

1992: The Preventive Health Amendments were enacted to enhance primary health care and prevention.

1996: The Health Insurance Portability and Accountability Act (HIPAA) provided protection for employees enrolled in group insurance plans as well as protection of personal health information.

2002: The Nurse Reinvestment Act was designed to address the nursing shortage by offering various financial incentives aimed at training nurses and nursing faculty.

2003: The Medicare Prescription Drug Improvement and Modernization Act added the option of coverage through a private insurance plan. It is referred to as Medicare Part D.

The Omnibus Budget Reconciliation Act of 1981

The Omnibus Budget Reconciliation Act of 1981 (OBRA) grew out of President Ronald Regan's Program for Economic Recovery. It was intended to give more spending discretion to the states through the creation of block grants from the federal government focusing on targeted areas. OBRA included cuts in funding and spending restrictions; in particular, it drastically cut funding for public health, resulting in a decrease in services.

The Personal Responsibility and Work Opportunity Reconciliation Act of 1996

As part of his platform as a presidential candidate, Bill Clinton campaigned on the promise to "end welfare as we know it." His subsequent signing of the Personal Responsibility and Work Opportunity Reconciliation Act of 1996 (PRWORA) accomplished that goal by replacing Aid to Families with Dependent Children (AFDC), popularly known as "welfare," with Temporary Assistance to Needy Families (TANF). This legislation placed a time limit on the eligibility for assistance, with the intent of incentivizing employment. Additionally, it restricted eligibility for food stamps and required recipients to actively seek employment. Ultimately PRWORA resulted in a deepening of poverty among the most vulnerable populations, such as single mothers, because they were forced into minimum-wage jobs while losing their benefits. "Nearly one-quarter of families who left welfare more than a year ago (before PRWORA) and had a full-time worker went without housing, food, or necessary medical care, while 29.9% of those in families that left welfare more recently did so" (Boushey, Gundersen, Brocht, & Bernstein, 2001). While PRWORA resulted in a decrease in the number of welfare recipients, it also produced an increase in the number of homeless families.

Healthcare Reform of 2010

What is popularly referred to as "healthcare reform" actually comprises two pieces of legislation: the Patient Protection and Affordable Care Act and the Health Care and Education Reconciliation Act of 2010. Both were signed into law by President Barack Obama in March 2010. "The health care law seeks to extend insurance to more than 30 million people by expanding Medicaid and providing federal subsidies to help lower- and middle-income Americans buy private coverage" ("Health Care Reform," 2011). It also

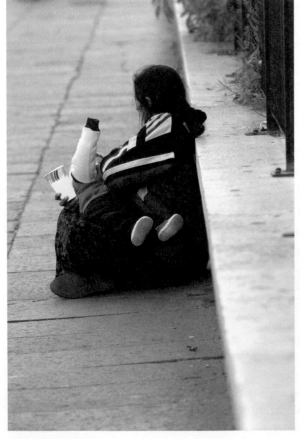

prohibits insurance companies from denying coverage due to preexisting medical conditions and allows children to remain on their parents' health insurance until the age of 26, among many other provisions. The provisions were to be phased in over a 4-year period. The legislation is massive and complicated, however, and since its ratification several of its conditions have been challenged in the courts. The constitutionality of the requirement for individuals to purchase health insurance or be assessed a fine is currently under review by the courts, with the U.S. Supreme Court hearing arguments on the matter in March 2012.

Opponents of the 2010 healthcare reform legislation claim that the cost of its implementation is prohibitive, while supporters direct attention to the report by the bipartisan Congressional Budget Office that estimates it will reduce the federal deficit by $138 billion over the next decade. Regardless of the final form that the legislation eventually takes, it has tremendous importance. Since at least the 1980s, the majority of the American public has supported creation of a government-sponsored insurance plan that would cover all citizens of the United States (Sack & Connolly, 2009). Every Democratic president since Franklin Roosevelt has—unsuccessfully so far—attempted to implement some kind of healthcare reform that included health coverage for all Americans. Time will tell exactly what kind of healthcare reform has been achieved with the latest plan.

Ethical and Philosophical Concerns

Debate surrounding health policy can be roughly divided into two main concerns: ethical and philosophical concerns, and financial concerns. Ethical and philosophical concerns question the view of health as a fundamental right of each American and the obligation of a society to provide for the health, and consequently the health care, of its people. Financial concerns revolve around the cost of health care and who should be obligated to pay for it. The American people seem to be sharply divided on these issues, and the debate can become quite heated, as was seen in the summer of 2009 during the debate over healthcare reform and in its subsequent evolution.

Health policy is of vital importance to the profession of nursing, as it determines in large measure how nurses care for the health of both individuals and communities. It affects nurses' practice directly by regulating who may practice and in what capacity. Health policy also determines what kind of health care, if any, is provided to the public. It affects health directly, in that lack of health care is directly correlated with poor health outcomes. Nurses should care about health policy because it affects them both professionally and personally.

The Policy Process

Health policy sits squarely within the domain of nursing, but to date nursing has been largely absent in forming, influencing, and evaluating health policy ("RWJF Gallup Survey," 2010). One reason often cited for nurses' reluctance in participating in this area is that the **policy process** is complicated, is complex, and varies depending upon the policy in question. In reality, the policy process is surprisingly like the nursing process. **FIGURE 4-2** compares the steps of the nursing process and the steps of the policy process. The policy process is the same for all types of public policy, such as environmental policy and national defense policy. This discussion, however, focuses specifically on the policy process as it applies to health policy.

Policy process: The process of forming, influencing, and evaluating policy; it includes the steps of identification, formulation, adoption, implementation, and evaluation.

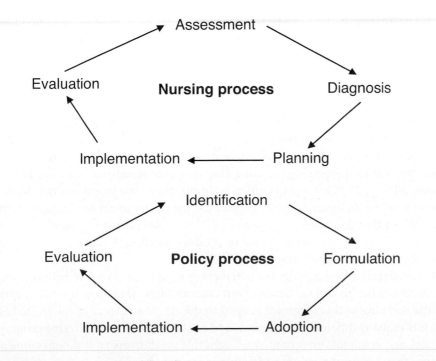

Figure 4-2 The nursing process and the policy process.

Identification Phase

During the identification phase, a health problem or the potential for a health problem is identified. An example of an actual problem might be an increase in adolescent smoking in the fictional town of Eastville. A potential health problem (or need) may also be identified, such as the need for a prenatal clinic for poor women in the town of Eastville. This phase correlates with the assessment and diagnosis phase in the nursing process.

Formulation and Adoption Phases

The formulation and adoption phases of the policy process mirror the planning phase of the nursing process. During these phases, various policies are considered and all known and possible consequences are examined. Questions asked at these stages include the following: Who is affected by the problem? How are they affected? Which ethical and legal principles are involved? What are the obstacles to the success of the policy? What are the costs and where is funding to be found? While many questions are discussed, the main focus of any health policy should be the needs and the demands of the community itself. After a thorough investigation, a policy is decided upon (adopted) and is written.

Implementation and Evaluation Phases

Implementation is the phase in which the health policy is put into use. The success or lack of success of the new policy is directly reflective of how well the questions were addressed in the formulation phase. As in the nursing process, the evaluation of a health policy compares the actual results of the policy with what the policy was supposed to do. It is during this phase that a decision is made about whether the policy should be revised, continue on as is, or be terminated completely. This assessment includes, but is not limited to, process evaluation, outcome evaluation, and cost-effectiveness evaluation. Process evaluation examines the implementation of the policy and whether it reached its target population; outcome evaluation determines whether the policy actually worked as intended; and cost-effectiveness evaluation seeks to determine whether the results of the policy justified the cost of implementing it. The final evaluation of a health policy must consider whether it contributes to health services that are assessable, acceptable, and affordable to all members of the community (Porche, 2004).

Politics and Power

So far the policy process appears to be straightforward and simple. In reality, however, the policy process involves politics—and politics implies power and the use of power. Here is where the process becomes complicated and complex. **Politics** can be described as "the process of influencing the allocation of scarce resources" (Mason, Leavitt, & Chaffee, 2007, p. 4). While the definition is simple, the actual practice is not. Merriam-Webster's online dictionary defines **power** as "the ability to act or produce an effect" (n.d.). When that definition is applied to politics, **political power** might be defined as the ability to influence others to act or produce an effect. Politics is the stage upon which the healthcare debate plays out.

As noted earlier, health policy is a statement of what we, as a society, believe is important about our health and the health of our communities. Therefore, it is not surprising that the meaning of this statement is open to debate. The citizens of the United States are a mix of many different backgrounds and cultures, who live in differing geographic, political, and economic environments. Given this great diversity, it should come as no surprise that Americans' beliefs and opinions are also diverse.

Politics: "The process of influencing the allocation of scarce resources" (Mason, Leavitt, & Chaffee, 2007, p. 4).

Power: "The ability to act or produce an effect" (Merriam Webster Online, n.d.).

Political power: The ability to influence others to act or produce an effect.

People of like beliefs and opinions on a certain issue may come together to form a special interest group. These groups consist of individuals who share political, religious, economic, or ethical views on either a specific issue or on a range of issues. The purpose of a special interest group is to advance the interests of its members. Examples of special interest groups include the American Medical Association, the National Rifle Association, Mothers Against Drunk Driving, the American Nurses Association, and the National Black Nurses Association. In a discussion of the need for a health policy, a special interest group will use advocacy to try to convince others of the validity of their opinions; **advocacy** is defined as the act of pleading for another's cause.

When it uses advocacy to try to influence policy makers, a special interest group becomes an advocacy group or a lobbying group. **Lobbying** is the act of influencing the allocation of resources and the political decisions of public policy makers (Gelak, 2008). Thus a special interest group such as the American Nurses Association, comprising people with a common interest (health care), can become a lobbying group when policy makers are considering a vote on a health policy issue. Because democracy is a form of government in which power is derived from the people being governed, this is truly an example of democracy in action.

Health policy legislation is vitally important to the healthcare system in the United States because it establishes the services that are provided and because it allocates funding mechanisms to pay for those services. It is no wonder, then, that lobbying groups hire professional **lobbyists** to try to influence politicians and other decision makers to vote the way the special interest group would like them to. Lobbyists have been popularly depicted in a rather sinister and negative light; they have often appeared in movies and other media as representing big tobacco or big pharmaceutical companies. In reality, most special interest groups employ professional lobbyists to represent their views and to try to influence the outcome of legislation. Lobbying is a way to use the power of a group to influence the political system.

Advocacy: The act of pleading for another's cause.

Lobbying: The act of influencing the allocation of resources and the political decisions of public policy makers.

Lobbyist: A professional who represents the views of his or her client before lawmakers and tries to influence the outcome of legislation.

How a Bill Becomes a Law

To understand how all of these forces come together to produce health policy, one must understand how a bill becomes a law. The law-making process is similar at both the state and federal levels, with the only difference being the names of the state and federal houses and representatives. To demonstrate this process, this section presents the path taken by an imaginary bill that would provide Lamaze training at no charge to all residents of the state of New York, through the steps of becoming a New York state law. The proposal will be called the "NY Delivers Bill." The actual steps of the process can be found on the New York state government website ("How a Bill Becomes a Law," n.d.).

1. The first step of the process is for someone to decide that a new law is needed to provide for Lamaze training at no charge to all residents of the state of New York. This instigator can be a legislator, an individual, or a group. In this case, a CHN through the New York State Nurses Association (NYSNA) originated the idea and then formed a coalition with Planned Parenthood and the Citizens for Home Birth to promote its adoption.

2. All bills must be sponsored by an official in the state government—for instance, the governor, the attorney general, or a legislator. In this case, Representative Big from Little County has offered to sponsor the bill.

3. The bill is read by a representative (although, in reality, an administrative aide reads the bill) and then sent to the Legislative Bill Drafting Commission (LBDC) to be written in the necessary proper and legal style. After it is returned to the representative, the representative looks for co-sponsors among his or her colleagues.

4. NY Delivers is introduced—that is, it is taken to the Index Office, assigned a number, printed, and distributed to all interested parties.

5. NY Delivers goes to the appropriate committees of the Senate or the Assembly (in this case, the Assembly, as the representative is an assemblyperson) for review, revision, and (its sponsors hope) passage.

6. Each time NY Delivers goes through a committee, it can be revised (amended); each time it is amended, it must go back to the LBDC to make sure that it is still properly and legally written. This step can take a very long time. If any one of the committees decides not to vote on NY Delivers, it "dies in committee." In this case, all of the committees eventually pass NY Delivers and it is "reported out" to the Assembly floor for a vote.

7. Because NY Delivers involves financing, it must first pass the Assembly Ways and Means Committee. It must repeat this whole process from step 5 in the Senate and go through the Senate Finance Committee at this point.

8. NY Delivers is voted on by the representatives in the Assembly. If it does not pass, it "dies on the floor." If it passes, it goes to the appropriate Senate committees in step 5 and then goes through steps 6–8 in the Senate.

9. After NY Delivers passes both houses, it must go to the governor to be signed into law. If the governor does not sign the bill (vetoes it), the bill will not become a law unless both houses of the legislature override his or her veto with a two-thirds majority vote. Because NY Delivers is considered a vital bill, the governor signs it and it becomes a law.

Assessing the Policy Environment and Getting Involved

There are many opportunities throughout the law-making process for lobbyists to try to influence politicians to vote in favor of the groups they represent. Nevertheless, a person does not need to be a professional lobbyist to lobby for a bill. Each individual citizen has the right to approach his or her representative at any level in the U.S. government—local, state, or federal. As noted earlier in this text, policy development is one of the core public health functions. It can be argued that a CHN has not only the right, but also the obligation, to participate in the political process. A humorous yet important approach to political involvement is provided in "Dodd's 10 Commandments of Politics and Reasons to Obey Them," presented in **Table 4-2**.

The CHN is required to advocate for the community, but sometimes the issues at hand may be difficult to understand. When two sides are arguing for and against a proposed health policy, it is the responsibility of the CHN as an expert in the field of community health to investigate the issues and translate them so that the public will have a clearer understanding of what their legislators are attempting to do. This is part of the core public health function of advocacy. To assist with this task, the questions shown in **Table 4-3** have been posed as a framework for assessing the policy environment.

How can you, as a CHN, get involved? First and foremost, join your professional organization. The American Nurses Association (ANA) represents more than 3 million American nurses. "The ANA advances the nursing profession by fostering high standards of nursing practice, promoting the rights of nurses in the workplace, projecting a positive and realistic view of nursing, and by lobbying the Congress and regulatory agencies on health care issues affecting nurses and the public" (ANA, n.d.). State and district membership is available in affiliate organizations of ANA.

Also in the United States, the National League for Nursing (NLN) promotes excellence in nursing education to build a strong and diverse workforce to advance the nation's health (http://nln.org). Nurses concerned with the critical relationship between basic and advanced nursing education and the art of developing skills of political action might consider NLN membership. The NLN serves nurse educators, preparing the next

TABLE 4-2
Dodd's 10 Commandments of Politics and Reasons to Obey Them

	Commandment	Reason to Obey The Commandment
1	The personal is political. Each of us is just one personal or social injustice away from being involved in politics.	Each person can make a difference with his or her vote, and many who participate in political action do so because of a personal experience or tragedy.
2	Friends come and go. But enemies accumulate.	Be careful to keep your friends, and realize that someone who opposes you on one issue may join you on another.
3	Politics is the art of the possible. Count votes in advance. The majority rules.	Politics is a compromise, and to be successful you must attempt what is possible. A bill is passed by majority vote, and it often takes only one vote to reach a majority.
4	Be polite, be persistent, be persuasive, be polite. Send thank you notes, write, write, write, ghost write, and write.	Communicate with your legislators and remember to be polite. Write letters to your legislators, letters to the editor, and op-ed pieces. When your legislator supports a bill you support, remember to write a thank you note.
5	Ignore your mother's rule. Talk to strangers, or network. Carry business cards. Flaunt your professional credential proudly.	Go to fundraisers and political meetings, and talk to everyone. You never know when you will need their support.
6	Money is the mother's milk of politics. Give it early and if you don't have it, raise it. Even if you do have it, raise it!	It takes money to campaign for office. Donate to your candidate of choice, if you have money. If you do not, help to raise money.
7	Negotiate visibility. Take credit, take control.	Nurses have valuable expertise, and it is time for us to take credit for our accomplishments.
8	Politics has a "chit" economy. So keep track. Seniority counts.	If you help a candidate in an election, he or she will owe you—so keep track.
9	Reputations are permanent.	It is difficult to rebuild a good reputation once it is lost, so take care of yours.
10	Don't let 'em get to ya.	Remember that politics can sometimes be painful.

Source: Dodd, C. (2004). Making the political process work. In C. Harrington & C. Estes (Eds.), *Health policy: Crisis and reform in the U.S. health care delivery system* (4th ed., pp. 19–28). Sudbury, MA: Jones and Bartlett.

generation of nursing care providers. The power to affect health legislation by 3 million nurses is reason to get involved in professional organizations.

Evidence-Based Research

For most of history, nurses have used specific interventions because they knew those measures worked and because "that is what we have always done." In other words, nurses have used what has been handed down from one generation to the next—their clinical

TABLE 4-3
Ten Questions to Ask When Assessing the Policy Environment

1. What is the problem?
2. Where is the process?
3. How many are affected?
4. What possible solutions could be proposed?
5. What are the ethical arguments involved?
6. At what level is the problem most effectively addressed?
7. Who is in a position to make policy decisions?
8. What are the obstacles to policy intervention?
9. What resources are available?
10. How can I get involved?

Source: Malone, R. (2005). Assessing the policy environment. *Policy, Politics and Nursing Practice, 6*(2), 135–143.

expertise. However, many forces have combined to demand that nursing empirically justify nursing practice. There is now an increased emphasis on quality care that is also cost-effective. The cost of health care has escalated to a level that most agree is unsustainable, and cost containment has become a much debated issue. Meanwhile, the quality of health care received by Americans has been called into question. In 2001, the Committee on Quality of Health Care in America (CQHCA) published a landmark study documenting the discrepancy between technology and quality that exists in the healthcare system in the United States and calling for efforts to cross the chasm that exists between knowledge and practice.

Definitions

Evidence-based practice, simply stated, is just that—practice that is based upon best evidence. While many definitions of EBP exist, the one used here goes as follow: EBP in nursing combines patient preferences with best practices that have been validated by evidence-based research and clinical expertise to formulate the plan of care for clients (Rector, 2010). **FIGURE 4-3** relates evidence-based practice to evidence-based research.

Research is the systematic collection and analysis of data related to a particular problem or phenomenon. Research can be understood from two perspectives: scientific research and clinical research. In nursing, **scientific research** is accomplished by a nurse investigator with the purpose of generating knowledge. **Clinical research** is conducted to determine what the literature has concluded is the best practice in a specific area.

An example of the two types of research might be useful in distinguishing between them. Scientific researchers might choose to investigate the growing epidemic of childhood obesity in the United States. Individual studies may examine perceptions of childhood obesity, pharmacological interventions, nonpharmacological interventions, interventions aimed at dietary control, interventions aimed at increasing physical activity, health problems related to childhood obesity, and many other aspects of the

Evidence-based practice (EBP): Nursing that combines patient preferences with best practices that have been validated by evidence-based research and clinical expertise to formulate the plan of care for clients.

Research: The systematic collection and analysis of data related to a particular problem or phenomenon.

Scientific research: Research accomplished for the purpose of generating knowledge.

Clinical research: Research conducted to determine what the literature has concluded is the best practice in a specific area.

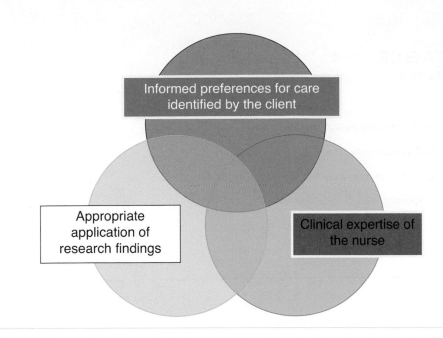

Figure 4-3 Three major components of evidence-based practice and evidence-based research.

phenomenon with the intention of increasing existing knowledge about it. In contrast, clinical research might be conducted by a clinician to determine what the literature says (or does not say) is the best approach to use to combat childhood obesity. Such research focuses on a specific clinical question with the intention of finding the best evidence to be used to formulate evidence-based practice.

Scientific Research

An understanding of EBP starts with an understanding of the scientific research process and the way in which it can be used to determine best practice. Nursing research, like all scientific research, follows the same basic steps, shown in **Table 4-4**.

While the processes involved in scientific research are mastered at the postgraduate level of nursing education, all nurses should be familiar with them so that they can critically appraise the evidence to assess its validity. To determine best practice from the literature, it is necessary to know whether a study was well designed and well controlled. It is beyond the scope of this chapter to offer a thorough explanation of the steps in the scientific process; you will learn about it in more detail in your research course. For our purposes, we will describe the different types of studies and the concept of control. The concept of control might best be understood through an example of a hypothetical study. First, however, a discussion of variables is necessary.

A variable is, simply stated, something that varies—the item being studied in a research study (LoBiondo-Wood & Haber, 2010). It may be either dependent or independent. The independent variable is the variable that is being manipulated (the intervention), and the dependent variable is the variable that is affected by the manipulation. The point of the study is to explore whether manipulation of the independent variable will affect the dependent variable (LoBiondo-Wood & Haber, 2010).

For example, suppose a nurse scientist wants to explore the effects of guided imagery (the independent or intervention variable) on the perception of pain (the dependent variable) during labor in pregnant women who have completed Lamaze training and have opted to not

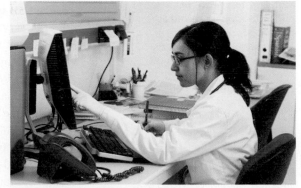

© La Vieja Sirena/Shutterstock.com

TABLE 4-4
The Steps of the Research Process

1. Identify the phenomenon of interest.
2. Review the literature.
3. Formulate research questions, goals, and objectives.
4. Develop a theoretical framework.
5. Design a research methodology.
6. Collect, analyze, and interpret the data.
7. Develop a conclusion and recommendations.

Inclusion/exclusion criteria: A means of controlling variables in research that aims to ensure that participating groups are as much alike as possible.

Randomization: A means of controlling variables in research that aims to ensure that any differences within the entire patient population in the study that existed before the intervention will be distributed evenly between the two groups and will not affect the outcome.

Control (in research): "The introduction of one or more constants (something that does not vary) into the experimental situation" (LoBiondo-Wood & Haber, 2010, p. 180).

receive pain medication during labor and delivery while experiencing at-home childbirth. If there is a difference in the perception of pain between women who have only the Lamaze training and those who have both Lamaze training and guided imagery during labor and delivery, it is possible that the difference may arise because of an unknown factor or simply because of chance and is not actually an effect of the intervention. This would mean that manipulation of the independent variable may not be the only thing that affects the dependent variable.

To increase the likelihood that the difference in the perception of pain in the two groups following the intervention is due to the intervention, the scientist uses various methods to control the variables. One method is to make sure the two groups are as much alike as possible, a feat accomplished through **inclusion/exclusion criteria** and **randomization** (LoBiondo-Wood & Haber, 2010). For instance, in the study on pain during labor and delivery, the inclusion/exclusion criteria might be that the patient is female, between the ages of 21 and 40, in her first pregnancy, speaks English, plans to deliver at home, and has no known complications. The scientist would next randomly assign the patients to either the control group (those who will not receive the intervention) or the intervention-experimental group (those who will receive the intervention). Randomization is important because it makes it more likely that any differences within the entire patient population in the study that existed before the intervention will be distributed evenly between the two groups and will not affect the outcome.

Control is defined as "the introduction of one or more constants (something that does not vary) into the experimental situation. Control is acquired by manipulating the independent variable, by randomly assigning subjects to a group, by using a control group, and by preparing intervention protocols that maintain a consistent approach" (LoBiondo-Wood & Haber, 2010, p. 180). In the previously described study of the effect of guided imagery (the independent variable) on the perception of pain (the dependent variable), the "constant" is the control group of women who had Lamaze training but were not subjected to guided imagery and, therefore, do not vary. The women who had Lamaze training and were subjected to guided imagery are the intervention or the experimental group. If the perception of pain was different for the experimental group than it was for the control group, we would have reason to believe that this effect is due to the intervention.

The strength and quality of evidence (**Table 4-5**) are judged by the amount of control that was built into the research study and described as levels of evidence descending from Level 1 (the strongest) to Level 7 (the weakest).

Types of Studies

Research studies are either quantitative or qualitative in nature, although some studies include both types. **Quantitative studies** use mathematical principles and statistics to measure phenomena or test hypotheses. **Qualitative studies** explore the subjective experience of a phenomenon in an attempt to interpret it; they strive to understand the lived experience in coping with life (Polit & Beck, 2008).

Quantitative studies are categorized as experimental, quasi-experimental, and non-experimental in design, depending on the degree of control that they exert. **Experimental studies**, also known as randomized controlled trials (RCTs), are considered Level 2 evidence because they include randomization, control, and manipulation of at least one variable. **Quasi-experimental studies** provide Level 3 evidence. They are like experimental studies except that they lack one of the three essential elements, which usually is randomization. Therefore they contain less control than experimental studies. **Nonexperimental studies** provide Level 4 evidence; they usually lack randomization and manipulation. The nonexperimental design is used often in nursing research to examine conditions that naturally exist. For instance, if you wished to study the effects of miscarriage on emotional well-being, you would not randomly assign a population of pregnant women to a control group and an intervention group and then induce miscarriage in the intervention group—that would obviously be unethical. Many studies on human beings are not amenable to randomization and manipulation.

Qualitative studies provide Level 6 evidence. While they provide for a rich and deep understanding of a phenomenon, they are "ranked lower on a hierarchy of evidence, as a 'weaker' form of research design" (LoBiondo-Wood & Haber, 2010, p. 95). Such research is considered "weaker" because most of the hierarchies that rate evidence are based on the strength of an intervention, and many qualitative studies do not examine

Quantitative studies: Research studies that use mathematical principles and statistics to measure phenomena or test hypotheses.

Qualitative studies: Research studies that explore the subjective experience of a phenomenon in an attempt to interpret it.

Experimental studies: Research studies that include randomization, control, and manipulation of at least one variable, and that produce Level 2 evidence; also known as randomized controlled trials.

Quasi-experimental studies: Research studies that lack one of the three essential elements (randomization, control, and manipulation of at least one variable), usually randomization; they produce Level 3 evidence.

Nonexperimental studies: Research studies that usually lack randomization and manipulation of at least one variable, but do include control; they produce Level 4 evidence.

TABLE 4-5
Control Built into the Research Study

Level 1 (strongest) → Level 7 (weakest)
Level 1: Systematic review or meta-analysis of all relevant randomized controlled trials (RCTs), or evidence-based clinical practice guidelines based on systematic reviews of RCTs
Level 2: Evidence from at least one well-designed RCT
Level 3: Evidence from a well-designed controlled trial without randomization
Level 4: Evidence from well-designed case-control and cohort studies
Level 5: Evidence from systematic reviews of descriptive and qualitative studies
Level 6: Evidence from a single descriptive or qualitative study
Level 7: Evidence from the opinion of authorities and/or reports of expert committees

Source: Melnyk, B., & Fineout-Overholt, E. (2005). *Evidence-based practice in nursing and healthcare: A guide to best practice*. Philadelphia, PA: Lippincott Williams & Wilkins, p. 10.

the effects of an intervention (LoBiondo-Wood & Haber, 2010). The low ranking of qualitative studies is actually a bit misleading, because the questions that are addressed by qualitative methods can only be answered by these methods.

Clinical Research and Evidence-Based Practice: An Example

The practice of CHN to find the scientific evidence upon which evidenced-based practice is built includes five fundamental steps that are clearly like the nursing process (**Table 4-6**). A theoretical example of a nurse working in a rural community illustrates how the process works with an intervention such as Lamaze preparation.

In this example, a CHN practices in a rural community of recent immigrants to the United States. In the CHN's practice, the nurse assists the women with childbirth. Because most of the families in the community are poor and have no health insurance, they labor and deliver at home without the benefit of pain medication. During the years the CHN has practiced in this community, the nurse has experienced many alternative methods for alleviating pain in the client population. The nurse believes that Lamaze training combined with guided imagery is the most successful approach.

The community health nurse wants to establish the Lamaze approach as "best practice" procedure within the agency. To do so, the nurse decides to undertake a clinical study of the problem.

Step 1: Assessment of the Problem

The first step involves an assessment of the clinical problem that is to be investigated and the formulation of a well-built clinical question. While many methods may be used to accomplish this step, one effective method is the PICO process (Fineout-Overholt & Stillwell, 2010):

P = Patient/Problem
I = Intervention
C = Comparison/Control
O = Outcome/Effects

The PICO process is a very effective way to organize the researcher's thinking around a clinical problem. In the example of pain during at-home labor and delivery, the "patient" is women in the community experiencing labor during at home childbirth and the "problem" is pain. The "intervention" is guided imagery combined with Lamaze training. The CHN will "compare" the effectiveness of the chosen intervention with the other

---

TABLE 4-6

Five Fundamental Steps of Evidence-Based Practice

Step 1: Formulate a well-built question.
Step 2: Identify articles and other evidence-based resources that answer the question.
Step 3: Critically appraise the evidence to assess its validity.
Step 4: Apply the evidence.
Step 5: Reevaluate the application of evidence and identify areas for improvement.

methods the nurse has experienced during practice in this community. Ideally, the chosen intervention would be compared to a single alternative intervention; however, it can be compared to several or none at all, if there are no known alternatives. The "outcome" the nurse expects to find is that women who labor and deliver at home following Lamaze training combined with guided imagery report that they experience less pain than women using other interventions or no interventions at all.

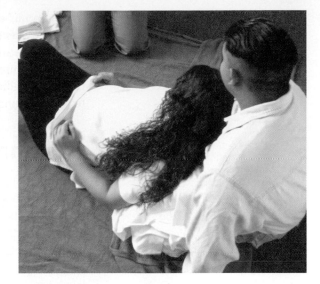

© Bill Crump/Brand X Pictures/Alamy Images

Steps 2 and 3: Literature Review

The next step in the process is to do a literature review of the evidence-based resources that explore the question. This is actually a two-step process. First, the CHN reads widely on the subjects of pain during childbirth and delivery, delivery at home, and any other topics that are related to the subject. Second, this cursory review is followed by an in-depth examination and critical appraisal of the literature that is relevant to the problem. This appraisal is based on an understanding of the scientific research process and the levels of evidence discussed earlier in this chapter.

Step 4: Organization and Presentation of Findings

In step 4, the CHN organizes his or her findings and presents them to the organization. In this example, the nurse discovered that the preponderance of evidence supports the practice of combining Lamaze training with guided imagery in relieving the perception of pain in women experiencing labor and delivery in an at-home environment. Additionally, the literature supports the contention that it is the most cost-effective intervention. After being presented with this evidence, the organization established the intervention as a best practice protocol and began to implement it in actual community practice.

Step 5: Reevaluation and Revision

As in the nursing process, the next step is reevaluation and revision as warranted. However, because the nurse is a community health nurse, he or she does not stop with establishing the intervention as a protocol for only his or her (employing) organization. Community health nursing is concerned with the larger community. In this case, the CHN feels that all women who decide to experience labor and delivery at home should have the benefit of best practice as established by evidence-based research. The CHN supports the phenomenon of client-centered decision making by offering choices that reflect best practices.

A Return to the Idea of Health Policy

Because many of the families who choose home delivery are poor and without health insurance, the CHN believes that education on Lamaze training and guided imagery as a means of reducing pain during childbirth should be provided at no charge to all residents of the state. To accomplish this, the nurse begins the political process by forming a coalition with the New York State Nurses Association (NYSNA), Planned Parenthood, and the Citizens for Home Birth. This same scenario was described in the beginning section of this chapter, on how a bill becomes a law.

In the current example, the CHN has addressed all three core functions of public health: assessment, policy development, and assurance. The nurse assessed the community and discovered a need. The CHN searched and critically appraised the literature to find evidence to support an intervention that was both the best practice and cost-effective. After helping to establish the evidence-based intervention in the community where the nurse worked, the nurse advocated for the even larger (state) community. This advocacy was completed at the state level, and influenced the formation and implementation of a new health policy. The public can now benefit from the formation of a health policy that supports a service that is cost-effective, accessible, and acceptable to them. Of great significance is the growing trust and confidence the client will develop related to the emerging healthcare delivery system.

Summary

Health policy and research are related because of their close fit. Health policy informs which research questions need to be answered; research findings serve as the basis for establishing health policy. The relationship between these concepts supports the concept of the evidence-based practice of nursing.

This chapter began with a review of how health policy is defined and how the policy process works in the clinical setting. Because health policy on the state and national levels involves legislation, understanding how an idea about health becomes a bill, and how a bill becomes law, is critical to be an effective advocate for health care.

To explain the process by which a CHN assesses the policy environment and becomes involved in the health policy formulation process, this chapter presented an example of a fictitious bill on providing support to women choosing the Lamaze process of childbirth preparation. In the example, the idea to improve birthing services for women came from the most recent information representing best practice, or evidence-based practice. In this case, evidence-based practice was identified through information gleaned from client preferences, expert clinical practice, and quality research.

To be an effective advocate for evidence-based practice, the CHN must understand the basic precepts of scientific research, including the types of studies used in community health nursing. Research models can be classified as either qualitative or quantitative in nature. The PICO process is one valuable technique for the study of clinical problems; its utilization in research can result in findings that may be used to set health policy, reconnecting the concepts of research and health policy.

REFERENCES

American Nurses Association (ANA). (n.d.). *About ANA*. Retrieved from http://www.nursingworld.org/FunctionalMenuCategories/AboutANA.aspx

Blakemore, K., & Griggs, E. (2007). *Social policy: An introduction* (3rd ed.). New York, NY: McGraw-Hill.

Bourne, L. (2010). Policy making and community health advocacy. In J. A. Allender, C. Rector, & K. D. Warner, *Community health nursing: Promoting and protecting the public's health* (7th ed.). New York, NY: Lippincott Williams & Wilkins.

Boushey, H., Gundersen, B., Brocht, C., & Bernstein, J. (2001). *Hardships in America: The real story of working families*. Washington, DC: Economic Policy Institute.

Committee on Quality of Health Care in America (CQHCA). (2001). *Crossing the quality chasm: A new health care system for the 21st century*. Institute of Medicine. Washington DC: National Academy Press.

Dodd, C. (2004). Making the political process work. In C. Harrington & C. Estes (Eds.), *Health policy: Crisis and reform in the U.S. health care delivery system* (4th ed., pp. 19–28). Sudbury, MA: Jones and Bartlett.

Fineout-Overholt, E., & Stilwell, S. (2010). Asking compelling clinical questions. In C. Mazurek Melynk & E. Fineout-Overholt (Eds.), *Evidence-based practice in nursing and healthcare: A guide to best practice* (2nd ed.). Philadelphia, PA: Lippincott Williams & Wilkins.

Gelak, D. (2008). *Lobbying and advocacy*. Alexandria, VA: Capital.Net, p. 5.

Gerber, D., & McGuire, S. (1995). Understanding contemporary health and welfare services: The Social Security Act of 1935 and the Public Health Service Act of 1944. *Nursing Outlook, 43*(6), 266–272.

Hanley, B., & Falk, N. (2007) Policy development and analysis: Understanding the process. In D. Mason, J. Leavitt, & M. Chaffee (Eds.), *Policy and politics in nursing and health care* (5th ed., pp. 75–93). St. Louis, MO: Saunders Elsevier.

Health care reform. (2011, March 4). *New York Times*.

How a bill becomes a law. (n.d.). New York State Government. Retrieved from http://www.bcnys.org/inside/sb/billlaw.htm

Institute of Medicine. (1988). *The future of public health*. Washington DC: National Academy Press.

LoBiondo-Wood, G., & Haber, J. (2010). *Nursing research: Methods and critical appraisal for evidence-based practice* (7th ed.). New York, NY: Mosby.

Malone, R. (2005). Assessing the policy environment. *Policy, Politics and Nursing Practice, 6*(2), 135–143.

Mason, D., Leavitt, J., & Chaffee, M. (2007). *Policy and politics in nursing and health care* (5th ed.). St. Louis, MO: Saunders Elsevier.

Melnyk, B., & Fineout-Overholt, E. (2005). *Evidence-based practice in nursing and healthcare: A guide to best practice*. Philadelphia, PA: Lippincott Williams & Wilkins.

Merriam-Webster Online. (n.d.). *Power*. Retrieved from http://www.merriam-webster.com/dictionary/power?show=0&t=1295728379

Polit, D., & Beck, C. (2008). *Nursing research: Generating and assessing evidence for nursing practice* (8th ed.). Philadelphia, PA: Lippincott Williams & Wilkins.

Porche, D. (2004). *Public and community health nursing practice: A population-based approach*. Thousand Oaks, CA: Sage.

Porter-O'Grady, T. (1994). Building partnerships in health care: Creating whole systems change. *Nursing and Health Care, 15*(1), 34–38.

Porter O'Grady, T., & Malloch, K. (2011). *Quantum leadership: Advancing innovation, transforming health care* (3rd ed.). Sudbury, MA: Jones & Bartlett Learning.

Rector, C. (2010). Evidence-based practice and ethics in community health nursing. In J. A. Allender, C. Rector, & K. D. Warner, *Community health nursing: Promoting and protecting the public's health* (7th ed.). New York, NY: Lippincott Williams & Wilkins.

RWJF Gallup survey finds nurses should have more influence. (2010). *American Nurse Today, 5*(1). Retrieved from http://www.americannursetoday.com/Article.aspx?id=6180&fid=6116

Sack, K., & Connolly, M. (2009, June 20). In poll, wide support for government-run health. *New York Times*. Retrieved from http://www.nytimes.com/2009/06/21/health/policy/21poll.html?bl&ex=1245729600&en=d44716a77315c19c&ei=5087%0A

Sudduth, A. (2008). Program evaluation. In J. Milstead (Ed.), *Health policy and politics: A nurse's guide* (3rd ed., pp. 171–194). Sudbury, MA: Jones and Bartlett.

World Health Organization (WHO). (2010). *Health policy*. Retrieved from http://www.who.int/topics/health_policy/en

ADDITIONAL RESOURCE

Allender, A, Rector, C., & Warner, K. (Eds.). *Community health nursing: Promoting and protecting the public's health* (7th ed.). Philadelphia, PA: Lippincott Williams & Wilkins, pp. 353–370.

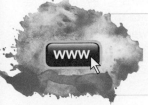

For a full suite of assignments and additional learning activities, use the access code located in the front of your book to visit the exclusive website: http://go.jblearning.com/Holzemer/. If you do not have an access code, you can obtain one at the site.

LEARNING ACTIVITIES   www

1. A nurse is aware that the main concern of healthcare policies should be which of the following?

   A. Identifying the concerns of a community
   B. Decreasing the cost of health care
   C. Clarifying the political beliefs of the society
   D. Providing a voice for the needs of healthcare providers

2. Which of the following is a priority for the community health nurse when developing healthcare policies?

   A. The cost of the needed programs
   B. The client(s) who is (are) affected by the policy
   C. The obstacles to success in program planning
   D. The history of the community with similar policies

3. What is the major factor that influences the success or failure of the implementation of health policy?

   A. The laws that are currently in place in the community
   B. How the community adopts and uses the policy
   C. The popularity of the legislators introducing the policy
   D. The support of the medical community

4. Place the five fundamental steps of evidence-based practice in the order a nurse would use them (1–5):

   _____ Applying the evidence
   _____ Critically appraising the evidence to assess its validity
   _____ Identifying articles and other evidence-based resources that answer the question
   _____ Formulating a well-built question
   _____ Reevaluating the application of evidence and areas for improvement

ADDITIONAL QUESTIONS FOR STUDY

1. For each of the following special interest groups, identify the implications the group has for health policy.

   A. American Medical Association
   B. National Rifle Association
   C. Mothers Against Drunk Driving
   D. American Nurses Association
   E. National Black Nurses Association

2. The following is another example of how a bill becomes law. Answer the questions about the legislative process, and how evidence-based research could be used to improve the understanding of the problem.

The Active Children Bill

An imaginary bill that would mandate 60 minutes of physical activity weekly for children in kindergarten through sixth grade in all schools in the state of Hawaii will be followed through the steps of becoming a Hawaii state law. The proposal will be called the "The Active Children Bill" (Active Children).

Step 1. The first step of the process is for someone to decide that Hawaii needs a new law to require all schools in the state to provide 60 minutes of physical activity weekly for all children in kindergarten through sixth grade.

A. Who could develop such a bill?

Step 2. The bill is sponsored by an official from the Hawaii state government.

Step 3. The bill is read by a representative or administrative aide, and then sent to the Legislative Bill Drafting Commission (LBDC) to be written in the necessary proper and legal style. After it is returned, the representative looks for co-sponsors among his or her colleagues.

Step 4. Active Children is introduced; that is, it is taken to the Index Office, assigned a number, printed, and distributed to all interested parties.

Step 5. Active Children goes to the appropriate committees of the Senate or the Assembly (in this case, the Assembly, as the representative is an assemblyperson) for review, revision, and passage.

Step 6. Each time Active Children goes through a committee, it can be revised (amended).

B. Where does the bill go when it is amended?

Step 7. Because Active Children involves financing, it must first pass the Assembly Ways and Means Committee. It must repeat this whole process from step 5 in the Senate and go through the Senate Finance Committee at this point.

Step 8. Active Children is now voted on by the representatives in the Assembly.

C. What happen if the proposal does not pass?

Step 9. After Active Children passes both houses, it must go to the governor to be signed into law. If the governor does not sign the bill (veto), it will not become a law unless both houses of the legislature override his or her veto with a two-thirds majority vote.

3. **Research Development: Childhood Obesity in an Urban Community**

A community health nurse practices in an inner-city community in the northeast United States that comprises a socioeconomically disadvantaged minority population. During the years the CHN has practiced in this community, she has noticed an increase in childhood obesity. She has also noticed a corresponding decrease in the time allocated to physical activity by the local schools. While she understands that many factors contribute to childhood obesity, the CHN believes that including at least 60 minutes of physical activity during school hours each week is a cost-effective intervention that will result in a decrease in childhood obesity in this population.

A. Why would the community health nurse be concerned with control of variables in exploring the effects of 60 minutes of physical activity weekly (the independent or intervention variable) on the body mass index (BMI—the dependent variable) of children in kindergarten through sixth grade?

B. Which inclusion/exclusion criteria would you suggest in this study sample?

C. How would you assign children to either a control group or an intervention group?

D. How would you proceed with the five steps of evidence-based practice? List your actions in each step.

CHAPTER OUTLINE

- ▶ Introduction
- ▶ The Importance of Clarity in Communication
- ▶ Communication with Clients to Ensure a Safe Environment
- ▶ Communication with Other Providers to Ensure a Safe Environment
- ▶ Use of a Huddle to Communicate Clearly
  - A Communication Huddle in the Community
  - Members of a Huddle in the Community
- ▶ SBAR/ISBARR Communication
- ▶ Electronic Health Records
- ▶ Communication and the Internet
- ▶ The Impact of Informatics and Social Networking on Nursing
- ▶ The Loss of the Ability to Communicate
- ▶ Summary

OBJECTIVES

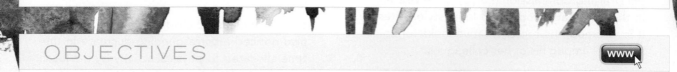

1. Explain the importance of communication when working with clients of various ages.

2. Identify and describe problems in communication within the fast-paced healthcare delivery system.

3. Practice SBAR and ISBARR communication techniques to foster confidence in communication.

4. Describe the benefits and limitations of Internet and social media venues as they relate to clear and accurate communication.

KEY TERMS

Electronic health record (EHR)

Huddle

Informatics

ISBARR (identify–situation–background–assessment–recommendation–read back)

SBAR (situation–background–assessment–recommendation)

Sentinel event

Social network sites

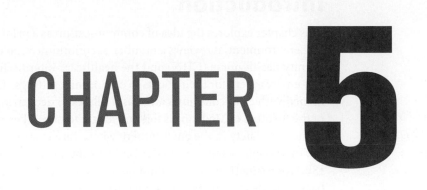

CHAPTER 5

Clear Communication and Information Management in the Community

Patricia F. Garofalo

Deborah J. Murphy

Introduction

This chapter explores the idea of communication as a priority concern in maintaining a safe environment. It reviews a number of communication concepts that assist the community health nurse (CHN) and the healthcare interdisciplinary team with creating a safe environment for their clients in community settings. The Joint Commission is concerned with clear communication as it relates to decreasing human error. The position of the Institute of Medicine is that nurses are to have a key role in using communication to increase safety in the environment where care is provided.

This chapter examines methods of communication, such as the huddle and SBAR/ISBARR (situation–background–assessment–recommendation/identify–situation–background–assessment–recommendation–read back) communication techniques. Additionally, methods for communicating using the Internet, such as social media tools, are explored. An example of a nurse using the Internet successfully to help a client to cope with a problem is presented to illustrate the use of high-technology communication and information management. This chapter ends with a vignette related to a therapist-turned-client who is having special problems with communication: communication is key to her living with a debilitating neurological illness.

The Importance of Clarity in Communication

Communication in nurse–patient relationships is an important part of nursing practice (Sheldon, Barrett, & Ellington, 2009). The power of effective community nursing care is strengthened and enriched by good communication skills. The exchange of information, feelings, and concerns is vitally important in therapeutic relationships in health care (Sheldon et al., 2009). Nurses need to voice their clients' needs and to articulate them well. Communicating well is a skill that can be learned. To communicate well, the nurse needs to be organized to send and receive the information needed for good decision making.

The key to successful nursing care delivery, education, and research is communication. Nurses and healthcare providers often feel that high-technology interventions are the most important. In reality, without clear communication, all other therapeutic interventions may be of limited use. **FIGURE 5-1** relates the three key concepts of communication—listening, reflecting back, and clarifying information that is communicated. This continuous process is part of every client–nurse interaction. The listening–reflecting back–clarifying triad supports the efforts of the CHN in using communication effectively in meeting the needs of individuals, families, groups, and communities.

Communication with Clients to Ensure a Safe Environment

Communication with individual and family clients is key to maintaining a safe environment. When providing direct care, the CHN is in continuous communication with the client, family, and others in the community, as well as the agency in which the nurse is employed. In any client care situation, the CHN may make multiple contacts—for example, to durable medical equipment providers, distant relatives, pharmacy staff, the physician of record, and support services such as "meals on wheels." Communication with the client and support networks promotes safety by making the environment for recovery one that is both well constructed and safe.

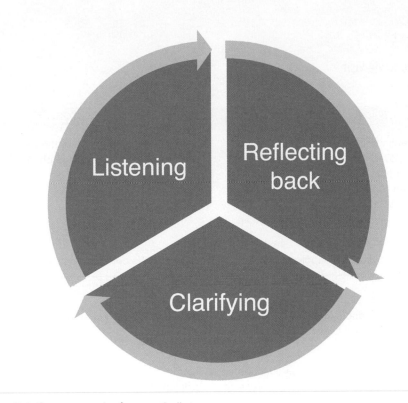

Figure 5-1 Key components of communication.

The following scenario is an example of poor planning on the part of the CHN. In this situation, the CHN should have put more time into planning the discharge process from hospital to home. Nurses (and other providers) from the acute care setting and the home care facility should have communicated more effectively to prepare for the client's, return home after surgery.

Lack of Complete Communication for a Home Care Visit

The CHN is scheduled to make a home visit. The client is a 65-year-old female who was discharged from the hospital yesterday, eight days post abdominal surgery. The postsurgical course was complicated by abdominal dehiscence, poor nutritional absorption, and wound infection. The client's mid-abdominal wound requires daily packing with wet gauze, followed by application of a sterile outer dressing. In addition, client teaching needs to include dressing application, medication regime adherence, and signs and symptoms of infection reoccurrence.

The CHN arrives at the client's house 20 minutes late because the nurse failed to obtain clear directions to the client's home. When the nurse arrives, the primary caretaker, the client's husband, has already left to return to work. The CHN discovers that dressing supplies were not delivered to the client's house as ordered. The box that the client thought contained supplies for the dressing change contained a foam pillow that the client used while she was in the hospital.

TABLE 5-1
A Preferred Conversation Before a Home Visit

Conversation	Interpretation
Visiting Nurse: "Ms. Smith, [identify self]. I will be coming to your house around 1:00 P.M.; if I am delayed, I will call you. Please keep your cell phone with you. Will your husband be available, as we discussed, to review your dressing change and nutritional status? Please give me his phone number in case I need to call him." **Client:** "Around 1:00 P.M. is fine. I will make sure my husband can stay until around 2:30 P.M."	Establish the parameters of the visit; encourage the client to have phone with her.
Visiting Nurse: "Did the pharmacy deliver the supplies for your dressing?" **Client:** "Yes, it is all here, in a box."	Verify that the correct supplies are available.
Visiting Nurse: "Please look in the box and tell me what you see." **Client:** "It is a pillow! That nice doctor in the hospital said I could have it. I thought it was the supplies."	Verify that the correct supplies are available.
Visiting Nurse: "Please call the pharmacy, or have your husband do so before tomorrow. I need the supplies so I can review the dressing change with you and your husband." **Client:** "Don't worry about him; he knows about dressings."	Instruct client on how to resolve problem. Reestablish the need for the caregiver to be present.
Visiting Nurse: "I am sure he does, Ms. Smith, but you both need to learn about your special dressing change. Did you take your temperature this morning?" **Client:** "No, I forgot. I will do it this afternoon."	Monitor the client's participation in self-care.
Visiting Nurse: "Remember, if your temperature is higher than 101°F (38.3°C), you need to call your doctor. Do you have your doctor's number? Please read it to me to make sure you have the correct number."	Reinforce the proper action.

In this scenario, the CHN should have been better prepared for the home visit with the client returning home from surgery. Although preparing for every problem and concern is impossible, **Table 5-1** describes a conversation that, if it had taken place before the home visit, might have made the visit more productive. The CHN should use every opportunity to communicate clearly and effectively to improve client outcomes.

Communication with Other Providers to Ensure a Safe Environment

Client safety has always been a priority in nursing care, and recent literature points to the important connection between communication and positive safety outcomes. Miscommunication is a major factor cited in the literature in error reports (Hughes, 2008; Institute of Medicine [IOM], 2001, 2002). The Joint Commission (2011) has identified that poor communication is one of the root causes of serious medical errors. The use of electronic medical records with electronic provider orders as well as medication administration through the use of bar-code scanning offer promise in reducing the number of errors due to poor communication. Miscommunication during "handoff" transfer of clients has also been identified by The Joint Commission (2011) as a serious error potential. Transfer of client care in the community setting requires the diligent handoff of information to decrease the risk of omission of necessary client care.

According to Boynton (2009), communication does not just involve a message between a sender and a receiver, but—at least in health care—can be influenced by such variables as power dynamics, clinical urgency, personalities, time limitations, and fatigue. The goals of communication in health care are to establish a relationship that will influence the behavior of others and to nurture and sustain working relationships.

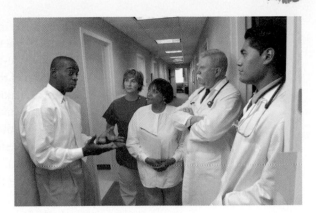

© Thinkstock Images/Comstock/Thinkstock

The current challenge in health care is to make open and transparent communication the norm rather than the exception. Chapman (2009) describes a team approach to establish a patient-centered healing environment with mutually beneficial partnerships between patients (clients), families, and healthcare providers. In this author's study, bedside rounds assisted both the caregivers and the patient with putting the puzzle together to improve the quality of information given.

Recent findings by the IOM (2002) have identified poor communication and lack of teamwork as the cause of the majority of medical errors. Healthcare personnel need to hone their technical and communication skills to improve team dynamics (Wolfson, 2009). Nurses need to practice and become comfortable with their communication and roles to become strong patient advocates. Two communication strategies used to improve safe care outcomes—the huddle and SBAR or ISBARR communication—are described next.

Use of a Huddle to Communicate Clearly

Huddle is the latest buzzword in communication. Merriam-Webster defines this term as "to gather in a close-packed group; to hold a consultation" (Huddle, n.d.). The notion of huddle communication may encompass face-to-face meetings of providers or meetings using technology to create a team. The use of huddle technology makes a team more diverse, and can include anyone almost anywhere connectivity is available. Such a strategy offers a particular advantage in the community.

Communication in nursing is the core of the nursing process. A communication huddle involves the interchange of knowledge, attitudes, and skill between members of the healthcare team and the clients in the community and, therefore, can promote safety in the healthcare environment. In an acute care setting, a huddle refers to a brief meeting, lasting 5 to 10 minutes, with all members of a team. It can be performed both at the beginning of the nursing shift and at the end of the shift. All caregivers are included in this huddle. The main purpose of the huddle is for offgoing staff to report critical information on each patient that everyone needs to know (Chapman, 2009). It gives oncoming staff some idea of the status of all clients who require care and their treatment plans, as well as the pulse of the unit.

Huddle: To gather in a close packed group or to hold a consultation. In an acute care setting, it consists of a brief meeting, lasting 5 to 10 minutes, with all members of the healthcare team; in the community setting, it may involve a telephone conference call.

A Communication Huddle in the Community

A conference telephone call huddle can achieve the same results in the community as the huddle on the hospital unit. The CHN can use a call huddle when he or she cannot physically be in the same place with other team members. The call huddle still serves to communicate to the team the important information needed to provide up-to-date client care. Face-to-face huddles in the community setting also occur, but usually include only some of the players in the healthcare decision-making team. The CHN is often in charge of making sure that all information obtained in a "smaller huddle" is passed on to everyone involved in decision making.

In a hypothetical example, a CHN might call for a huddle to assist a client with strong religious beliefs who is recovering in the community from a cerebrovascular accident (brain attack). After assessment of who is closely involved in the client's care, the CHN calls a huddle. Special concerns of privacy and confidentiality exist in the community because the CHN works with lay caregivers and providers from a number of organizations.

Included in the huddle in this example are the client, decision-making family members, the physician/nurse practitioner supervising the client's care, significant others from the client's house of worship, and the CHN and other team members in the field. As the health of the client unfolds, individuals may be added or subtracted from the huddle. The huddle should be called to improve communication, and to provide coordinated and realistic care. Lay and professional care providers may need to huddle many times throughout the care of a client in the community.

Members of a Huddle in the Community

FIGURE 5-2 is a diagram of the people who may be called into a communication huddle in the community.

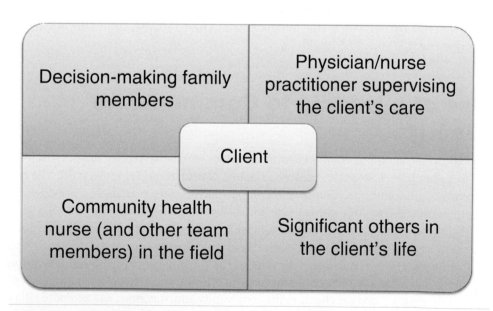

Figure 5-2 People who may be called into a communication huddle in the community.

The Client

The client is central to the huddle. Although many discussions can occur without the client being present, the huddle is held to meet the needs of the client; thus the client is the central member. When the client is an entire community, the key representatives or stakeholders would become part of the huddle. The only time that the client (individual) is not central to the process is when the person is neurologically compromised and cannot participate. The client is also included because of the need to know client preferences—a key aspect of evidence-based practice. The preferences of the client are considered key to decision making in many, if not all, healthcare decisions.

Decision-Making Family Members

Family members who choose to work with the healthcare team in the community need to participate in the huddle. The huddle should not include family members who are not willing to serve in the best interest of the client. The client identifies helpful significant family members and others to participate in the huddle.

The Physician/Nurse Practitioner Supervising the Client's Care

The medical primary care provider is a necessary member of the huddle. In multi-problem situations, multiple medical providers may be included in the group. The CHN will also communicate individually with providers supervising care, especially as a final plan of care is developed. Specialists may participate in a communication meeting during the period in which their services are being used by the client.

Significant Others in the Client's Life

The client identifies significant others to include in the huddle, and gives the CHN permission to invite them into the huddle. In this example, the client has identified two people from St. Agatha's Church as most supportive of the care she receives at home, so they are included in the huddle.

The Community Health Nurse and Other Team Members in the Field

The CHN, the occupational and physical therapists, and the medical social worker are key members of the huddle in this example. The healthcare team members are those able to provide support to the client in this hypothetical situation.

SBAR/ISBARR Communication

In 2011, The Joint Commission observed that approximately 100,000 deaths in the United States each year are attributed to medical errors resulting from ineffective communication: "Communication problems are the root cause for nearly 66% of all sentinel events." A **sentinel event** is an unexpected event or occurrence involving death, or serious or permanent physical or psychological injury. A timeline recording the concerns of The Joint Commission as they relate to communication appears in **Table 5-2**.

With U.S. facilities being held accountable for meeting National Safety Measures, improvements in effective communication materialized in the form of the framework for a process known as **SBAR**: situation–background–assessment–recommendation. The SBAR process deals with communication between members of the healthcare team about a patient's condition. The SBAR acronym is an easy-to-remember, concrete mechanism useful for framing any conversation, especially critical ones, requiring a clinician's immediate attention and action. It provides a standard method for communicating

Sentinel event: An unexpected event or occurrence involving death, or serious or permanent physical or psychological injury.

SBAR (situation–background–assessment–recommendation): A framework for communication between members of the healthcare team about a patient's condition.

between members of the team, which is essential for developing teamwork and nurturing a culture of patient safety. Using SBAR is illustrated by the vignette in **Table 5-3**, which pairs each SBAR stage with a clinical example of what information the nurse would communicate during that stage.

TABLE 5-2
Concerns of the Joint Commission Related to Communication

In 2003, the Joint Commission enacted the first two National Safety Measures to address communication concerns:
1. The read back of verbal and telephone orders
2. The use of approved standard abbreviations

In 2005, the Joint Commission added a third National Safety Measure:
3. Timely and accurate reporting of critical lab results

In 2006, the fourth National Safety Measure was identified:
4. Requirement for standardizing "handoff" communication

TABLE 5-3
SBAR Stages and Clinical Examples

SBAR Stage	Example
Situation: When communicating with healthcare providers, the nurse will report on the client's condition. Details such as the nurse's name, unit, time of day, location (room number), and the client's name, age, sex, and problem are identified.	**Situation Example:** "Dr. Pause, this is Nurse Murphy from the Orthopedic Unit. Your patient, Joe Jones, experienced chest pains this evening at 10 P.M. Mr. Jones is an 88-year-old male."
Background: Relevant background information is provided that is specific to the situation. Information such as vital signs, mental and physical status, ability to communicate, pain level complaints, and physical assessment is part of this scope.	**Background Example:** "As you know, Mr. Jones was admitted for reconstructive surgery of the knee yesterday and was stable since being admitted. As of the last nursing rounds at 9:00 P.M., his vital signs were stable. Mr. Jones was alert and oriented to person, place, and time and was comfortable. At 10 P.M., Mr. Jones complained about tightening in his chest and the on-call resident was notified."
Assessment: Here, the nurse has the ability to offer an analysis of the problem. Clarity in determining the issue at hand may require the ability to isolate the issue to the body system affected and the degree of severity. For assessment, critical thinking is key, and the nurse should expect to deliver more extensive details.	**Assessment Example:** "I have noticed that Mr. Jones is visibly in pain and is experiencing a shortness of breath. His blood pressure is 175/90 and his pulse is 65, with an O_2 saturation of 87%. His prior assessment at 9:00 P.M. was stable."
Recommendation: Here, the nurse identifies the steps that he or she believes are necessary to address the situation.	**Recommendation Example:** " I believe we should draw blood chemistry, a CBC, and blood enzymes to determine the risk for a heart attack. A bedside EKG is in order, along with the placement of oxygen and continued monitoring. Do you agree that this is a plan you would support?"

TABLE 5-4
ISBARR Stages and Clinical Examples

ISBARR Stage	Example
Identify: State name and title.	**Identify Example:** "Dr. Pause, this is John Paul, Mr. Jones's home care nurse."
Situation: When communicating with healthcare providers, the nurse will report on the client's condition. Details such as the client's name, age, sex, and problem are identified.	**Situation Example:** "Your patient, Joe Jones, age 88, is not able to complete his physical therapy exercises. He is complaining of knee pain (5 on a 10-point scale) and is taking aspirin for pain. He has no allergies to food or medication."
Background: Relevant background information is provided that is specific to the situation. Information such as vital signs, mental and physical status, ability to communicate, pain level complaints, and physical assessment is part of this scope.	**Background Example:** "As you know, Mr. Jones has been home for 10 days since his knee surgery. The dressing on his knee is clean, and when I changed the dressing there was no drainage. His temperature is normal, pulse 68, and blood pressure 160/80. Mr. Jones is alert and oriented to person, place, and time and is otherwise comfortable. His gait is steady."
Assessment: Here, the nurse has the ability to offer an analysis of the problem. Clarity in determining the issue at hand may require the ability to isolate the issue to the body system affected and the degree of severity. For assessment, critical thinking is key, and the nurse should expect to deliver more extensive details.	**Assessment Example:** "I have noticed that Mr. Jones is guarding his knee. He says that he stays in his chair most of the day. He told the physical therapist last week not to return because he understands his exercises. He is not able to explain them to me today."
Recommendation: Here, the nurse identifies the steps that he or she believes are necessary to address the situation.	**Recommendation Example:** "I believe we should change Mr. Jones's pain medication to ibuprofen; he says that he has obtained relief in the past from this medication. Do you think having the physical therapist return once to review exercises before he sees you in your office next week is necessary?"
Read Back: Restate medical orders, changes in vital sign monitoring, and the circumstances in which to call back.	**Read Back Example:** "I will tell Mr. Jones to take two ibuprofen, no more than four times a day if he needs it, and to expect a call from the physical therapist to review his exercises. I will tell Mr. Jones to call 911 if he feels any chest pain or shortness of breath, and to call your office if he has questions about his upcoming appointment."

A variation of the SBAR construct is **ISBARR**, meaning identify–situation–background–assessment–recommendation–read back. This acronym adds "identify" to begin the communication, meaning that the CHN would identify his or her name and the location where the CHN is working. The ISBARR method ends with "read back," in which the nurse restates medical directives, clarifies the need for changes in collecting vital sign measurements, and clarifies when a report back to the primary provider will be necessary (Enlow, Shanks, Guhde, & Perkins, 2010). Table 5-3 presents an example of SBAR communication with a client, Mr. Jones, in the hospital; **Table 5-4** provides an example of ISBARR communication when Mr. Jones goes home and is cared for by a CHN.

In many settings, students who are learning SBAR/ISBARR cannot be involved in the transcription of verbal orders or execution of medical orders. SBAR/ISBARR restrictions

ISBARR (identify–situation–background–assessment–recommendation–read back): The SBAR framework for communication between members of the healthcare team about a patient's condition, extended by a beginning stage in which the care provider identifies himself or herself, and an ending "read back," in which the care provider restates and clarifies instructions and expectations.

vary from state to state, and it is important to know your state regulations regarding the nursing student's role within the hospital and community setting when medical directives are involved. Students must report findings to the primary nurse and observe the SBAR/ISBARR process in many other settings. The simulation laboratory is an excellent venue to illustrate the SBAR/ISBARR process to students and allow them to practice this technique of communication (Kesten, 2010).

Electronic Health Records

Electronic health record (EHR): A digital medical record that is intended to allow access and updating of clients' medical records wherever they receive care and to make data available to the next healthcare team wherever the client seeks care.

The **electronic health record (EHR)** is mandated to be used by all U.S. healthcare agencies by 2014 (Simpson, 2007). The goal of adopting the EHR is to allow access and updating of clients' medical records wherever they receive care and to make data available to the next healthcare team wherever the client seeks care. The EHR is the future—not just of health care, but also of nursing (Simpson, 2007). The automation of the EHR will simplify work and reduce errors. The EHR also provides an opportunity for better communication between professional nursing practice, other health professionals, and the client.

More than 10 years agent, a report from the Committee on the Quality of Health Care in America (IOM, 2001) made an urgent call for fundamental changes to close the quality gap in health care and outlined key steps to promote evidence-based practice and clinical information systems (EHRs). According to the report, two of the major advantages of the EHR are that it provides nurses and other health care professionals with immediate access to information and that it improves the flow of that information (Trossman, 2009).

The American Nurses Association (ANA) position statement (2009) regarding EHRs notes that the public has a right to expect health data to be centered on patient safety and improved outcomes for all segments of the healthcare system. The ANA (2009) strongly supports efforts to refine the creation of standards-based EHRs and promote efficient and effective interprofessional and patient communication and decision-making. Poon, Wright, and Simon (2010) concluded that having an EHR is not sufficient to improve care quality; it must be complemented by specific features that are used on a regular basis by the healthcare team.

Communication and the Internet

The process of communicating with families and communities involves an array of skills, ranging from simple skills such as data acquisition to more complex skills such as consulting and negotiating care goals (Zavertnik, Huff, & Munro, 2010). According to Zavertnik et al. (2010), it is of utmost importance for nurses (and nursing students) to practice simple communication skills so as to build and advance to complex nurse–client–family (and community) interactions. Using Internet resources wisely can assist with this communication process.

The Safe Healthcare blog on the Centers for Disease Control and Prevention (CDC) website (http://blogs.cdc.gov/safehealthcare) is one way for community nurses to obtain information and communicate

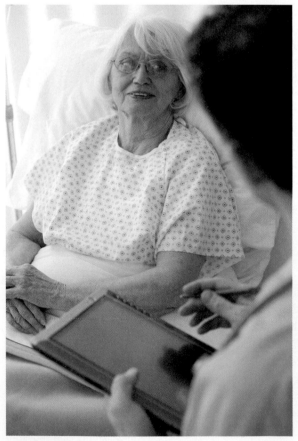

© Comstock/Thinkstock

information. This blog contains information about drug-resistant infection communications, clinical guidelines, community clinics, and other timely topics. Blogging online with this website from the CDC is a 24 hour per day, 7 day per week opportunity for all healthcare professionals to communicate nationally as well as globally.

The Google search engine (www.google.com) is a layperson's way to obtain information. Community nurses need to use this search engine to ascertain which information their clients are reading, to determine the validity of this information, and to be able to correct errors and guide clients to valid websites and information. "Googling" the search term "methicillin-resistant *Staphylococcus aureus*" (MRSA), for example, produces more than 7 million hits. The first result might lead the searcher to an article from the PubMed Health website; the sixth result might lead him or her to the CDC website. The CHN needs to read these results to advise the client who has MRSA, and to assist the client with making health choices.

The Impact of Informatics and Social Networking on Nursing

Informatics is a multidisciplinary study of the application of information technology to any field. Informatics has helped generate and develop advanced information systems for education and business. Through the storage and manipulation of information digitally by computer, the rapid sharing of information has changed lives. The ability to handle vast amounts of information cheaply and quickly has, for example, revolutionized the way CHNs share knowledge. This collaborative means of sharing information and knowledge has led to new forums such as eBay, Facebook, Twitter, YouTube, blogs, podcasts, MySpace, and vast entertainment networks.

Social network sites (e.g., Facebook, various blogs, and Twitter) are online communities where people can meet, interact, and exchange information, including photos and videos. These social networks connect communities both locally and internationally. Hundreds of Web tools are available for individuals to use for networking, collaborating, information seeking, and communicating. Social networking tools have the ability to support and provide informational content and resources.

Students and professional colleagues have the responsibility to evaluate the various network sites as viable sites for use by their clients. When seeking valid healthcare websites, it is helpful to talk with colleagues and professionals in specific areas to obtain tips on useful sites. In addition, social networking tools are valuable because they allow for interactions among users and create a forum on which to post questions and concerns. The vignette at the top of the following page reflects the experience of a nurse-as-client navigating the information available on a healthcare blog.

Informatics has had a tremendous impact on nursing. Nurses have the ability to use social networking to aid clients in obtaining current information, or to provide clients with a forum for communication on a broad spectrum of topics. Nurse educators use social network tools to post items and discussion boards for their students and clients when appropriate. The healthcare professional who posts or shares information on social media sites, however, must remember key risk management principles. Specifically, these posts should never contain confidential information from the work or clinical setting. No information should identify any client, whether in the form of a post, photograph, or video feed. The CHN must always remain professional and communicate in an ethical manner.

Informatics: A multidisciplinary study of the application of information technology to any field.

Social network sites: Online communities where people can meet, interact, and exchange information.

facebook

Facebook helps you connect and share with the people in your life.

© Tomislav Pinter/Shutterstock, Inc.

A Nurse Who Is Also a Client Navigates a Website on Lymphedema

The client is an experienced nurse, post unilateral mastectomy and lymph node dissection since 2007, who develops an aggressive cellulitis of her affected arm with no apparent source. In the past, the client has not had any problems with lymphedema. Since her infection has cleared, however, the client has experienced lymphedema that is very difficult to control.

While the client is at the lymphedema clinic for treatment, the certified lymphedema therapist suggests a blog site that could help answer the client's questions, allow her to talk to other clients experiencing the same issues, and serve as a resource tool for when the client is at home. The hope is that the client can view the information provided at any time, have the capability to talk about the problem, and be able to speak with someone about the problem through blogging.

The client is able to navigate the site with ease. Information about the client's current condition of cellulitis, along with resources from a physician, is provided. The client is able to find more than adequate information regarding lymphedema, along with links to other facets of lymphedema management. The site has a blog section for each link, and current information can be shared instantly this way. One of the advantages of social networking is the nearly instantaneous sharing of information and the ability to communicate with people all over the world. The disadvantages relate to the fact that the site has to have valid information, which can be difficult to verify sometimes. Nurses and other professionals need to refer their clients only to sites that provide reliable information.

When the Therapist Becomes the Patient

For 32 years, I served as a speech therapist for patients with a variety of backgrounds. I loved my profession and my patients, but was saddened to witness the deterioration of those with Parkinson's disease. Getting diagnosed with Parkinson's disease in 1994 at the age of 47 left me in shock and disbelief. The idea of transitioning from therapist to patient felt impossible. But that very journey led me to a level of growth and rediscovery of life unlike anything I could have imagined.

As a speech therapist, I was highly in demand, and often struggled with the luxury problem of being offered too much work. I had published therapy materials that were in circulation for decades. I was well respected for my extensive experience in the field, my honesty, my integrity, and the interest I took in my patients. Witnessing the growth and progress in my patients' conditions as a result of our sessions felt very satisfying. I loved my work, and I was good at it.

I provided home health therapy, which allowed me to learn about each patient's family, interests, and previous work, and gave me a special insight into my clients' individual struggles and conditions. Based on that discovery, I developed programs to meet their customized needs, and made it a goal to never put people in labeled boxes. Despite the compassion and empathy that I displayed, it never occurred to me that I myself might one day be put into a labeled box—Parkinson's disease.

It took two years to receive a diagnosis from the time I began showing symptoms. Watching my own professional performance deteriorate so drastically while having no idea what was wrong with me felt traumatic and terrifying. I became sleepy, nervous, and tense, and I cried very easily. My handwriting became almost illegible, and as a result I had to ask my 16-year-old daughter to write my nightly reports for me as I dictated them. I drooled at times, had hand tremors, and began to shuffle while walking. Worst of all, I sometimes fell asleep during sessions in the homes of my patients. I even occasionally hit the floor when my elbow left the table.

Some of the nurses, aides, and therapists in the agencies I worked for felt I might just be suffering from emotional problems or going through menopause. I knew this wasn't the case, and that there was definitely something more wrong with me. I furiously exercised at the gym but made no progress. I began to fear I might have amyotrophic lateral sclerosis (ALS), multiple sclerosis, or a brain tumor. I went from doctor to doctor, and visited psychologists and specialists, but received no real answers. I felt extreme frustration with their attitudes, and my fears grew.

When I finally received the diagnosis of Parkinson's disease, I was somewhat relieved. However, my relief didn't last long. I had worked with many patients with Parkinson's disease, and had watched many of them helplessly and hopelessly deteriorate. Like me, they had once been active, vibrant individuals, and they slowly lost their ability to be heard or speak clearly, write legibly, walk, or function. I became angry and fearful before I could begin the slow climb up the hill of acceptance.

I finally had to come to accept that I could no longer work. I spent years joking that I would give anything to retire early, but never did I mean it, particularly if it meant giving up my health. At 49 years of age, I had to file for Social Security and disability benefits. I had partially defined myself by my profession, and I had to learn who I was without it.

As a part of the process of accepting my illness, I read voraciously on the subject. I learned more than I desired about the progression, debilitation, and compounding of symptoms, with special insight from my professional experience. My husband and I joined a self-help group, and started a Young Parkinson's group. I also soon found that I could express my feelings through journaling and writing poetry. I later began to paint. Having an outlet for expression was imperative in my journey.

I had to begin to use the methods I had taught for decades as a speech therapist on myself. I constantly reminded myself to close my mouth, stand up straight, move my lips, breathe, and project my voice. I had swallowing problems, and I needed to slow my eating. My work with dysphasia patients provided me with the tools to help control my oral motor problems. I practiced facial exercises throughout the day, either in front of a mirror or by making faces while at traffic stops.

I finally accepted the fact that I had fully transitioned from the therapist to the patient. Ironically, I have even worked with a speech therapist whose publications I used for years in my own profession. She was someone whom I had always admired, and when she was assigned to me as my therapist, I realized I had truly come full circle.

My challenges as a Parkinsonian patient extended beyond the problems I experienced with my speech. My toes permanently and painfully curl under from dystonia. If I don't think about balance while walking or reaching, I fall. While walking, the forward propulsion of my feet accelerates to the point where I can't catch up with myself and I crash to the ground. I had to complete 3 months of physical therapy on land and in water, and have done work in several long-term rehabilitation stints. I have to use tricks to complete everyday tasks like walking such as singing, counting, chanting, or focusing on taking steps heel to toe.

In an attempt to slow down the effects of Parkinsonian dementia, I do everything I can to keep my mind sharp, and follow the old adage, "Use it or lose it." I discuss the news with my husband, read every night, do crossword puzzles, write poetry, and use the computer with a special interest in reading the daily posts from the National Parkinson's Federation, as well as my email.

Despite having fully transitioned into being a patient, it is still important for me to keep that therapist side of myself alive. I have had a wonderful neurologist, but consider it critical to keep alert, and to monitor all of my own medical changes in conjunction with my doctor. I know my body better than anyone, and must describe side effects to my physician to receive adequate treatment.

The patient in me looks at the entire picture and says, "Oh, I am getting worse." The therapist in me looks for each individual problem and works on them independently from the others. This is imperative, for if I look at all of my problems at once I am incapable of handling any of them.

I keep my expectations high and look for creative solutions. When one door closes, another opens, and when I lose one skill, I create another. I very much miss camping, horseback riding, sledding, ice skating, and dancing. I have substituted writing, poetry, art, and gardening. I have difficulty calling myself a senior or disabled. I have so much to do and want to enjoy my family and my present life. I will not allow myself to become a just a Parkinsonian or just a patient. I am now, yours truly, a woman, 63, who happens to have Parkinson's disease.

Source: Betty Jo Blauner, January 21, 2011.

The Loss of the Ability to Communicate

Clients sometimes lose the ability to communicate. The CHN needs to be vigilant in assessing the client's ability to communicate. The preceding story , "When the Therapist Becomes the Patient," provides insight into the case of a client who experiences the loss of the ability to communicate, as she was once able to do as a professional. Although this chapter has focused on the communication between professionals, it is critically important to view the humanity of nurses and other providers as clients with communication defects. Understanding and empathizing with clients who are losing the ability to communicate is critical because of their central role as the recipient of care.

Monitoring the client's ability to communicate should be a priority in every nurse–client interaction. The dynamics of communication change the relationships between the client and their lay caregivers and professional providers. The experience of losing part, or all, of the ability to communicate complicates the nurse–client relationship. Frequent "communication checks" to make sure that the client's voice remains central to the communication process is a particular challenge for the CHN.

Summary

Communication is a key concern in maintaining a safe environment. This chapter reviewed a number of communication concepts that assist the nurse in the community setting, and the healthcare interdisciplinary team in general, in creating a safe environment for their clients. The Joint Commission has taken a special interest in clear communication as it relates to decreasing human error. The Institute of Medicine reinforces the notion that nurses have a key role in using communication to increase safety in the environment where care is provided.

Methods of communication such as the huddle and SBAR/ISBARR techniques are valuable strategies for healthcare providers. The Internet as a social medium also has great value for enhancing communication, although the validity of information found via this means must always be evaluated critically. Finally, the CHN must routinely monitor how clients maintain their communication ability, thereby enabling clients to actively participate in their care as long as possible.

REFERENCES

American Nurses Association (ANA). (2009, December 11). *Position papers on electronic health record*. Retrieved from http://www.nursingworld.org/MainMenuCategories/HealthcareandPolicyIssues/NAPositionStatements/practice.aspx

Boynton, B. (2009). How to improve your listening skills. *American Nurse Today, 4*(9), 50–51.

Chapman, K. (2009). Improving communication among nurses, patients, and physicians. *American Journal of Nursing, 109*(11), 21–25.

Enlow, M., Shanks, L., Guhde, J., & Perkins, M. (2010). Incorporating interprofessional communication skills (ISBARR) into an undergraduate nursing curriculum. *Nurse Educator, 35*(4), 176–180.

Hughes, R. G. (2008). *Patient safety and quality: An evidence-based handbook for nurses*. AHRQ Publication No. 08-0043. Rockville, MD: Agency for Healthcare Research and Quality.

Institute of Medicine (IOM). (2001). *Committee on Quality of Health Care in America: Consensus report. Crossing the quality chasm: A new health system for the 21st century*. Washington, DC: National Academy Press.

Institute of Medicine (IOM). (2002). *Speaking of health: Assessing health communication strategies for diverse populations*. Washington, DC: National Academies Press.

The Joint Commission. (2011). *Facts about advancing communication, cultural competence, and patient-and-family centered care*. Retrieved from http://www.jointcommission.org/assets/1/18/Advancing_Effective_Comm.pdf

Huddle. (n.d.). In *Merriam-Webster online dictionary*. Retrieved from http://www.merriam-webster.com/dictionary/huddle

Kesten, K. S. (2010). Role-play using SBAR technique improves observed communication skills in senior nursing students. *Journal of Nursing Education, 50*(2), 79–87. Retrieved from http://www.slackjournals.com/article.aspx?rid=79001

Poon, E., Wright, A., & Simon, S. (2010). Relationship between the use of the electronic health record features and health care quality. *Medical Care, 48*(3), 203–209.

Sheldon, L., Barrett, R., & Ellington, L. (2009). Difficult communication in nursing. *Journal of Nursing Scholarship, 38*(2), 141–147.

Simpson, R. L. (2007). Easing the way for the electronic health record. *American Nurse Today, 2*(2), 48–50.

Trossman, S. (2009). The benefits of electronic health records. *American Nurse Today, 4*(2), 31–32.

Wolfson, W. (2009). AJN reports: Saving SimBaby. *American Journal of Nursing, 109*(11), 24–25.

Zavertnik, J., Huff, T., & Munro, C. (2010). Innovative approach to teaching communication skills to nursing students. *Journal of Nursing Education, 49*(2), 65–71.

ADDITIONAL RESOURCE

World Health Organization (WHO). (2003). *Choosing the channels of communication*. Retrieved from http://www.wpro.who.int/internet/resources.ashx/TFI/choosing+the+channels+of+communication.pdf

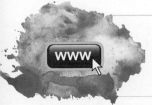

For a full suite of assignments and additional learning activities, use the access code located in the front of your book to visit the exclusive website: http://go.jblearning.com/Holzemer/. If you do not have an access code, you can obtain one at the site.

LEARNING ACTIVITIES   `www`

1. Which of the following statements, made by a nurse, reflects "listening" to a client who has questions about his or her care?

   A. "Repeat what you said to me about your leg pain, so I better understand you."
   B. "You need to be on time for your appointment next week."
   C. "In the event of an emergency, call 911."
   D. "Do not use over-the-counter drugs, unless you tell your nurse practitioner."

2. Which of the following statements, made by a nurse, represents "reflecting back" after the client says, "I am so angry—my daughter never listens to me!"?

   A. "Anger is not healthy for your relationship with your daughter."
   B. "Maybe anger management should be a goal for us to work on."
   C. "You feel angry when your daughter does not listen to you."
   D. "Most mothers feel the same way when their children do not listen to them."

3. A client who is pregnant asks a nurse, "Which Internet sources are best for me to look at, from the list you gave me?" Which of the following statements would be the best response by the nurse?

   A. "You need to find out that information on your own; you are the client."
   B. "All the suggestions may be helpful."
   C. "Look at a few, and we can discuss the sites that seem best for you."
   D. "Pick the sites that you and your partner find most interesting."

4. Identify all of the people whom you would include in a huddle concerning a married male who is not following the plan of care. The client's wife states, "He listens to only his best friend." Choose all that apply.

   A. The client
   B. The client's best friend
   C. The client's employer
   D. The client's wife
   E. The client's physician

5. A nurse is communicating with a physical therapist, using the SBAR technique. The therapist says, "Just use plain language; you are giving me too much information." Which of the following statements is the best response for the nurse to make?

   A. "You need to listen to me to get all the important information."
   B. "The communication technique I am using is required by The Joint Commission."
   C. "I am trying to provide all the necessary information so that you can fully participate in the client's care."
   D. "Please let me speak to your supervisor; that person will appreciate my communication efforts."

ADDITIONAL QUESTIONS FOR STUDY

1. Write your response to the following three beliefs about communication. Are there other beliefs about communication that are important to you? Discuss these beliefs with a classmate.

    A. Therapeutic communication is the most important skill a nurse will ever use in providing nursing care.

    B. Therapeutic communication is an intimate exchange between the nurse and the client; therapeutic communication is not casual communication.

    C. Therapeutic communication is learned, and will develop throughout one's professional career.

2. A community is concerned about safety in their neighborhood in the evening. There are few streetlights, and no "safe place" for children and adolescents to play or congregate after school. The community has a school, a church and a synagogue, and five stores in the area. A small group of residents have met with the police three times about the problem, with no success in making the neighborhood "feel safer." How would the CHN use the idea of a huddle to work toward solving this problem?

Assessment and Diagnosis of the Voice of the Client, by People Who Provide Care to Them

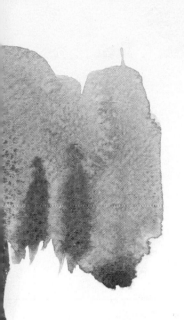

SECTION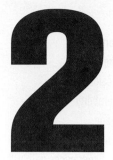

SECTION OUTLINE

CHAPTER OUTLINE

- ▶ Introduction
- ▶ Voice of the Client
- ▶ Clients Speaking
  - • Vulnerability
  - • Courage
  - • Transcendence
  - • Lived Experiences within the Community
- ▶ The Voices of Families, Groups, and Communities
  - • Voices of Families
  - • Voices of Groups
  - • Voices of Communities
  - • Common Voices
- ▶ Coping with Loss
- ▶ Nurses Listening
  - • Spirituality
  - • Cultural Awareness
  - • Caring
  - • Meaning
  - • Technology
  - • Presence
- ▶ Communities Supporting
  - • Care Structures: A Place of Power
  - • Community Health Nurses as Caregivers
- ▶ Summary

OBJECTIVES

www

1. Explain the critical role of listening in being present to the client in community health nursing.

2. Identify resources that can assist the nurse in improving his or her ability to listen to the voice of the client as an individual, family, group, or community as a whole.

3. Define the role of loss in coping with variations in health status.

4. Identify ways in which the nurse and others can change the healthcare delivery system to be more attentive to the voices of clients.

KEY TERMS

www

Competence

Cultural competency

Cultural proficiency

Culture

Health status

Phenomenological research method

Population health paradigm

Relative risk

Resource availability

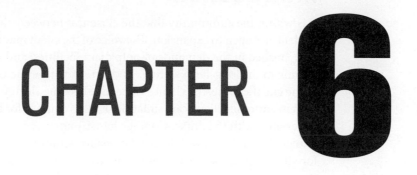

CHAPTER **6**

Narratives of Courage: The Voice of Clients in Community Health Nursing

Patricia Donohue-Porter

COURAGE

Yet the patient (client), for all the superb physical and technical improvements in his environment, feels lonely and even abandoned, because nobody cares for him as a person.

—Lanara, 1981, p. 6

Introduction

It is within the community that the closeness between client and nurse often becomes evident and open to expansion. The voice of the client may be lost in the flurry of hospital care, hushed in the demands of outpatient facilities, and unrecognized in the passages of time in the long-term setting. In contrast, within the community and, in particular, in the client's home, the client's voice may become clearer and be recognized more fully than in any other client-care situation. It takes courage for the client to disclose his or her experience with the nurse. Courage has strong interpersonal characteristics that foster knowledge of the nurse–client relationship. Community health nurses (CHNs) caring for clients within the personal setting of clients' homes, and in other community settings, are privileged to experience and listen to those individuals' life histories and honor their courage. The concept of courage is discussed in greater detail later in this chapter.

This chapter gives recognition to the voice of the client and the response by nursing and delineates areas of contemplation for improved nursing practice. Some of the skills take years to develop and need to be observed, reflected upon, and encouraged by mentors and colleagues. When clients speak about illness experiences, there are often connections to themes of experiencing vulnerability and moving toward courage and transcendence. Often these themes are expressed in qualitative pieces of nursing research in which clients are interviewed and their ideas and words are then formulated into narratives. Selected areas of that type of research are described in this chapter. Nurses have many skilled ways to listen to the voices of clients. Six guides to extend listening skills—spirituality, cultural sensitivity, caring, meaning, technology, and presence—are also addressed in this chapter.

The final section of this chapter addresses nurses as caregivers within social support structures of the community. Throughout the chapter you will find the narratives of clients—that is, their verbatim descriptions of their experiences—in block quotations. The chapter also includes vignettes of nurse and client narratives that arose from a clinical or research situation.

Voice of the Client

Why listen so closely to the voice of the client? There is really only one reason—to be a better CHN. Becoming a better nurse means being able to give better care, and giving better care comes out of understanding the experience of the client. Many of the experiences that nursing students learn about and that new nurses face are unique and challenging to understand. Many CHNs wish to gain a better understanding of these experiences not only to help individual patients, but also to gain more knowledge so that they can offer more help to more clients under a **population health paradigm**. This paradigm consists of integrated care that focuses on health promotion, illness prevention, and chronic condition management but with a special emphasis on patient centeredness and engagement (Sidorov & Romney, 2011). The bridge to communication with clients to promote patient centeredness lies in deliberately listening to, reading about, and perhaps writing narratives about this particular population—that is, clients isolated by their illnesses (Stanley, 2004). "These voices are crying in solitude if we choose not to listen" (p. 361). By consciously attending to these patients' descriptions of their illnesses, more understanding and community building directed to their inclusive care can begin.

Jeanine Young-Mason is a CHN author and long-time advocate of the role of the humanities in helping nurses better understand the full range of human experience. In her work as a clinical nurse specialist in a burn unit, she saw first-hand the differences in the

Population health paradigm: Integrated care that focuses on health promotion, illness prevention, and chronic condition management but with a special emphasis on patient centeredness and engagement.

great needs of clients and the resources necessary for their emotional care. "The devastating losses and grief, the profound remorse experienced by certain individuals at times staggered the nurses and myself" (Young-Mason, 1997, p. 196). "Staggered" is a strong term reflecting the strong response inherent in nurses and nursing as we help clients cope with unimaginable suffering. Vignette 1 expresses what it was like for a nurse to experience the suffering of a small child. The knowledge about experience of the client is deep in this experience, and able to be captured in the narrative.

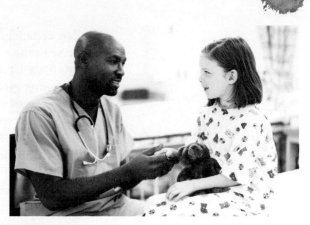
© Kzenon/Shutterstock.com

Young-Mason (1997) captures 16 accounts of children's and adults' experiences of illness in an effort to illuminate these experiences for nurses and help them better understand and care for others. The humanities—areas of study devoted to literature, poetry, drama, music, and art—are other sources of understanding of shared human experiences of suffering and loss, courage and determination. Bruner (1979) writes of the "shock of recognition" one may have when realizing that a poem, play, piece of music, or other aesthetic lesson can fill a gap in experience or bring a concept to life better than a textbook description.

Clients Speaking

If you open your nursing practice to hearing and then value what you are hearing from clients, you will elevate your practice of nursing, feeling comfortable and competent in your growing skills. Your knowledge of nursing science is essential, of course—but it is equally essential that you listen to the voice of the clients, to assess the content and meaning of the other's experience. Your close listening will help you to apprehend vulnerability, courage, and transcendence—all themes related to the experience of the clients in the community. Certain research methodologies such as phenomenology lend themselves to an exploration of client experiences. Nurses have explored these experiences and searched for meaning in what the community-dwelling client and family are experiencing. You will find the path to understanding these experiences by reading research that describes these experiences.

Vulnerability

There are multiple perspectives through which nurses can view vulnerability in the community health setting. For example, people may be considered vulnerable because they have poor physical, psychological, or social health (Aday, 2001). Another view suggests

---

Vignette 1: Care of a Suffering Small Child

As a graduate nursing student in a burn unit, I had to give the first shower to a small child after he had been deliberately burned in a bathtub by his mother. I felt fear and anxiety in this experience, concerned that I would reintroduce the trauma of the event to this defenseless child. Could I be of help? Would I do the right thing? The immediate setting of the high-acuity, critical care area also widened to me as I thought beyond the burn unit to how this child would return to the community and perhaps to a family that would repeat or recover from violent patterns. Where was the knowledge I could gain about these complex and contrasting intersections of care?

Resource availability: The availability of socioeconomic and environmental resources including human capital, social connectedness, and social status as well as access to health care and quality of care.

Relative risk: Exposure to risk factors across age groups.

Health status: Age- and gender-specific morbidity and mortality, including patterns of disease.

that certain groups within the community have increased risk or susceptibility to adverse health outcomes (Flaskerud & Winslow, 1998). These groups may be vulnerable by virtue of their age and comorbid health conditions. They also may be vulnerable due to their engagement in risk-related behaviors, lack of access to care, and other factors of great complexity.

The conceptual framework of Flaskerud and Winslow can help CHNs investigate the experience of vulnerability and discover ways to intervene to diminish clients' vulnerability. The concepts in their model include **resource availability**, which refers to the availability of socioeconomic and environmental resources including human capital, social connectedness, and social status as well as access to health care and quality of care. Another concept is **relative risk**, which refers to exposure to risk factors across age groups. **Health status** refers to age- and gender-specific morbidity and mortality, including patterns of disease. These concepts are useful to help the student nurse and the CHN to identify selected aspects of the larger concept of vulnerability and to see how it can be broken down and analyzed so interventions can be offered. Sellman (2005), in analyzing vulnerability, reminds us that the concept applies not only to exposure to harm, but also to capacity for self-protection. Nursing is vitally involved in this aspect of vulnerability. Although all persons may be thought of as vulnerable as part of being human, Sellman points out that clients who are experiencing illness are often more vulnerable, and nurses can be helpful in recognizing and attending to their needs.

Nurses in the community can be alert to those special groups whose members are more than usually vulnerable owing to the nature of their underlying state, the nature of their illness, and the complicated means of coping they develop in response to illness. For example, an elderly woman may be frail due to weight loss, poor nutrition, and weakened bone density. If she falls and incurs a fracture, she may have difficulty coping with recovery due to her already compromised state. Because she is not in generally good health and resilient, she may develop complications, both physical and mental. She may become frailer due to the fall and develop a fear of falling again. This description is not to say that this individual client does not have inner strengths and resources that may allow her to accomplish full recovery. The nurse should look for these resources and use vulnerability as a way of viewing the client's potential problems—but not a way of identifying her as being in a weak, passive, or negative state.

Look for the client and family strengths first, and be aware that they may be under the surface you see at first glance. Hildegard Peplau, who is considered the mother of psychiatric nursing and the creator of the term "nurse–client relationship," advises us that we will never know, and should never expect to know, the totality of the clients we care for; a natural reserve of their identity and independence helps the relationship from being symbiotic or dependent. Nurses need to see the client's vulnerability as a condition that may be transitioned to strength whenever and wherever possible.

Courage

The investigation of courage provides a framework through which nurses can understand the experience of the client. Research interests in caring for clients with disabling complications of diabetes, for example, can lead the nurse to an exploration of the lived experience of individuals whose complications are progressive and life-threatening, requiring treatments that are often painful and exhausting and at times unsuccessful. These clients have multiple tasks to perform to cope with this devastating physical illness, and the research honors the courage necessary to complete these tasks.

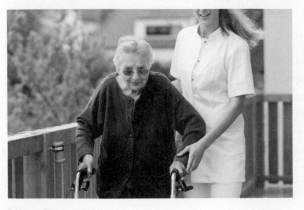

© Kzenon/Shutterstock.com

The **phenomenological research method** is an inductive, descriptive research method concerned with the investigation and description of all phenomena; it has been widely used to examine the issue of courage. For example, a small sample of diabetic clients with disabling complications ranging in age from 30 to 55 years were interviewed in their home settings. The transcripts of the client interviews were analyzed for themes and used to generate a descriptive profile of the role of courage in their experience. The word "courage" brings to mind many different meanings. An earlier dictionary definition from the *World Book Dictionary* (1963) provides a short description of a highly comprehensive concept—the moral strength that allows a person to face any danger, trouble, or pain steadily. A contemporary definition from Dictionary.com (2011) states that courage allows the difficulty to be faced without fear.

Many philosophers focusing on the area of courage would disagree with the latter definition, because fear is often part of the experience of courage but can be diminished through the love and support of others. This is the link to community health nursing: The support of others is central to the goals of a healthy population within a community health model. The bridges that are built that show care and concern for a group of individuals can influence and help sustain courage in clients. Nurses may recognize clients' experiences of courage and support the development of courage as a foundational task. Nurses can help develop patients' courage through actions such as listening, being genuinely and fully present in a helping, caring relationship, interpreting technology, entering into dialogue, and helping to support clients during times of health, suffering, and recovery.

> *Courage is rightly esteemed the first of human qualities … because it is the quality which guarantees all others.*
>
> —Winston Churchill (1874–1965)

Transcendence

The concept of transcendence may be viewed as the final goal of excellence in nursing care. Assisting a client to transcend the immediate situation of suffering may help him or her to become more fully integrated within the world around the client. This clearly does not mean that the nurse pushes the client to strive to overcome suffering in a way that sets up an additional burden in the already stressful client situation. It does mean that if the client wishes to discuss changes in worldview and in self-perceptions due to the challenges of illness, the nurse is ready and open to hear those views.

Hope, patience, positive thinking, and humor were some of the ways that clients with disabling complications of diabetes transcended the experience of suffering. Finding beauty in nature, leisure activities, and the simple joys of family life became more important to some clients who were interviewed. Rather than feeling debilitated owing to the complications, they instead felt more open and alive to the world around them. A profound change occurred in their perceptions of themselves and of others.

Transcendence is particularly important for CHNs because these nurses are with clients during transitional time periods of recovery and in intimate home settings that hold great meaning for individuals and families. These nurses are deeply involved with the restoration of health. "Transcendence is probably the most powerful way in which one is restored to wholeness after an injury to personhood. When experienced, transcendence locates the person in a far larger landscape" (Cassell, 2004, p. 43). Nurses are part of the community—the healthcare community as well as the human community—that supports the individual client through recovery or release from suffering.

Phenomenological research method: An inductive, descriptive research method concerned with the investigation and description of all phenomena.

Lived Experiences within the Community

Some of the following experiences are examples derived from literature and studies that illuminate the client's voice during periods of aging, loss, and stress and adjustment of caregiving for an ill family member. The aging voice of the client can be heard directly or by readings in literature and poetry that speak to the stillness of loss. Florida Scott-Maxwell describes this poignantly in her memoirs of the experiences of life and aging:

> Old people can seldom say "we"; not those who live alone, and even those who live with their families are alone in their experience of age, so the habit of thinking in terms of "we" goes, and they become "I." It takes increasing courage to be "I" as one's frailty increases. (Scott-Maxwell, 1968, p. 130)

The Voices of Families, Groups, and Communities

The voice of families, groups, and communities (collectives) are heard as they complete their responsibilities to their members. Collectives have the responsibility to complete at least five functions:

1. Collectives open their boundaries to allow new members to enter, and other members to leave.
2. Collectives meet the physical, emotional, and spiritual needs of members, and foster growth and development of their members.
3. Collectives seek and allocate resources to meet the needs of their members.
4. Collectives instill values, beliefs, and an ethical–cultural orientation to foster collective cohesion.
5. Collectives use communication to promote positive interaction within the collective, and with the larger community.

Voices of Families

Families are collectives of choice. People come together in fidelity to experience life together as a unit. Their boundaries change, for example, with the birth, adoption, and death of members. Adults leave the family voluntarily to live alone, go to school, seek employment, or enter new families. Sometimes, family members are removed from the family unit because the family cannot meet their needs because of a physical, emotional, or legal challenge. Some members are placed in a care setting because they need skilled nursing care, or psychiatric monitoring, or are incarcerated because of behavioral problems. A unique characteristic of families is that (ideally) they survive and thrive for many generations.

Voices of Groups

Groups are collectives with a shorter life span, and often exist only to get work done or a task completed. Depending on the constellation of the group, it can be characterized as healthy or unhealthy. Healthy groups are able to complete their assigned tasks—representing their voice. The role of the CHN, in working with groups, is to foster cooperative interaction of members so that the group can work productively. Often, the CHN has the responsibility to work with many lay and professional groups, each with unique needs, as they complete tasks of short and long duration.

Voices of Communities

Communities are defined by geographical boundaries (cities, states, nations), special interests (religious, political, educational), or a special health focus (lay and professional organizations). As with smaller groups, the voices of communities can be seen as a reflection of cooperative interaction. A unique characteristic of a community's voice is the responsibility to provide resources to meet the needs of families and groups that belong to the community.

Common Voices

The family that resolves problems, the group that accomplishes tasks, and the community that thrives despite all of its challenges demonstrates its uniqueness as well as its level of health. These collectives experience vulnerability, demonstrate courage, and may experience transcendence. They cope with loss, have needs for caring, and search for meaning. The role of the CHN is to be present to each of these collectives and to assist its members in their journey toward cooperation and demonstration of healthy behaviors.

Coping with Loss

Community health nurses see clients coping with losses of many kinds. These losses involve grieving and bereavement that may be difficult to understand and to cope with for the early-career nurse. In all aspects of the nursing profession, continued education and openness to new information about nursing science are necessary—but perhaps are even more essential when it comes to listening to the individual voice of the client who is grieving a loss.

For many years, nurses were taught that the grieving process includes distinct stages and that clients' responses emerged in a linear fashion. We know from evidence-based research that some of these assumptions were flawed and may now be considered myths (Wortman & Silver, 1989). Wortman and Silver helped to point out that coping with loss varies widely and that its many forms must be acknowledged: "Recognition of this variability is crucial in order that those who experience loss are treated nonjudgmentally and with the respect, sensitivity, and compassion they deserve" (p. 355). It is essential that nursing students and nurses respond to bereaved individuals and family with care that is based on the knowledge that there is great variability in response to grief. Clients are unique not only in their loss but also in their need for support and compassion.

Nurse researchers have examined the existence of long-standing myths of coping with loss in undergraduate psychiatric nursing books and have found instances where evidence has still not supplanted myths (Holman, Perisho, Edwards, & Mlakar, 2010). Positive areas of client strengths such as resilience, coping, and communication were identified in evidence concerning coping but often were not translated into interventions to aid coping. As a result, myths often drive care even when evidence does not support interventions. Holman et al. point out that because the role of nursing is critical in giving support to clients as they cope with loss, it is especially important that nursing education in this area be balanced, evidence based, and contemporary so as not to create false expectations among nurses about the trajectory of clients' grief responses. This relationship demonstrates how nurses must be constantly attuned to the evolution of knowledge and not rely on a singular view of how they care for others.

Backstrom, Asplund, and Sundin (2010) examined the meaning of middle-aged female spouses' lived experiences of the relationship with

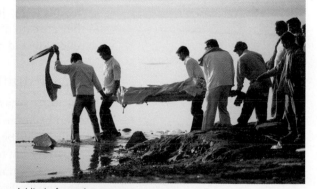

A Hindu funeral ceremony.

© Özgür Donmaz/iStockphoto

a partner who has suffered a stroke. In their study, interviews were conducted at 1, 6, and 12 months post discharge; the interviews were transcribed into a text and carefully interpreted for themes using a phenomenological method. Spouses came to identify and adjust to changes in their partners' conditions. Many experienced great grief and anxiety. The themes of loss and grief and the necessary transitions to be made in marital and life adjustments were predominant findings.

These descriptions helped to bring to life the real feelings and experiences that spouses have within the community and that nurses are often called upon to support. The implications of the changes associated with the stroke often become evident only after a period of time at home, during which the CHN may be the only source of support for the family. The themes and subthemes uncovered in Backstrom et al.'s (2010) study can help the inexperienced nurse make sense of some of the overwhelming emotions the spouse may be expressing. Themes such as being estranged, having to be hypervigilant of the spouse's fragility, losing one's own identity, keeping hold of the marital relationship, feeling lonely together, becoming aware of a permanently altered relationship, and suffering in silence are only a small selection of the richly detailed descriptions of the transitions these researchers discovered.

In this study, the spouses were suffering terribly and often in silence, but were ready to tell their life stories to a trusted listener. It is within the scope of nursing to help bear witness to this suffering through attentive listening. Listen to the fatigue in one of the participant's tone:

> It's tough, it's really tough … It is … now he has been home for 6 months, sometimes it feels to me like it's 10 years. I feel like I have not breathed in ages … as a close relative you need some form of relief. (p. 262)

Nurses Listening

The previous section focused on how clients have described their illnesses, suffering, and meanings in their journeys to health and recovery or their adjustment to a peaceful death. Other descriptions are also available in the research literature, particularly the qualitative literature that illuminates multiple areas of concern to nurses in the community: the new mother, the infirm elderly, the chronically ill child, the client with mental illness, and many more. Some of these situations involve joy mixed with stress or sorrow. How does a nurse develop the skills to listen to the voice of the client? Six lenses can be your guide to understanding the experience of the client and your guide to areas of further study necessary to develop your expertise: spirituality, cultural sensitivity, caring, meaning, technology, and presence. Although these are surely not the only lenses, they are carefully chosen for inclusion here because they give the CHN the resources for reflection and enrichment needed to move to a deeper level of nursing care.

Spirituality

Spirituality has traditionally been difficult to describe and measure, and nurses have often been unsure as to what their best course of action to help clients fulfill spiritual goals should be. Nursing research has addressed spiritual well-being and its investigation as paramount to excellent nursing practice (Florczak, 2010), yet this paramount area of concern for nurses "dwells on the periphery of the profession" (Carr, 2010). Carr notes that spirituality has been acknowledged in nursing theory and history but continues to be marginalized in education and practice, pointing out that often nurses' primary concern with spirituality is task oriented, such as making a referral to a chaplain or arranging for a religious practice.

Carr's research study focused on a phenomenological investigation of multiple individuals within the hospital organizational culture—oncology nurses, clients and their families, chaplains, and hospital administrators—to see which barriers are in place that diminish spiritual care. She found social distancing between nurses and clients, owing to nurses' compressed time constraints, their fear of implying doom by broaching subjects such as death, and their fears of not being adequately prepared to address topics of a spiritual nature with their clients. These same barriers may be in place in the community setting. Carr acknowledges the depth of these concerns but encourages nurses to use their intuition and their assessment of clients' needs to start these conversations: "We must, therefore, let the client take the lead in addressing topics of a spiritual nature and not be afraid to go on that journey if he or she should invite us" (p. 1387).

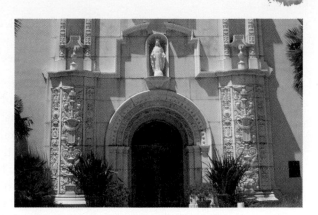

Courtesy of Deborah Murphy.

Others have noted that although spirituality definitions may be so vague as to seem almost meaningless, this is definitely not the case. Swinton (2010) argues that despite its vagueness, the language of spirituality remains useful and cautions us not to misinterpret a lack of clarity as a lack of significance. He notes that spirituality may be particularly helpful in times of chaos when important discussions come to the foreground. Because there is no set boundary for these discussions, an open space for nurses to enter into dialogue with clients develops. Often the unique relationship between nurse and patient in the community setting allows for highly permeable boundaries of communication. Yet how can students receive education about a topic as vast as spirituality?

Swinton (2010) argues that if spirituality is seen not as a single topic but rather as a response to a variety of human quests, nurses can be educated through an examination of literature that illuminates meaning, hope, and connections and can be encouraged to be flexible in seeking out knowledge in this area (p. 235). Spirituality can be viewed as an element of an individual's quality of life, as the basis to providing quality of life, as a source of meaning of experiences, as a coping mechanism, or as a relationship with a supreme being; for those who do not have a belief in a relationship with a supreme being or God figure, spirituality may enter into their relationship with themselves, others in the universe, and the environment (Tinley & Kinney, 2007, p. 72). Again, nurses are directed to return to the voice of the client, listening to the narratives of client experiences.

This author's research investigating courage in the lived experience of clients with diabetes complications identified clients' spiritual outlook as a theme (Donohue-Porter, 1987). All clients were able to discuss different aspects of spirituality in the development of courage. Several also said they were not religious and did not find any spiritual means helpful in developing courage:

> I think I've always not been a religious person. I grew up and went to Temple once in a while but I don't really have a religious outlook. I don't understand when so many things are happening and everybody says they are happening for a reason. I don't really believe it. No, really don't have faith. I guess, if anything, I just have faith in myself that I will get through it. But I don't think somebody up there is taking care of me.

This perspective stands in contrast to another person's view that derives strength from a spiritual focus when facing the disease:

> My religion has helped me get through the terrible things I was told in the beginning about my eyes, and facing blindness. I thought, "Oh

God, they said I could only have one child and you sent me this one. You would not have sent her if you did not mean for me to take care of her."

The differences in responses are to be expected, yet the nurse's question can always remain the same: "Would you like to speak about some spiritual issues?" "Would talking about spiritual concerns help you during this difficult time?" "I believe spiritual well-being is as important as your physical well-being; is there anything I could help you with, or talk to you about, or concerns I can listen to at this time?"

This topic is sensitive and sometimes you need to practice these kinds of questions with your instructors or peers to gain more comfort and experience. Remember, you do not have to be perfect as you begin your discussions with your clients. They are not expecting that—just a genuine desire to listen to them.

Mary Elizabeth O'Brien has long contributed to nursing work on spirituality through her studies on spirituality influences in adjustment to dialysis (1983) and HIV (1992) and through her classic book *Spirituality in Nursing: Standing on Holy Ground* (2003). In her long-term study of clients coping with renal failure and dialysis, she noted a shift in many of the clients' views of spirituality, with the importance of religious faith increasing as the clients learned to adjust to the demands of their chronic illness. For example, one client, who had stated that he had no faith in religion at all at the beginning of her study, explained three years later that religion helped him to have faith in the dialysis and the health professionals working with him (p. 36). It is important for nurses who work with clients for years in the community setting to realize and remain open to the many changes and transitions in faith and feelings that clients undergo.

O'Brien (2003) describes the "holy ground" as the posture a nurse assumes each time he or she gives comfort to a client, beyond the material world. She movingly describes how nurses sing to ill babies, shelter the bereaved in their arms, and wait during the vigil at the bedside of the dying, and how these actions take shape as we stand on holy ground.

Nurses are sometimes fearful of discussing spiritual issues with clients, thinking such concepts are too personal for general discussion. Yet nurses lose some of the most powerful information that they can gain about their clients when they overlook this dimension of their clients' lives. Individuals need a basis from which to derive strength and courage so that they can transcend their present situation. This can, at times and for certain individuals, flow forth from spirituality. Individuals also need other human beings to help them grapple with existential issues of life and death. Nurses can be the other half of an interpersonal dimension of transcendence, assisting the client to find and sustain the courage to do so.

Results from a small pilot study using spirituality-based interventions related to quality of life, depression, and anxiety in community-dwelling adults with cardiovascular disease (CVD) showed a significant modest increase in overall quality of life for 41 adult clients with CVD who received interventions. The interventions were individualized and included such techniques as meditation, prayer, and reflection. Clients kept a journal of their responses. Those who had used a self-discovery meditation described their experiences with words such as "comforting," "peaceful," and "calming." The authors pointed out that individualized spirituality-based interventions can aid and be added to traditional cardiac care to improve quality of life (Delaney, Barrere, & Helming, 2010).

Cultural Awareness

Cultural competency: A set of behaviors, attitudes, and policies that come together in a system, agency, or professionals that allow for effective work in cross-cultural situations.

A set of behaviors, attitudes, and policies that come together in a system or agency or, importantly, in professionals that allow for effective work in cross-cultural situations is defined by the Office of Minority Health of the United States as **cultural competency**

(U.S. Department of Health and Human Services, 2005). Two important definitions are given by this agency. **Culture** describes the integrated patterns of human behavior that include language, thoughts, communications, actions, customs, beliefs, values and institutions of racial, ethnic, religious, or social groups. **Competence** means having the capacity to function effectively as an individual and an organization within these needs. These are demanding tasks for the nursing student or new nurse within the community, yet cultural competency is directly tied to closing healthcare disparities or gaps. Nurses need knowledge about cultural aspects of clients' experiences as well as the ability to be aware and sensitive to the complexity of cultural situations.

A nurse researcher who has examined this issue in detail is Marcia Wells (2000). Wells encourages us to not stop at accepting cultural awareness, cultural sensitivity, and cultural competence as being enough to guide client care, but rather to aim for **cultural proficiency**. She describes this level of achievement as the mastery by the individual nurse of the cognitive and affective phases of cultural development. These would include a continuum of realizing there is a lack of knowledge about cultural implications of health behavior, learning the elements of culture and how they shape behavior, and recognizing the cultural implications of behavior (cognitive). Also included are the integration of knowledge and awareness into one's behavior and routine application of culturally appropriate health care (affective).

Wells's work builds on that of the nursing theorist Madeleine Leininger (1978), whose internationally recognized work on transcultural nursing has influenced generations of nursing scholars. Leininger historically views nurses as capable of deep reflection on their own biases so as to avoid stereotyping of groups and to remain open and accepting of other cultures. Her culture care diversity theory attests to this belief. Community health nurses who are committed to providing individual, holistic care will find that culturally responsive care is a priority.

The root of cultural sensitivity is respect. Respect for other cultures allows you to realize that you may not have enough knowledge about another's culture and to seek to gain more knowledge. Respect allows you to assign a high priority to culturally proficient care when planning your nursing practice. Respect helps you to fully enter into a conversation with another individual who is unlike you and to learn from each other. Hill (1999) cautions us to never presume that we will not discover something about the life of the mind and something valuable for all of us in a dialogue with the radically diverse other (p. 225).

Elements of respect have been identified and explored by Lawrence-Lightfoot (1999), who uses the West African word "tolani" as the foundation of her description. "Tolani" means "one who gives respect and one is who is respected" (p. 4). This symbol of respect demonstrates the energy inherent in the action of giving and receiving respect. Lawrence-Lightfoot describes the underlying character of respect, explains how it is nurtured into growth, and points to what she calls six windows on respect—empowerment, healing, dialogue, curiosity, self-respect, and attention. She begins her detailed descriptions with a story of a nurse–midwife caring for mothers experiencing the poverty of the South Bronx. The midwife describes how she wants to empower these women as a form of respect for them, in all aspects of their journey to becoming mothers:

> It is always a question of how to respect their pain without taking it in. If you just take in pain, you become the pain. You become paralyzed and powerless. So I give them the space, my full attention, and I listen. I acknowledge that I hear them

Culture: The integrated patterns of human behavior that include language, thoughts, communications, actions, customs, beliefs, values and institutions of racial, ethnic, religious, or social groups.

Competence: Having the capacity to function effectively as an individual and an organization to meet clients' needs.

Cultural proficiency: The mastery by the individual nurse of the cognitive and affective phases of cultural development.

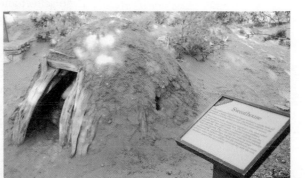

© Jeffrey M. Frank/Shutterstock.com

even though I don't always have solutions. Sometimes that is all I can do. (p. 47)

Other descriptions follow, not only of nurses, but also of educators, doctors, photographers, and ministers—an array of humankind whose stories represent respectful actions. As Lawrence-Lightfoot makes clear, respect is a cornerstone of cultural awareness.

Caring

How is caring expressed in nursing? Caring is fundamental to the discipline. Caring is in direct opposition to just carrying out appropriate interventions for clients (Bishop, 2010). It continually places the client at the center of the nurse's concern and continually places the pair in a movement together, a pattern. Watson (1999) has described this as a call and response, meaning that the calling allows nurses to show compassion and commitment to clients.

Caring is built on relationships and reflection. A nurse who is working at a level of excellence is always reflecting upon what the client experience means and how can he or she work to improve it. Examining client experiences and reflecting upon how they can improve your caring relationships with clients is the most important action a CHN can perform. The more you read about and live through client experiences, the more you can reflect upon your own judgments, presuppositions, intentions, actions, and reactions. The clearer your vision of yourself and your caring relationship with your clients becomes, the more natural it will become to build trust. Building trust in caring for families at risk for health problems in the community is another essential action the CHN can take.

Being nonjudgmental goes hand in hand with trust. In another qualitative study of specific actions used by public health nurses to care for families at risk, nursing interventions such as avoiding labeling, avoiding viewing parents through their past actions, purposefully identifying strengths, and including each family member in decision making were found to be powerful elements of planned nursing actions (Browne, Doane, Reimer, MacLeod, & McLellan, 2010). All of these actions were taken with a clear goal of preventing further trauma to the children in high-risk homes. The end results of success came about because of the relational aspects of the nurse–client relationship.

Meaning

An important part of the experience of human illness is a search for meaning within the client situation. Nurses can be viewed as partners during the journeys of their clients to reflect and gain understanding of their experiences. Because nursing is a profession that interacts with human beings during critical life periods, nurses are able to develop an awareness of intimate, individual human problems. Meaning is unique to each human's perception, and nursing has historically valued the uniqueness of the individual and his or her perceptions.

Nurses can help clients to find meaning in their suffering by inquiring and accepting what is meaningful to them in life in general. Within the client's beliefs and values, some meaning will be assigned to the present injuries. This may help to reduce the amount of suffering for the client, who then feels he or she has obtained some control over his or her own attitude toward the situation.

Clients are frequently asked by nurses, "How do you feel?" but less frequently are asked "How do you feel about this—your illness and its impact?" This question and others like it must now be asked by nurses if they are going to successfully care for clients, particularly in assisting the development of courage or coping skills.

Technology

Technology's role in the home and community has grown in its importance and placement. Equipment that might have been used only in hospitals in the past is now commonplace in the community system. Yet the nurse working within the community must realize that the attention paid to the technical aspects of the client environment competes with the attention paid to the human needs of clients. Concerns with technology are presented in Vignette 2.

The need for increased communication to balance the increased use of technology was identified as early as the 1970s. Due to the increasingly technical environment in which health care is delivered, it is important that the nurse and the client are able to come closer, in self-disclosure, to communicate and humanize depersonalized care (Jourard, 1971).

Technology is often viewed as an inevitable part of nursing and something that challenges the nurse–client relationship. Other nurse scientists dispute that view, instead perceiving nurses' competent use of technology as a way of demonstrating caring (Locsin, 2005), as the proximity of the technology affording the development of authentic presence of the nurse to the client (Sandelowski, 2002), and as a chance to focus and refocus on the client within the environment of technology (Barnard, 2009). This choice is reflected in the words of Barnard: "If you do not return to the person at an appropriate moment in their care, it is you, rather than the technology, that has made a choice to distance yourself from your client" (2009, p. 371).

Dehumanization has occurred within the healthcare environment, including the community, due to increasing use of technology. Such technology has become critical to saving lives, but it also causes stress to clients, particularly chronically ill individuals, who are continually battling for survival within the system, whether at the hospital or at home. It is the role of the nurse to interpret for and assist the client to effectively deal with a technological environment.

Society expects nursing to stand against the stream of dehumanization in health services (Lanara, 1981). The nurse can be viewed as a bridge, closing the gap between the client and the highly technical environment. It is always the nurse who has the vision of what a scientific discovery will really mean to the client, in regard to all of the

Vignette 2: Caring for a Young Girl in a Comatose State

I had the experience of caring for a young girl of 13 who was in a comatose state. Because she had a high fever, she was on a hypothermia blanket and other vital sign monitoring technology and attached to a ventilator for respiratory compromise. I had positioned her on her side about a half hour before going back to check her vital signs, so I did not need to touch her to reposition her. When I began to check the vital signs, I realized that I could read her temperature from the hypothermia blanket machine, see her respirations and cardiac rhythm on another readout, and check her blood pressure electronically as well— all done without touching her. In that moment I realized that I could interpret the health of my client without the use of touch that is integral to nursing care, so I purposely placed my hand on her arm and described to her my every step. This incident led to a research project that investigated the connections between technology and caring touch and how touch can help to fulfill the multiple stages of Maslow's hierarchy of needs.

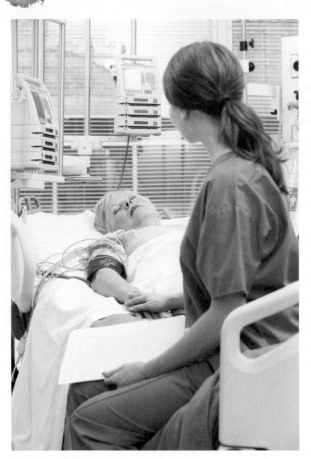

© LifesizeImages/iStockphoto

client's human dimensions, and who helps to interpret technology for the client. A client in a research study about diabetes complications and courage offers a striking example of this relationship, as described in Vignette 3.

Presence

Nursing is an active profession, and nurses are active agents—coordinating care, administering treatments and medications, talking to clients and families. Nurses are at clients' bedsides in hospitals and communities or sitting next to them in their kitchens and living rooms. Sometimes they are teaching, at other times they are actively listening, but they often can be found being present to the experience that is uniquely the client's human activity. Margaret Newman, nurse theorist and visionary, advises nurses to become even more fully present to their clients in her book *Transforming Presence: The Difference That Nursing Makes* (2008). She gently guides her readers to recognize that presence is characterized by a nurse's openness and sensitivity to the other (p. 52).

Presence is truly part of community health nursing, where often the nurse visits clients and families in a regular pattern of care. The CHN's presence is not only evident in the physical format, but may linger after a visit has occurred as the relationship becomes stronger and deeply genuine. Newman advises nurses to view the connection between the two individuals in the nurse–client relationship:

We need to view the relationship from within and recognize the shared consciousness that occurs. As the nurse is fully present with the client, the meeting forms a new rhythmic pattern of the combined fields. The nurse "hangs in there" and waits for insight to occur. When it does, the nurse can move away and allow the client to center in the resonating process without the physical presence

---

Vignette 3: Technology and the Human Dimensions of Care

A client explained that when he first learned that his kidneys had failed, he was told this by a group of doctors and nurses who surrounded his bed. They offered him three options: hemodialysis, peritoneal dialysis, and transplantation. They asked him to consider these technologies and they left the room. For the next 7 hours he felt that his life had fallen apart and he was overwhelmed with confusion and fear. The evening nurse in charge of his care came into his room after her shift was completed and sat with him, explaining again what the doctors had said, talking with him and reassuring him. The client realized that the nurse was giving him extra time that had not been available earlier in the evening and that the nurse had recognized his intense need for assistance. The client stated that he would never forget this nurse. He attributed his better understanding of the available technological choices to her nursing interventions.

Vignette 4: Transforming Presence

I recently had the experience of visiting at the bedside of a friend with a neurological illness that had caused total paralysis. Her only communication method
was through the blinking of her eyes. A nurse entered the room to administer a
tube feeding and medications and, without a look at the guests around the bed
and without any attempt at eye contact with the client, abruptly announced that
we needed to leave for a while during her tasks of giving a tube feeding and
administering medications. This nurse missed the opportunity to be fully present
in that moment with that client who had great needs. She could have mentioned
the joy of having visitors at the bedside. She could have asked us how we knew
the client and found out more of her humanness. She could have recognized to
the client and to the gathering that in the deep sorrow of the experience we had
all come together to divide the burden of deep grief.

of the nurse. The pattern of their transformation persists even though
they have moved apart. (Newman, 2008, p. 55)

Newman stresses that to be fully present, the nurse must be one with the client and
focus on that transforming presence to the exclusion of time and tasks. That is an admi-
rable goal, but one that may be difficult for the early-career nurse to achieve. Newman
helps to achieve that by reminding us that certain clients, such as those experiencing
dementia, may have no sense of past or future; for them, the present is all (p. 56). Other
clients, such as those in pain or in emotional crisis, may be oriented only to the present
and may value the nurse's transforming presence as he or she concentrates on being with
and understanding the client's experience.

Opportunities like this are often missed because nursing students and new nurses
have tremendous responsibilities to get the technology and the tasks "right." This problem is even more apparent in the home and community setting, where the nurse may be
the only professional seen by the client for weeks, and has grave responsibilities related
to tasks and technology. Yet it is just as essential for the nurse to be present to the entire
client, meeting his or her emotional and psychological needs in ways that will assist in
full recovery and restoration.

The "Nurses Listening" section of this chapter is an integral part of evidence-based
practice. An essential part of evidence-based nursing practice is assessing, honoring,
and fulfilling client preferences for their care. As Baumann (2010) points out, nurses
need to develop their own nursing perspective so they can synthesize knowledge from
diverse sources, including client values and preferences, and apply it to each individual
client encounter. He emphasizes that considering the experience and narrative of both
clients and practitioners is a central element of the process of evidence-based nursing
care (p. 229).

Communities Supporting

The previous two sections of this chapter separated out the client's voice and the nurse's
listening response as key elements in nurses' education about community health nursing.
Yet, there is really no division between the two concerns, because community nursing is

never about a client and a nurse as separate entities. Both are partners in a relationship that shifts back and forth, in motion and in dialogue. Central to that relationship is the circle of caregivers, whose presence expands the vast potential of relationships involved in community care. Other social support structures are in place, assisting in developing, assessing, and providing for client needs.

Care Structures: A Place of Power

Relationships between nurses and clients have certain power structures in place. Nurses have knowledge that they "give" to clients; clients' decisions may be either welcomed or marginalized. Caring professionals may not think consciously about the many areas in which hierarchies are built into the nurse–client relationship, but they certainly exist and as the nurse becomes more experienced they may become clearer. Such power-based structures are to be avoided in all healthcare arenas, but particularly in the community, where partnership and respect are privileged aspects of the nurse–client relationship.

Macurdy, in "Mastery of Life" (1997), a recollection of his adaptation to home health nursing, gives an example of crossing a street without the permission of his attending nurse as they are out walking together while he adapts to the use of a portable ventilator. He explains to the nurse that he needs her nursing competence but that he is not mentally incompetent and is still quite capable of making decisions for himself, particularly in crossing a street in a town in which he has lived for 10 years. He continues on to say that no one will make decisions for him, but finds the terminology of his care—describing him as "denying pain," "refusing medications," and the like—as representing authoritarian statements that make him seem childlike. Macurdy wants information provided directly from him in each supportive care structure that he encounters and, importantly, he wants health care viewed as part of his life, not all of his life:

> Health care is a means to a full and meaningful life; it is not an end in itself. But because the professionals deal only with the medical aspects of my life, they often lose sight of the impact of their recommendations on my career, home life, and relationships. If their efforts are not resisted, the medical agenda will overwhelm the human agenda—the tail will wag the dog. (Macurdy, 1997, p. 14)

This perspective is in keeping with contemporary nursing thought that is evolving from viewing the client as an object of care to viewing the client as a person who is a knowledgeable participant in his or her care (Locsin & Purnell, 2009, p. xix). If nurses can consciously reset the off-balance hierarchy of power in every community healthcare setting, then no matter where care is offered (e.g., home, nursing homes, clinics, day programs), clients will be valued as participants in their care.

Community Health Nurses as Caregivers

Community health nurses are asked to be independent and fearless in their care for clients in multiple areas where resources are limited and where they may be the only health professional directly responsible for the client's care. They have a tremendous opportunity to show their care and exquisite competence in an array of situations. At times nurses practicing in the community, particularly those at the advanced level of preparation, are not recognized for their preparation and scope of skills. White and Kudless (2008), in their study using participant action research, interviewed community mental health nurses who were found to highly value the autonomy of their role, but who struggled to have others recognize their role and nursing identity and felt frustrated when burdened with clerical work that took time away from important nursing interventions. Nurses' talent and energy may be constantly poured into the client care situation, leaving these caregivers overwhelmed and in need of support, too. Leaders of community health teams and administration must be aware that nurses as caregivers are under stress and need support. Their experiences need to be listened to and valued as well.

Summary

The coming together of clients and nurses in the community can arise from shared communication, which requires courage on the part of the client. Nurses' listening to the voice of the client will result in both partners coming together with one voice of respect, valuing and caring for the strength of community health nursing. This chapter focused on recognition of the voice of the client (both individual and collective) and the response by nursing, and delineated areas of contemplation for improved nursing practice. The skills to communicate and improve nursing practice take years to develop and need to be observed, reflected upon, and encouraged by mentors and colleagues.

When clients speak about their illness experiences, they often make connections to themes of experiencing vulnerability and moving toward courage and transcendence. Often these themes are expressed in qualitative pieces of nursing research, in which clients are interviewed and their ideas and words are then formulated into narratives. Selected examples of that approach to research were presented in this chapter. Nurses have many skilled ways to listen to the voices of clients, and six guides to extend listening skills include spirituality, cultural sensitivity, caring, meaning, technology, and presence. Finally, nurses operate as caregivers within social support structures of the community, though they may need support themselves to provide the best possible care to their clients.

REFERENCES

Aday, L. (2001). *At risk in America*. San Francisco: CA: Jossey-Bass.

Backstrom, B., Asplund, K., & Sundin, K. (2010). The meaning of middle-aged female spouses' lived experience of the relationship with a partner who has suffered a stroke, during the first year postdischarge. *Nursing Inquiry, 17*(3), 257–268.

Barnard, A. (2009). Vision, technology and the environment of care. In R. Locsin & M. Purnell (Eds.), *A contemporary nursing process: The (un)bearable weight of knowing in nursing* (pp. 357–377). New York, NY: Springer.

Baumann, S. (2010). The limitations of evidenced-based practice. *Nursing Science Quarterly, 23*(3), 226–230.

Bishop, V. (2010). The caring aspects of any health care discipline versus the enthusiasm for scientific precision: Is the evidence base in nursing flawed? *Journal of Research in Nursing, 15*(5), 383–384.

Browne, A., Doane, G., Reimer, J., MacLeod, M., & McLellan, E. (2010). Public health nursing practice with "high priority" families: The significance of contextualizing "risk." *Nursing Inquiry, 17*(1), 27–38.

Bruner, J. (1979). *On knowing: Essays for the left hand*. Cambridge, MA: Harvard University Press.

Carr, T. (2010). Facing existential realities: Exploring barriers and challenges to spiritual nursing care. *Qualitative Health Research, 20*(10), 1379–1392.

Cassell, E. J. (2004). *The nature of suffering and the goals of medicine* (2nd ed.). New York, NY: Oxford University Press.

Churchill, W. (n.d.). BrainyQuote.com. Retrieved from http://www.brainyquote.com/quotes/quotes/w/winstonchu130619.html

Delaney, C., Barrere, C., & Helming, M. (2010). The influence of a spirituality-based intervention on quality of life, depression, and anxiety in community-dwelling adults with cardiovascular disease: A pilot study. *Journal of Holistic Nursing, 20*(10), 1–12.

Dictionary.com. (2011). Retrieved from http://dictionary.reference.com

Donohue-Porter, P. (1987). *The role of courage in the experience of patients with diabetes complications.* Unpublished doctoral dissertation, Adelphi University, Garden City, NY (UMI No. 8715251).

Flaskerud, J., & Winslow, B. (1998). Conceptualizing vulnerable populations' health-related research. *Nursing Research, 47*(2), 69–79.

Florczak, K. (2010). Gathering information on spirituality: From whose perspective? *Nursing Science Quarterly, 23*(3), 201–205.

Hill, P. J. (1999). Multiculturalism: The crucial philosophical and organizational issues. In B. Pescosolido & R. Aminzade (Eds.), *The social worlds of higher education: Handbook for teaching in a new century* (pp. 220–232). Thousand Oaks, CA: Pine Forge Press.

Holman, E., Perisho, J., Edwards, A., & Mlakar, N. (2010). The myths of coping with loss in undergraduate psychiatric nursing books. *Research in Nursing & Health, 33,* 486–499.

Jourard, S. (1971). *The transparent self.* New York, NY: VanNostrand Reinhold.

Lanara, V. (1981). *Heroism as a nursing value: A philosophical perspective.* Athens, Greece: Sisterhood Evniki.

Lawrence-Lightfoot, S. (1999). *Respect: An exploration.* Reading, MA: Perseus Books.

Leininger, M. M. (1978). *Transcultural nursing: Concepts, theories, and practices.* New York, NY: Wiley.

Locsin, R. (2005). *Technological competence as caring in nursing: A model for practice.* Indianapolis, IN: Sigma Theta Tau International.

Locsin, R., & Purnell, M. (2009). *A contemporary nursing process: The (un)bearable weight of knowing in nursing.* New York, NY: Springer.

Macurdy, A. (1997). Mastery of life. In J. Young-Mason (Ed.), *The patient's voice: Experience of illness* (pp. 8–18). Philadelphia, PA: F. A. Davis.

Newman, M. (2008). *Transforming presence: The difference that nursing makes.* Philadelphia, PA: F. A. Davis.

O'Brien, M. E. (1983). *The courage to survive: The life career of the chronic dialysis client.* New York, NY: Grune & Stratton.

O'Brien, M. E. (1992). *Living with HIV: Experiment in courage.* Westport, CT: Auburn House.

O'Brien, M. E. (2003). *Spirituality in nursing: Standing on holy ground* (2nd ed.). Sudbury, MA: Jones and Bartlett.

Sandelowski, M. (2002). Visible humans, vanishing bodies and virtual nursing: Complications of life presence, place and identity. *Advances in Nursing Science, 24,* 58–70.

Scott-Maxwell, F. (1968). *The measure of my days.* New York, NY: Penguin Books.

Sellman, D. (2005). Toward an understanding of nursing as a response to human vulnerability. *Nursing Philosophy, 6,* 2–10.

Sidorov, J., & Romney, M. (2011). The spectrum of care. In D. Nash, J. Reifsnyder, R. Fabius, & V. Pracilio (Eds.), *Population health: Creating a culture of wellness* (pp. 3–19). Sudbury, MA: Jones & Bartlett Learning.

Stanley, P. (2004). The patient's voice: A cry in solitude or a call for community. *Literature and Medicine, 23*(2), 346–363.

Swinton, J. (2010). Moving beyond clarity: Towards a thin, vague, and useful understanding of spirituality in nursing care. *Nursing Philosophy, 11,* 226–237.

Tinley, S., & Kinney, A. (2007). Three philosophical approaches to the study of spirituality. *Advances in Nursing Science, 30*(1), 71–80.

U.S. Department of Health and Human Services, Office of Minority Health. (2005). W*hat is cultural competency?* Retrieved from http://minorityhealth.hhs.gov/templates/browse. aspx?lvl=2&lvlID=11

Watson, J. (1999). *Postmodern nursing and beyond.* Edinburgh, Scotland, UK: Elsevier.

Wells, M. (2000). Beyond cultural competence: A model for individual and institutional cultural Development. *Journal of Community Health Nursing, 7*(4), 189–199.

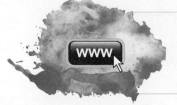

For a full suite of assignments and additional learning activities, use the access code located in the front of your book to visit the exclusive website: http://go.jblearning.com/Holzemer/. If you do not have an access code, you can obtain one at the site.

White, J., & Kudless, M. (2008). Valuing autonomy, struggling for an identity and a collective voice, and seeking role recognition: Community mental health nurses' perceptions of their roles. *Issues in Mental Health Nursing, 29*(10), 1066–1087.

World book dictionary. (1963). Chicago, IL: World Book, Inc.

Wortman, C. B., & Silver, R. (1989). The myths of coping with loss. *Journal of Consulting and Clinical Psychology, 57*(3), 349–357. doi: 10.1037/0022-006X.57.3.349

Young-Mason, J. (1997). *The patient's voice: Experiences of illness.* Philadelphia, PA: F. A. Davis.

LEARNING ACTIVITIES

www

1. Which statement is most accurate about the concept of vulnerability?

   A. Some clients are born vulnerable, and will not live a normal life.
   B. Health teaching is an antidote for vulnerability.
   C. People of wealth are rarely vulnerable.
   D. Multiple conditions may contribute to vulnerability of clients.

2. In which of the following ways would a CHN view a family as unique? Choose all that apply.

   A. The way a family experiences loss
   B. The way a family seeks support
   C. The way a family accepts compassion
   D. The way a family is willing to change
   E. The way a family shares its experience

3. Which of the following statements, made by a CHN, correctly describes the concept of courage?

   A. "Courage is a personal characteristic, not influenced by the behavior of others."
   B. "Courage is evident only in the behavior of adolescents and adults."
   C. "Courage is experienced uniquely as people face difficult situations."
   D. "Courage is absent when people decide to 'terminate further treatment.'"

4. Which of the following approaches is the most effective way the CHN can foster courage in clients?

   A. Allow clients to "figure out" their choices privately
   B. Explain that "fear" is not related to the concept of courage
   C. Provide encouragement to develop lay and professional support systems
   D. Identify the plan of care as a safe process that does not require courage

5. Which of the following concepts relates to the experience of "moving beyond a crisis, and viewing the event within the context of being and feeling alive"?

   A. Hope
   B. Transcendence
   C. Acceptance
   D. Health

ADDITIONAL QUESTIONS FOR STUDY

Review the four vignettes presented in the chapter, and respond to the questions.

Vignette 1: Care of a Suffering Small Child

1. What role do you think preprocedure pain medication administration would play in this situation?

2. Which resources should the nurse seek to cope with the care of a complex client situation?

3. What are your thoughts about communicating with family members who might visit the child in this situation?

Vignette 2: Caring for a Young Girl in a Comatose State

1. What is the value of touch in every nursing care situation?

2. What would you say to visiting family members who might be afraid to touch the young girl?

Vignette 3: Technology and the Human Dimensions of Care

1. How do you provide care to a client (individual and collective) who is overwhelmed with confusion and fear?

2. Which sorts of activities would you use to meet the needs of a group of clients experiencing concerns with chronic illness?

Vignette 4: Transforming Presence

1. Which measures can the CHN take to be "fully present" when there are so many tasks that need to be completed?

2. What would a community look like, and act like, if it operated in transforming presence?

CHAPTER OUTLINE

▶ Introduction
▶ Compassion on the Part of the Nurse in Community-Based Care
▶ Cognitive–Affective–Psychomotor Skills of the Nurse (and Client)
  • Cognitive Skills
  • Affective Skills
  • Psychomotor Skills
▶ Mentoring and Developing Evidence-Based Practice Roles
  • Nurse as Care Manager/Advocate Role
  • Leader/Follower Role

  • Teacher/Learner Role
  • Consumer of Evidence-Based Research Role
▶ Compassion Fatigue
  • Definition
  • Developing Therapeutic Relationships in the Community to Offset Compassion Fatigue
▶ Nurses Supporting a Culture of Care for Nurses in the Community
▶ Summary

OBJECTIVES

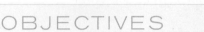

1. Explain the need for a nurse to have a complete cognitive, affective, and psychomotor skill set in community health nursing.

2. Define the various roles of the nurse working in the community.

3. Discuss the similarities and differenced of compassion fatigue in both the nurse and other care providers in the community.

4. Describe the essential nature of therapeutic relationships that need to be developed with others in the community.

KEY TERMS

Affective skills   Cognitive skills   Compassion fatigue   Psychomotor skills

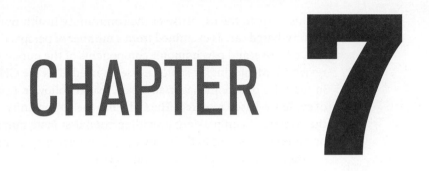

CHAPTER 7

Expertise of the Compassionate Nurse in Community-Based Care

Stephen Paul Holzemer

Anne Belcher

Introduction

In this chapter, the expertise of the community health nurse (CHN) working in community-based care is examined from a number of perspectives. In particular, the cognitive, affective, and psychomotor components of the nursing roles in the community are reviewed. Mentoring by senior nurses is needed as the CHN develops expertise in the in the roles of care manager/advocate, leader/follower, teacher/learner, and consumer of evidence-based research. The CHN has the opportunity to develop these roles within the context of compassion; providing compassionate nursing care allows the nurse to be especially present to the many competing needs and demands of the community.

The CHN develops a therapeutic relationship in the community using principles of leadership and management, team building, and referral. Such a nurse can enter into a compassionate partnership with the community to improve its health and to maintain wellness. Another aspect of nursing in the community relates to nurses caring for other nurses so that mature nurses can provide safe, effective, and competent care to the community. Older nurses in all areas of nursing need support, but the more mature CHN may have special needs.

Compassion on the Part of the Nurse in Community-Based Care

Providing care to clients in the community is complex. Clients leave the hospital with multiple needs and often may not have the requisite personal and material resources for a successful recuperation. There is proven value in nurses' acting with compassion in providing care to these clients. Compassion is both intentional and central to the success of the work of the CHN. The nurse is dedicated to understanding the complexities of care in the community, and takes an *active, community-based approach* to provide care that will have lasting positive results.

Compassion suggests that the approach to meeting the needs of the community should be continuous, not episodic. The commitment to an ongoing monitoring of the community, to meet changing and emerging needs, suggests that the CHN is working with the community in a way that reflects compassion. Vigilance in using the nursing process with the community, from a local-to-global perspective, gives the CHN the opportunity to provide care that has a significant impact on the relief of suffering.

When the community is the client, the CHN acts to relieve suffering on a scale much different than that observed when caring for an individual. Compassion requires a larger view of the impact of suffering on clients' ability to participate in care and to seek solutions to their many problems. It humanizes the care needed to foster lasting change and recovery from distress (Schantz, 2007; van der Cingle, 2009). Compassion is central to the therapeutic relationship that the nurse (and others) enters into with the community to assist in meeting complex, multiple-problem concerns. The CHN provides care with a clear perspective of what the nurse needs to think, feel, and do—to meet the needs of the community.

Cognitive–Affective–Psychomotor Skills of the Nurse (and Client)

All care providers find themselves somewhere on the novice-to-expert continuum when providing care (Benner, 1982, 2001). The skills needed for community health nursing work are cognitive, affective, and psychomotor in nature, and are provided by novice and expert nurses. These three domains do not stand in isolation. Indeed, almost every problem a client experiences draws on a combination of cognitive, affective, and psychomotor skills on the part of the nurse. Clients develop full or partial independence from skilled nursing services as they develop their own cognitive, affective, and psychomotor skills.

Once the CHN develops a set of cognitive–affective–psychomotor skills, the nurse can assist others (clients and less experienced nurses) to develop their own skill set. **FIGURE 7-1** illustrates the movement from a lower level to a higher level of cognitive–affective–psychomotor skills for both the nurse and the client. The upper part of the diagram suggests that at the beginning of an interaction, the nurse and the client may have skill limitations, with fewer complementary skills (less overlap of circles). Over time (lower part of the figure), the nurse and the client develop more complementary skills; they work in a coordinated, successful way (more overlap of circles). Spending quality time with the individual, family, group, or community client fosters skill development.

Nurses need to identify the cognitive–affective–psychomotor skills they are proficient in performing, as well as those that need development. The CHN develops the ability to use anticipatory guidance with the client, just as the nurse develops other needed skill sets. In addition, the CHN plans on developing those skills that may be needed in the future to keep the client moving toward health and wellness. It takes time and experience for the CHN to be able to anticipate the needs of clients, and to assist them in meeting their needs.

The following vignette , "Anticipatory Guidance and Employment Change in a Group in the Community," demonstrates how the CHN uses anticipatory guidance when working with a group of clients who are employed by a company having financial difficulties. In this situation, an occupational health nurse (OHN)—a specialized community health

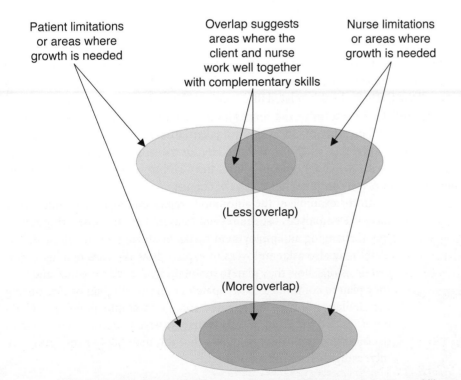

Patient limitations or areas where growth is needed

Overlap suggests areas where the client and nurse work well together with complementary skills

Nurse limitations or areas where growth is needed

(Less overlap)

(More overlap)

Over time the client and the nurse develop a more complementary skill set.

Figure 7-1 Strengths and limitations in the cognitive–affective–psychomotor skill set of the nurse and the client.

Anticipatory Guidance and Employment Change in a Group in the Community

An OHN is working with a group of clients on "on-the-job work safety" at an automobile repair plant. A recent financial downturn for the company is followed by the corporate decision to lay off 10 employees. The management of the company asks the nurse to assist in setting up a job retraining program, which is intended to assist the soon-to-be-terminated employees to secure other work in the community. The OHN is working with the human resources department of the company to focus on the psychosocial issues related to their change in job status. The OHN is aware that the group of employees will first need to discuss their feelings about their upcoming termination, and express their feelings about the loss of their jobs.

Using anticipatory guidance, the OHN allows the group to begin to reflect on and discuss the information related to their changing employment status. Once the process begins, the workers are able to begin to see and prepare for their changing futures. In time, the majority of the group members begin the process of job retraining without resistance, and are able to prepare for change with a positive approach. At the time the employees are released from their jobs, three decide to retire, two decide to work in information management technology, and five decide to remain in the automobile repair field. The OHN focuses on ways that the employees can maintain health insurance and cope with ongoing health-related concerns during their employment transition.

Cognitive skills: "Knowing" skills that encompass knowledge, critical thinking, and comprehension of particular topics.

Affective skills: "Feeling" skills that describe the way people react emotionally or empathize with others.

nurse—is working with a group of clients on "on-the-job work safety," when a crisis occurs with an anticipated layoff of employees.

Cognitive Skills

Cognitive skills are *knowing* skills. There is evidence of cognitive learning when the client knows when to take medications, knows when to call 911 for assistance, or knows when to call the CHN for health-related information. "Knowing," however, is difficult to measure or validate. To determine the client's level of cognitive learning, the CHN may ask the client to explain when medications are taken, discuss when to call emergency services, or give examples of when to call the CHN for consultation. An ongoing presence of the CHN with the client (group) allows the CHN to observe behavior change and signs of readiness to continue the process of change.

In the example of the automobile repair employees, the nurse may have the employees list the resources available for considering retirement, changing an employment focus, or staying in the job field. The CHN may also ask employees to explain how they are making financial decisions, how they plan to maintain insurance coverage, and how they plan to continue to participate in their health plan of care during the challenge of their anticipated change in employment. The CHN observes that the group moves from a passive to a more active role in decision making, which suggests that the members of the group are increasing their cognitive skill set.

Affective Skills

Affective skills are *feeling* skills. Feeling skills include accepting limitations in care, and sharing on an emotional level what it means to

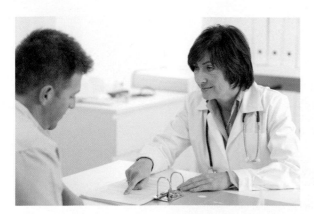

experience illness or to get well. In some situations, affective skills need additional time to be developed. Trust in the nurse–client relationship, or trust among group or family members, needs to be established before clients can comfortably share how they "feel" about a particular situation.

In the example of the automobile repair employees, the CHN begins to search for the meaning of the upcoming change with the group. Group members may need to share their concerns, fears, and disappointments about their current and future employment situation. The CHN is aware that this "work" is necessary before decisions can be made concerning the group's changing employment status, including decisions about retiring from work versus seeking ongoing employment. Group members, in sharing their concerns with one another and experiencing empathy for one another, may be a reflection of affective skill development.

Psychomotor Skills

Psychomotor skills are *doing* skills. They include skills of observation and manual dexterity. Clients are evaluated for their ability to do the activities necessary to stay well. For example, clients need to complete prescribed exercises for rehabilitation and demonstrate proper injection technique to self-administer insulin for treatment of diabetes mellitus. Psychomotor skills also involve time management—for example, when one person must provide or coordinate the care of other family members. Children and older persons with cognitive problems need another person to assist them in getting the care they need.

In the example of the automobile repair employees, some group members had to meet with their financial planners to plan for their retirement. Others had to find and sign up for training and education in information management technology. The remaining employees needed to find out which new skills they would need to develop to remain competitive in the automobile repair field. In this example, workers also need to continue to participate in getting the care they need for medical and emotional problems evident before the employment crisis. Following a recovery plan, developed by the group with the CHN, represents movement in developing psychomotor skills.

Psychomotor skills: "Doing" skills that involve the physical ability to manipulate tools or instruments.

Mentoring and Developing Evidence-Based Practice Roles

There are multiple roles for the nurse to assume in community health nursing—roles both similar to and different from those assumed by nurses working in more structured settings such acute and subacute care environments. Some of these roles are care manager/advocate, leader/follower, teacher/learner, and consumer of evidence-based research. Roles of the CHN are performed in various traditional and emerging community settings, such as home care agencies, assisted living locations, and schools.

As noted earlier in this text, the majority of nurses working in the community do so in acute care home care, care of the chronically ill, and other settings where treating illness is the focus of care. CHNs may also work in areas of special interest or with a defined focus such as faith community nursing or occupational health nursing. The area where nursing has the least presence in the community is in public health. These ideas are represented in **FIGURE 7-2**.

A preferred involvement by nurses in community-based care is provided in **FIGURE 7-3**. This approach is preferred if one accepts the benefits of primary prevention of problems developing in the community. In this representation, the majority of CHNs would direct their dedication toward public health nursing. If the priorities in

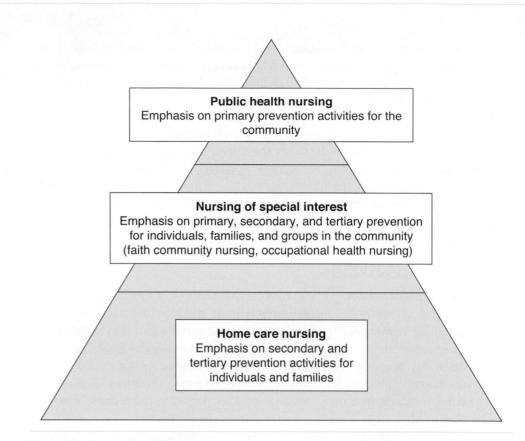

Public health nursing
Emphasis on primary prevention activities for the
community

Nursing of special interest
Emphasis on primary, secondary, and tertiary prevention
for individuals, families, and groups in the community
(faith community nursing, occupational health nursing)

Home care nursing
Emphasis on secondary and
tertiary prevention activities for
individuals and families

Figure 7-2 Community health nursing: nursing specialties working in the community.

health care shift in the future, and this change is anticipated by many providers in the community, the shift will require a different focus of care in community health nursing, and a different cognitive, affective, and psychomotor skill set.

In addition to the skill set that is needed to assist the client to move toward physical, emotional, psychosocial, and spiritual health as a care provider, the CHN needs to develop a skill set that complements the roles of care manager and advocate, leader and follower, teacher and learner, and consumer of evidence-based research. The challenge of learning and balancing these multiple roles places the CHN at risk for compassion fatigue, as discussed later in this chapter.

Nurse as Care Manager/Advocate Role

Nurses working in the community must work from a written plan of care, with specific goals, if the care is managed by a physician, as with Medicare-reimbursed home care. In contrast, nurses in independent practice create their plan of care autonomously. All care provided by nurses in the field should be informed by professional standards and ethical underpinnings (American Nurses Association, 2010a, 2010b; Fowler, 2010). Safety in the provision of care and confidentiality of sensitive health-related information are of primary concern in every client–nurse interaction (Hughes, 2008).

Nurses need to ready themselves for every client interaction so that they can provide competent care. Review of nursing and medical diagnoses, medication and treatment regimens, and client responses to care delivery interventions represents the minimal preparation needed to ensure safe practice. Special data collection and manipulation

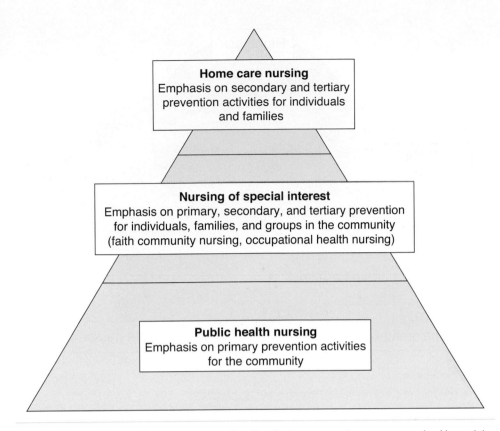

Figure 7-3 Theoretical emphasis on resource allocation if primary prevention were more valued by society.

resources exist in the community, and are used to monitor the use of resources in the community (DecisionHealth, 2011). Using consultation skills with more senior nurses, and referral skills with other health-related disciplines, allows the nurse to provide competent care, as required by the Nurse Practice Act of every state and commonwealth.

Basic delegation and supervision responsibilities are similar in all care settings. The unique delegation and supervision responsibilities of CHNs, however, come from their unique practice settings. The CHN often delegates and supervises care that is provided by a number of laypersons, with often unspecified dedication to the established plan of care. The CHN must clarify that lay caregivers understand the plan of care and are willing to participate in the plan. The five components of delegation in any setting are depicted in **FIGURE 7-4**.

In addition to direct observation, the CHN uses telephone and Internet follow-up with clients to monitor the delegation process. Developing and maintaining a therapeutic relationship with clients is the best way to monitor success with delegation. Clients need to feel empowered to assist with directing the care they receive and to notify the CHN when questions or problems arise. The nurse acts for or advocates for each client in making sure that the plan of care is followed or adapted to the changing needs of the client.

Leader/Follower Role

The roles of leader and follower are linked; at any point in time, a nurse could be a leader in one area of work and a follower in another area of work. Rarely do individuals

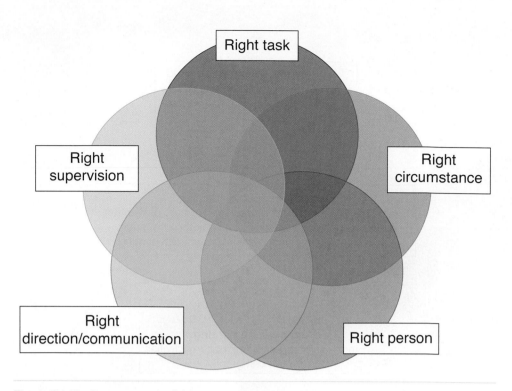

Figure 7-4 The five components of delegation in any clinical setting.

fill just one role exclusively. Leadership and followership roles change and may present unique challenges for the CHN. Although the CHN works with clients (families and groups) as a leader initially, he or she may shift into the follower role as the client gains more independence in self-care. Similar dynamics occur with the relationships among coworkers. The CHN may act as a leader in setting parameters for a physical therapy referral, then act as a follower in ensuring that the rehabilitation directions are followed correctly. According to a particular situation, sometimes the nurse leads and sometimes the nurse follows.

Flexibility in the leadership and followership roles allows the nurse to demonstrate personal skills that are developed in these areas as well as to learn from others who are more expert. Whether the nurse is working with clients or other care providers, the goal is always to foster independence and interdependence as necessary and appropriate to empower the individual, family, group, or community as a whole to move toward independence in self-care.

Teacher/Learner Role

> *Give a man a fish and you feed him for a day. Teach a man to fish and you feed him for a lifetime.*
>
> —Chinese proverb

The teaching and learning experience entered into by a CHN and client is one of the most significant professional and personal experiences that occurs in nursing practice.

It has the potential to empower the client to choose health and wellness alternatives. The most significant outcome of the teaching and learning experience is that clients become part of the solution to health-related problems. Every client–nurse interaction holds the potential for teaching and learning on the part of both the client and the nurse.

The teacher/learner dyad is also a part of the CHN's interaction with other providers. In an effort to maintain role competence, the CHN makes every effort to stay current in contemporary community health nursing practice. To do so, he or she participates in staff development and continuing education activities offered by the nurse's employing agency. In addition, the CHN seeks out professional activities to improve role competence, such as participation in certification and membership in professional organizations. The greatest responsibility related to role competence, second only to providing safe and effective care to clients, may be in fostering an environment in which nursing students are welcomed and enrolled in quality clinical experiences. These experiences may be specifically designed internships to promote their educational success, wherein the CHN assists them with skill-set development.

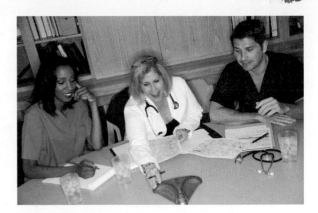

© Jupterimages/liquidlibrary/Thinkstock

Consumer of Evidence-Based Research Role

Community health nurses working in the community use research every day. In every client interaction, nurses use research evidence to assist their clients in developing, participating in, and evaluating their plan of care. As a consumer of research, the CHN assists in developing and maintaining "best practices." The CHN engages in the study of epidemiological trends and seeks to apply the most current understanding of primary, secondary, and tertiary prevention in the care of clients at all levels of acuity. The CHN has a role in creating an environment in which both qualitative and quantitative research outcomes are respected, and research is conducted using ethical principles in a culturally sensitive manner.

Compassion Fatigue

Definition

Compassion fatigue is a phenomenon that can be experienced by both CHNs and lay caregivers. Becoming exhausted from the many demands of caregiving is insidious and can affect everyone providing care in some way (Aycock & Boyle, 2009; Bush, 2009). Compassion fatigue is also embarrassing. It is difficult for CHNs and close family providers to admit to, and to cope with, their fatigue from caring for others. Compassion fatigue is closely associated with the concept of burnout and has physical, behavioral, psychological/emotional, and spiritual components (Aycock & Boyle, 2009).

For the CHN, compassion fatigue can affect multiple roles. The roles of care manager/advocate, leader/follower, teacher/learner, and consumer of evidence-based research can all be at risk. **FIGURE 7-5** depicts the components of compassion fatigue and potential solutions for recovery. There is no universal approach to resolving compassion fatigue. Instead, nurses should seek support from one another, and from other providers, to develop a plan for compassion fatigue that is specific to their situation. Professional assistance from a mental health provider may be necessary and should be approached as a positive option for maintaining professional competence.

Compassion fatigue: Exhaustion from the many demands of caregiving.

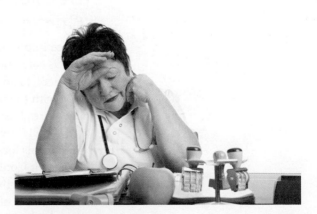

© Robert Kneschke/Shutterstock, Inc.

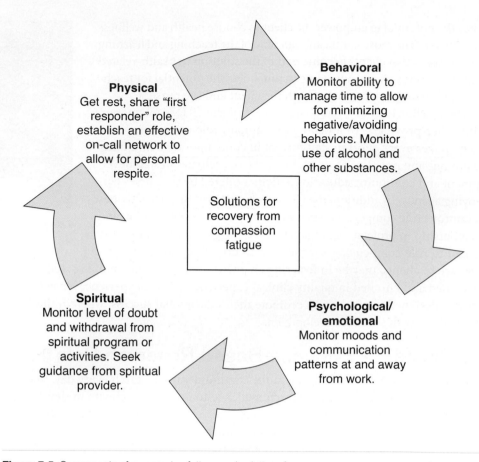

Figure 7-5 Components of compassion fatigue and solutions for recovery.

One antidote for compassion fatigue can be found in establishing a therapeutic relationship with the community that is served. A therapeutic relationship with the community allows the CHN to use resources (e.g., time, energy, commitment to compassion) wisely and at a less personal cost. When the CHN focuses on this therapeutic relationship, relying on the leadership and management, team building, and referral components of this process, effective care delivery in the community can be maintained.

Developing Therapeutic Relationships in the Community to Offset Compassion Fatigue

Three important components provide structure to the therapeutic relationships that CHNs enter into with communities. In community health nursing, leadership and management, team building, and referral are all used to strengthen the therapeutic relationship with the community. These relationships allow the nurse to experience success in the more global aspects of caring for the community as a whole.

The CHN works with the community to establish a working relationship with agreed-upon goals for community action. In the following vignette, "Negotiating Community Needs for Confronting Childhood Obesity and the Availability of Resources for Recreation," the CHN and community members must agree on how to proceed in implementing a variety of community programs. Discussion of the leadership and management, team building, and referral components of this process follows.

Negotiating Community Needs for Confronting Childhood Obesity and the Availability of Resources for Recreation

A CHN working with community leaders identifies HIV/AIDS education and diabetes education as the most important programs for implementation in the community. The CHN decides on this focus after a thorough review of epidemiological trends and interviews with nurse specialists working in the local hospital. When the CHN introduces these ideas to community leaders in an open forum, the leaders reject the CHN's initial proposal. The community leaders identify childhood obesity and a lack of recreational facilities available during the evening hours for the children in the community to use as the most important problem to resolve. The parks and playgrounds are locked after dusk in the evening due to the fact that the city budget does not have money with which to hire additional recreational staff.

Working with the Parks Commission and local businesses, the CHN and other members from the community develop a plan to keep the recreational facilities open for two additional hours in the evening. The local utilities company partners with a home improvement business to provide appropriate lighting. The businesses decide to provide personnel to staff the park as part of their employees' community service program. The local legislature provides for needed insurance coverage to assist with maintaining a safe environment.

The CHN, along with other providers, develops an on-site educational program related to proper exercise and healthy eating; the program is staffed by students from the local schools of human nutrition and exercise physiology. Along with students from the local school of nursing, they also provide information on diabetes and HIV/AIDS prevention and awareness. The CHN involves community members in every step of developing the comprehensive educational program.

After the immediate needs of the community, as identified by community leaders, were met, the community leaders were fully supportive of a more comprehensive program for obesity, diabetes, and HIV/AIDS screening, and program planning. In fact, the community's request for extended recreation services became a central motivator for children and adolescents to lose weight, learn more cooperative play, respect others, and begin the process of accepting more responsibility for their health.

Leadership and Management

Nurses working in the community assume various leadership and management roles. In program development, for example, the CHN may lead the process initially, and then move into a more managerial role once the community leadership function is established. In the example of the CHN negotiating with the community related to the community's need to confront childhood obesity and availability for recreation, the CHN wisely let the community leaders "take the lead." The CHN negotiated a way to meet the priority needs as identified by the community and to enfold additional, related concerns, supported by the epidemiological trends of morbidity and mortality in the community, within the overarching program.

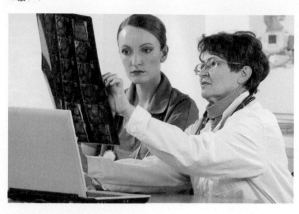

© iStockphoto/Thinkstock

A commitment to community-based leadership and management has the potential for evolving the care provided in the community into an innovative and transformative way of working with clients at all levels (Porter-O'Grady & Malloch, 2011). Leadership and management can embrace change, and guide it toward best practices and positive care outcomes. Securing the roles of both the CHN (and other providers) and the client as part of the emerging needs for sound leadership and management has the potential for strengthening compassion in community-based care.

Team Building

The role of the CHN in the community is a particular challenge due to the various special interest groups that may make up a team in the community. The CHN represents the expert in community nursing but is not an expert in the role of the client living in the community. Clients as a group in the community may, for example, identify programs that are more important to them than the programs identified as a priority by the CHN. The CHN needs to join the group and work with others to identify the problems in the community and to negotiate their priority for resolution.

In the example of negotiating with the community to confront childhood obesity and availability for recreation, the CHN was aware that to ignore the needs of the community from community members' perspective would severely damage team building. The CHN shares responsibility for applying the nursing process in the community with the client as full partner in the team. The "give and take" in decision making is a necessary aspect of conflict that assists in conflict resolution. The CHN and the client both have unique and important perspectives that relate to problem solving, and they deserve the respect of having their views included in any final decision about healthcare delivery.

Referral

The CHN working in the community uses referral on a daily basis. Knowing where to refer clients and their families for additional services is a delicate process. Handing a list of addresses and phone numbers to a client and advising him or her to seek additional help on his or her own is not proper referral. Every effort must be made to avoid making the referral process a negative experience for the client or the supportive family and friends, who often are needed to support the referral.

The nurse should have assurance that the referral is appropriate and will be handled efficiently by the individual or organization receiving the referral. It is the responsibility of the CHN to follow up with the individual, family, or group that enters the referral process. Even though some referrals may not work out for clients, the effort on the part of the CHN to monitor the process will potentially make the next referral more helpful.

In the example of negotiating with a community to confront childhood obesity and the availability of recreation, the actions by the CHN to respect the priorities of the community would now allow the nurse to refer clients with potential and actual problems with obesity, diabetes, and HIV/AIDS to obtain the necessary screening and care they may need.

Nurses Supporting a Culture of Care for Nurses in the Community

Nurses in the community have the opportunity to support the needs of CHNs working in the community. With the predicted shift in national priorities toward more community-based care, the nurses providing that care need their own healthcare needs met as well.

The CHN needs to be an active participant in supporting a culture of care for nurses (and other providers) in the community, so that clients can be successful in getting their healthcare needs met (Holzemer, 2010).

The workforce of nursing is changing, with the potential loss of a mature, experienced core of nurses. The older segment of the nursing profession represents a wealth of professional wisdom that has made a unique contribution to the nursing profession and, more importantly, a contribution to the public health. Mature nurses, acting in the role of care provider, educator, and researcher, need to preserve their physical and psychosocial integrity so that they can continue to contribute to the profession. The profession of nursing is in the position to create environments to meet the needs of the public while supporting the special needs of the mature nurse.

The Alliance for Health Model places the nurse in a central role in co-creating a healthcare system, in conjunction with the client, to meet their healthcare needs. **FIGURE 7-6** provides a visual representation of this idea. When approaching the concern of supporting a culture of care for nurses (and other providers) in the community, the model is adapted to place the nurse in the position of "client." The CHN and other providers have needs that must be met for them to be effective care providers. **FIGURE 7-7** depicts the adaptation of the Alliance for Health Model with the five key components of the model.

In this model, the first component, "community-based needs," relates to the needs of the maturing nursing workforce. The second component, "systems of care management," relates to the systems of support for the maturing nursing workforce. It is followed by "influences on resource allocation decisions," or identifying and securing the resources

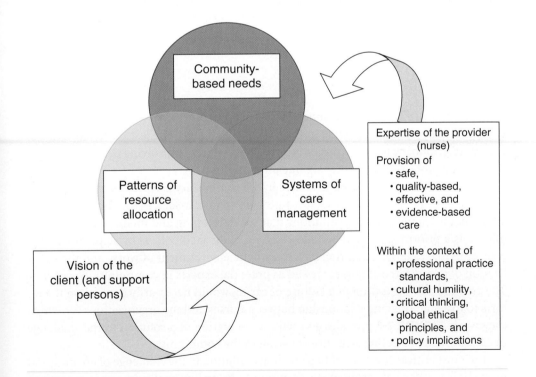

Figure 7-6 Alliance for Health Model of community health assessment.

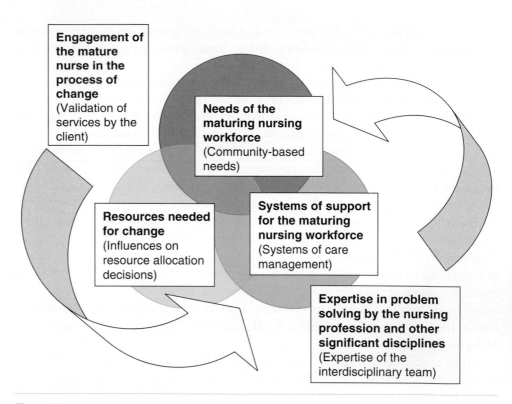

Engagement of
the mature
nurse in the
process of
change
(Validation of
services by the
client)

Needs of the
maturing nursing
workforce
(Community-based
needs)

Resources needed
for change
(Influences on
resource allocation
decisions)

Systems of support
for the maturing
nursing workforce
(Systems of care
management)

Expertise in problem
solving by the nursing
profession and other
significant disciplines
(Expertise of the
interdisciplinary team)

Figure 7-7 Alliance for Health Model: creating and protecting a culture of care for all nurses.

needed for change. The fourth component, "validation of services by the client," requires engagement by the mature nurse in the process of change. The last part, "expertise of the interdisciplinary team," includes the expertise in problem solving demonstrated by the nursing profession and other significant disciplines.

Caring for nurses and other providers in the community involves creating a culture of caring that begins with securing institutional support. In fact, in the community, this effort requires a network of institutions that see developing and maintaining a culture of care as a priority. It should be followed on a multi-facility level by steps directed at exploring role redesign, attention to the aesthetic environment of work, and the stabilization of a workforce of nurses viewed as potential experts in community-based care. The creation and protection of a culture of caring would necessarily depend on the efforts to foster an ongoing relationship between nurses and the organizations for which they work. **FIGURE 7-8** provides a visual representation of a solution to the challenge of creating and protecting a culture of caring in the community.

The most critical component in providing a solution to the challenge of creating and protecting a culture of caring in the community is institutional support. In a network of institutional support, the employing organization needs to address issues related to the nursing skill set, aesthetics and quality of the work environment, human resources practices, collegial support, and the vision and actions of the nurse-executive team (**FIGURE 7-9**). Institutional support is evident when funds are provided for changing the material and human resources necessary to support the work of CHNs working in the community.

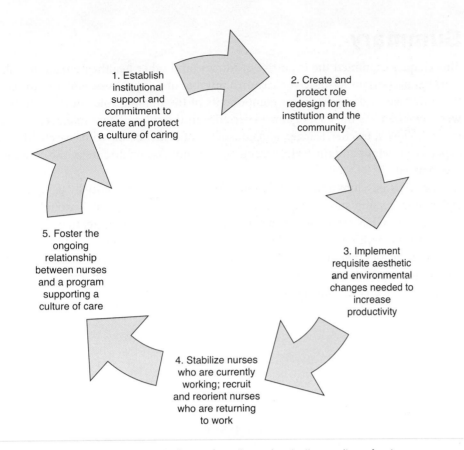

Figure 7-8 Exploring a solution to the challenge of creating and protecting a culture of caring.

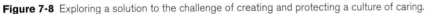

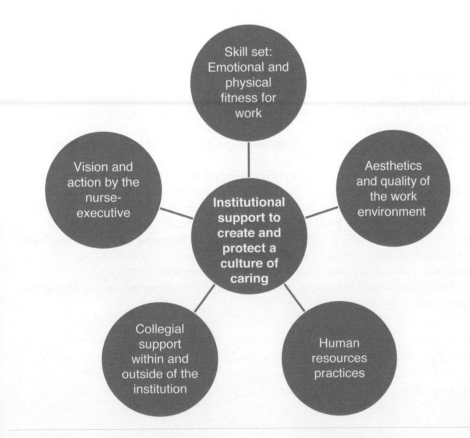

Figure 7-9 Institutional support to create and protect a culture of caring for all nurses.

Summary

This chapter examined the expertise of nurses (and other healthcare team members) working in community-based care from a number of perspectives. Notably, the cognitive, affective, and psychomotor components of the nursing roles in the community were reviewed. As the CHN gains experience in the roles of care manager/advocate, leader/follower, teacher/learner, and consumer of evidence-based research, his or her expertise develops and the CHN's influence on compassionate care in the community is enhanced.

The CHN develops a therapeutic relationship in the community by using the principles of leadership and management, team building, and referral. Through these approaches, the CHN can enter into a partnership with the community to improve health and wellness of the community. Another aspect of nursing in the community relates to nurses caring for other nurses, so that competent care can be delivered to the community on an ongoing basis. Ideally, CHNs will assist older, more mature nurses in the community practice safely and effectively, by creating and maintaining a culture of caring.

REFERENCES

American Nurses Association. (2010a). *Nursing: Scope and standards of practice* (2nd ed.). Silver Spring, MD: Author.

American Nurses Association. (2010b). *Nursing's social policy statement: The essence of the profession.* Silver Spring, MD: Author.

Aycock, N., & Boyle, D. (2009). Interventions to manage compassion fatigue in oncology nursing. *Clinical Journal of Oncology Nursing, 13*(2), 183–191.

Benner, P. (1982). From novice to expert. *American Journal of Nursing, 82*(3), 402–407.

Benner, P. (2001). *From novice to expert: Excellence and power in clinical nursing practice.* Upper Saddle River, NJ: Prentice-Hall.

Buddha. (n.d.). BrainyQuote.com. Retrieved from http://www.brainyquote.com/quotes/quotes/b/buddha133535.html

Bush, N. J. (2009). Compassion fatigue: Are you at risk? *Oncology Nursing Forum, 36*(1), 24–28.

DecisionHealth. (2011). *OASIS-C resource guide.* Retrieved from http://www.decisionhealth.com/oasisresourcestraining/guide.html

Fowler, M. D. (Ed.). (2010). *Guide to the code of ethics for nurses: Interpretation and application.* Silver Spring, MD: American Nurses Association.

Holzemer, S. P. (2010). Creating a culture of care for the maturing nurse. In M. Klainberg & K. M. Dirschel (Eds.), *Today's nursing leader* (pp. 277–290). Sudbury, MA: Jones and Bartlett.

Hughes, R. G. (2008). *Patient safety and quality: An evidence-based handbook for nurses.* AHRQ Publication No. 08-0043. Rockville, MD: Agency for Healthcare Research and Quality.

Porter-O'Grady, T., & Malloch, K. (2011). *Quantum leadership: Advancing innovation, transforming health care* (3rd ed.). Sudbury, MA: Jones & Bartlett Learning.

Schantz, M. L. (2007). Compassion: A concept analysis. *Nursing Forum, 42*(2), 48–55.

van der Cingel, M. (2009). Compassion and professional care: Exploring the domain. *Nursing Philosophy, 10,* 124–136.

ADDITIONAL RESOURCES

Baumann, S. L. (2010). The limitations of evidence-based practice. *Nursing Science Quarterly, 23*(3), 226–230.

Hudacek, S. S. (2008). Dimensions of caring: A qualitative analysis of nurses' stories. *Journal of Nursing Education, 47*(3), 124–129.

Pacquiao, D. F. (2008). Nursing care of vulnerable populations using a framework of cultural competence, social justice and human rights. *Contemporary Nurse, 28*, 189–197.

Running, A., Woodward, L., & Girard, D. (2008). Ritual: The final expression of care. *International Journal of Nursing Practice, 14*, 303–307.

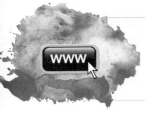

For a full suite of assignments and additional learning activities, use the access code located in the front of your book to visit the exclusive website: http://go.jblearning.com/Holzemer/. If you do not have an access code, you can obtain one at the site.

LEARNING ACTIVITIES

1. The most important concept in providing support to the older (mature) CHN is reflected in which of the following statements?

   A. Increased skill assessments to ensure safety in the mature nurse

   B. Decreased work expectations and regulation of the practice for all nurses

   C. Creation of an environment for caring for all nurses working in the community

   D. Implementation of programs to move mature nurses into management positions

2. Which of the following statements reflects a CHN working with compassion?

   A. The CHN takes steps to move beyond basic expectations to be present to families experiencing distress.

   B. The CHN delegates tasks to family members that they feel comfortable completing on their own or with others.

   C. The CHN divides the time spent with each family in a case load equally.

   D. The CHN allows the client to identify care goals independently.

3. A newly employed CHN is assigned to a nurse mentor as part of the orientation process. The primary reason for a CHN to work with a mentor is represented by which of the following statements?

   A. A mentor assesses the CHN's readiness to learn more complex tasks.

   B. A mentor evaluates the CHN's ability to complete basic skills.

   C. A mentor shares responsibility for actions if the CHN makes a clinical error.

   D. A mentor guides the CHN in developing his or her roles in providing comprehensive care.

4. Which of the following statements is true about the leader/follower role of the CHN?

   A. A CHN is a follower while on orientation, then becomes a leader once orientation is complete.

   B. Depending on the situation, the CHN is sometimes a leader, and sometimes a follower.

   C. Some CHNs (like other professionals) are born leaders, or have special leadership traits.

   D. Graduate education is required for the CHN to assume official leadership status.

5. Which of the following behaviors represents the nursing role of "consumer of evidence-based research"?

   A. The CHN devotes primary attention to quantitative methods of inquiry.

   B. The CHN participates as a researcher in using basic research designs.

   C. The CHN is informed of research trends, and maintains openness to how problems can be solved.

   D. The CHN applies the approach presented by senior nurses as they identify "best practices" in clinical situations.

ADDITIONAL QUESTIONS FOR STUDY

Special Interest Groups

Mothers Against Drunk Driving (MADD) and Students Against Destructive Decisions (SADD) are two special interest groups that the CHN may use when making referrals. To make a proper referral, the CHN must know the potential of the organization for serving the public. Answer the following questions about MADD and SADD.

Mothers Against Drunk Driving:
http://www.madd.org

Mission: Stop drunk driving and support the victims of this violent crime.

Students Against Destructive Decisions: http://www.sadd.org

Mission: Provide students with the best prevention tools possible to deal with the issues of underage drinking, other drug use, risky and impaired driving, and other destructive decisions.

1. Examine the scope of MADD and/or SADD as they relate to resolving problems of alcohol and drug use, and the effects of these behaviors on others.

2. Identify the chapter of MAAD and/or SAAD located closest to where you live. Identify the public transportation available to get to these offices or meetings.

3. Identify the role(s) of the professional nurse in working with MAAD and/or SAAD.

Compassion Fatigue

For many CHNs, an antidote for compassion fatigue is becoming involved in nursing and multidisciplinary organizations. The CHN can come together with other nurses for needed support. Review the information on the following organizations and answer the related questions.

American Association of Diabetes Educators (AADE): http://www.diabetes educator.org

The AADE is a multidisciplinary organization representing more than 10,000 healthcare professionals who provide diabetes education and care. Membership is open to all health professionals with an interest in helping people who have diabetes live full and productive lives.

Mission: Driving practice to promote healthy living through self-management of diabetes and related chronic conditions.

Academy of Medical–Surgical Nurses (AMSN): http://www.amsn.org

The AMSN is the only national professional nursing specialty organization dedicated to adult health/medical–surgical nurses.

Mission: Promote excellence in adult health.

American Public Health Association (APHA): http://www.apha.org

The APHA is the oldest and most diverse organization of public health professionals in the world; it has been working to improve public health since 1872.

Mission: Improve the health of the public and achieve equity in health status.

APHA Public Health Nursing Section:
http://www.apha.org/membergroups/
sections/aphasections/phn

The APHA's Public Health Nursing Section advances this specialty through leadership in the development of public health nursing practice and research; it assures consideration of nursing concerns by providing mechanisms for interdisciplinary nursing collaboration in public health policy and program endeavors.

Mission: Enhance the health of population groups through the application of nursing knowledge to the community.

1. Examine the websites for the American Association of Diabetes Educators (AADE), Academy of Medical–Surgical Nurses (AMSN), and American Public Health Association (APHA) Public Health Nursing Section. How would membership in these organizations benefit the nurse working in the community?

2. Find the chapters of AADE, AMSN, and APHA located closest to where you live. Identify the state or regional meetings that these organizations hold for interested nurses to attend.

3. Search the Internet for other nursing organizations that might be helpful for the nurse practicing in the community.

Assessment and Diagnosis of Community-Based Needs

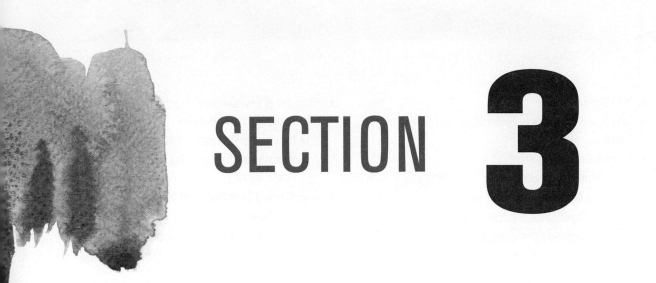

SECTION 3

CHAPTER OUTLINE

▸ Introduction
▸ Validity and Reliability in Epidemiology and Environmental Health
▸ Principles of Epidemiology
  • Calculating Illness Patterns in Populations
  • Data Collection in the Community
  • The Significance of Infant Mortality
▸ Types of Epidemiological Investigations
▸ The Natural History of Disease
  • Agent–Host–Environment Triad
  • Chain of Infection
  • The Visible Tip of the Iceberg
  • Web of Causation
  • Natural History of Disease and Levels of Prevention
▸ Health Information Systems

▸ Principles of Environmental Health: At Home, Work, School, and Houses of Worship
  • Expertise in Occupational Health
  • Educational Changes in the Field of Occupational Health Nursing
▸ Understanding Epidemiological Information
  • Life Expectancy
  • Response to Medical Advances
  • Transmission Categories and Morbidity in AIDS
  • Hospital-Acquired Infections
  • Nonfatal Occupational Injuries and Illnesses
▸ Revisiting Validity and Reliability in Epidemiology and Environmental Health
▸ Summary

OBJECTIVES www

1. Define validity and reliability as they relate to data collection and research in epidemiology and environmental health.

2. Explain the importance of observation in the process of making health care decisions related to patterns of health and illness.

3. Identify the importance of health information technology in the accurate monitoring of health and illness patterns.

4. Search for additional resources to assist in the analysis of patterns of behavior that relate to epidemiology and environmental health.

KEY TERMS www

Agent (in the disease process)

Age-specific death rate

Analytical epidemiology

Common morbidity rate

Crude rate

Descriptive epidemiology

Endemic

Environment (in the disease process)

Environmental health

Epidemic

Epidemiology

Ergonomics

Faith community nursing practice

Host (in the disease process)

Incidence

Infant mortality rate (IMR)

Natural history of disease

Nosocomial

Pandemic

Prevalence

Proportion

Rate

Ratio

Reliability

Validity

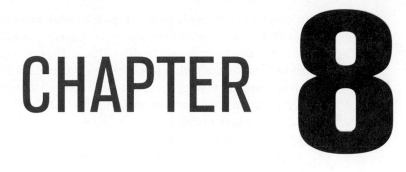

CHAPTER 8

Validity and Reliability in Epidemiology and Environmental Health

Patricia Eckardt

Patricia Facquet

Introduction

This chapter examines the topics of epidemiology and environmental health. The principles that guide epidemiology and environmental health are examined as they relate to the practice of community health nursing. The importance of sound data collection, analysis, and dissemination to healthcare providers is reviewed. Epidemiology is the process of inquiry making sense out of data related to patterns of disease and accidents, on a population level. Environmental health includes the more local patterns of health and disease where people live, work (employment), play (recreation), learn (schools), and pray (houses of worship).

Calculating patterns of illness in populations involves more than calculating total numbers of the sick or injured. Ratios, rates, and proportions are all potential options to present data in meaningful ways. Likewise, incidence rates and prevalence rates offer pictures of changing health and illness by providing related statistics.

Epidemiological investigations are descriptive, analytical, and experimental in nature. These activities will help the community health nurse (CHN) understand the natural history of disease, which may be described via concepts such as the agent–host–environment triad, the chain of infection, the visible tip of the iceberg, and the web of causation. The use of these data to better understand the ideas of primary, secondary, and tertiary prevention is covered later in this text.

Health information systems are important for the collection, analysis, and dissemination of critical health and illness patterns of information. National data systems are in place in the United States, but at times are incompatible with the data systems of other countries. The development of a universal set of data markers that will enable researchers to track illness on a global basis remains in an early stage.

Growing public discomfort with environmental conditions has supported closer monitoring of the environments where people work, play, and go to school, in part because these environments are usually public, shared environments. Where people live and where they pray seem to be connected to less regulation, because they are more private environments.

Validity and Reliability in Epidemiology and Environmental Health

Data provided from epidemiology and environmental health research provide the basis for the CHN to make decisions about who gets care and, among those who may need care, which individuals represent a priority for care. For this reason, the information collected must be valid. **Validity** suggests that the information is accurate and a reflection of reality—that is, the information is sound, unbiased, and well grounded (Polit & Beck, 2012, p. 175). Likewise, the information gathered must be reliable, meaning that repeated measurements agree and support each as being accurate. **Reliability** refers to the accuracy and consistency of information obtained over time (p. 175).

Questions about validity and reliability suggest that if a phenomenon of concern is not showing the patterns of behavior that people expect, or if it is changing in a way that is not understood, additional scientific investigation is necessary. For example, if influenza infection occurs in populations thought to be immunized, or if influenza is suddenly more evident in an unexpected age group, additional study is needed to understand how this virus and its means of transmission are changing in the human population. The principles of epidemiology and environmental health support the collection of data that are valid and reliable. Ongoing reevaluation of data and data collection techniques supports the maintenance of reliability and validity.

Validity: The idea that information is accurate and a reflection of reality—that is, the information is sound, unbiased, and well grounded.

Reliability: The demonstration of accuracy and consistency of information obtained over time—that is, repeated measurements agree and support each as being accurate.

Principles of Epidemiology

Nurses need to be prepared to care for populations within communities. Preparation to care for clients within certain populations involves the study of epidemiology. Epidemiology is concerned with phenomena related to health events in a population. More specifically, **epidemiology** is the measurement of the distribution and determinants of states of health, illness, and accidents in human populations. Much of the work of the epidemiologist is observational. Descriptive, analytical, and experimental trial studies are used as well. The discipline of epidemiology is based on a body of knowledge that includes population statistics and information developed about the natural history of disease, with an emphasis on prevention.

Epidemiology involves sound scientific investigation. Epidemiological investigations, like all statistical investigations, utilize descriptive and analytical methods that draw on statistical techniques for describing data and evaluating hypotheses, biological principles, and (at times) causal theory. Epidemiology consists of both descriptive and analytical (inferential) methodologies. **Descriptive epidemiology** involves characterizing the distribution of health- and disease-related events. **Analytical epidemiology** involves discovering and quantifying associations, testing hypotheses, and attempting to identify causes of health-related states of events (Merrill, 2010). Epidemiology, then, provides information about the type and size of the health problems with which a community must deal (Valanis, 1999).

Epidemiology also provides information that can be used as a predictor in health planning. The inclusion of issues related to wellness (such as those described in *Healthy People 2020*), in conjunction with improved technology for disease control (such as electronic detection and surveillance), has made epidemiology a viable and critical tool for the CHN to use on a daily basis. Using epidemiology in problem solving is similar to using the nursing process. A systematic approach to data collection and analysis is necessary to ensure the validity and reliability of findings. **Table 8-1** compares these methods of inquiry.

Epidemiology: The measurement of the distribution and determinants of states of health, illness, and accidents in human populations.

Descriptive epidemiology: A branch of epidemiology that involves characterizing the distribution of health- and disease-related events.

Analytical epidemiology: A branch of epidemiology that involves discovering and quantifying associations, testing hypotheses, and attempting to identify causes of health-related states of events.

TABLE 8-1
Comparison of the Nursing Process and the Epidemiological Process

Nursing Process	Epidemiological Process
Assessment: Establish database about client; gather related information from client and family; collect objective data	**Assessment:** Establish scope of problem; gather information from reliable sources; collect objective data related to problem (define problem)
Diagnosis: Interpret data; test subjective and objective hypotheses	**Develop hypothesis:** Analyze data
Planning: Develop plan to achieve level of wellness goals (clients included in development of plan)	**Planning:** Develop plan for prevention of condition or event (clients included in development of plan)
Implementation: Initiate plan with clients	**Implementation:** Implement plan with community as client
Evaluation: Determine achievement of goals with client and possibly redesign goals	**Evaluation:** Determine achievement of goals; reassess client; prepare report; conduct further research

Epidemiology combines principles and knowledge generated by the social and biological sciences and applied methodologies for quantitative and qualitative analyses. The transformation of the science of epidemiology has taken several centuries, and it can be viewed as a relatively young science, as is true of all other health-related sciences. The study of diseases and population phenomena is quite old, however. In fact, early descriptions of conditions that affect entire populations related to diseases of infectious nature have been found in writings of the Egyptians, Greeks, and Romans, as well as in many sacred scriptures (Lopez-Moreno, Garrido-Latorre, & Hernandez-Avila, 2000).

Calculating Illness Patterns in Populations

In the United States, census data are gathered about the population by the federal government every 10 years. These data provide information about changes within populations. They include information by age, sex, race, socioeconomic status, housing, and employment. The census data are used to compare trends in states and localities (census tract data). In the past few years, the accuracy of the census data regarding undocumented immigrants and the homeless population has been questioned. Migrant workers, for example, may be members of these populations and so may not be accurately documented.

Data are also gathered from physicians and nurse practitioners in the field, clinics, hospitals, and other institutions. Such data are sent to local health departments, state health departments, and eventually to the Centers for Disease Control and Prevention (CDC). After further analysis, the CDC reports information back to the state and local health departments. An ongoing process of data collection and reporting provides the CHN with the latest information. **FIGURE 8-1** reveals the sources and process for vital statistics collection.

Data Collection in the Community

A very basic way of collecting data is by simply counting the number of affected individuals. However, raw data (or numbers) can be misleading if they are taken at face value. For example, two cases of a disease in a population of 500,000 in a small town outside of Akron, Ohio, may not sound serious; however, if the disease in question is bubonic plague, these two cases are considered an epidemic. Conversely, 5,000 cases of varicella in a New York City community in which there is a large population of children 10 years of age and younger may not be unusual, but may be considered *endemic* (Valanis, 1999).

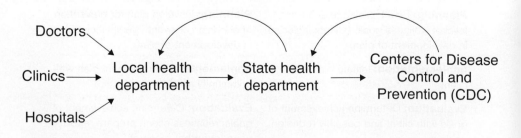

Figure 8-1 Sources and process for vital statistics collection.

Source: Friis, R. H., & Sellers, T. A. (2004). *Epidemiology for public health practice* (3rd ed.). Sudbury, MA: Jones and Bartlett.

Endemic refers to "the habitual presence of disease or infectious agents in a defined geographical area or population" (Valanis, p. 428). Moreover, the same 5,000 cases of varicella might be considered an epidemic on a college campus where there are 12,000 students. **Epidemics** are defined as rates of disease that are at a significantly higher level than the usual frequency (Valanis). The raw data, then, may be of little value. Epidemics are not defined by raw numbers, but rather by rates of disease. A disease epidemic occurs when there are more cases of that disease than normal. A **pandemic** is a worldwide epidemic of a disease (World Health Organization [WHO], 2009).

To quantify and provide an accurate description of health situations, rates and ratios are used by epidemiologists and public health professionals instead of raw number reports. A **rate** is a statistic used for describing an event or occurrence. In epidemiology, a rate is used to make comparisons between populations or between subgroups within populations. It is frequently reported as a fraction, where the numerator is the actual number of occurrences and the denominator is the total population at risk for the occurrence. In epidemiology, the rate is usually converted to a standard base denominator (such as 1,000 or 100,000) to allow for comparisons between groups. **Table 8-2** includes some additional definitions that relate to epidemiological investigation.

Endemic: "The habitual presence of disease or infectious agents in a defined geographical area or population" (Valanis, 1992, p. 428).

Epidemic: A rate of disease that is at a significantly higher level than the usual frequency.

Pandemic: A worldwide epidemic of a disease.

Rate: A statistic used for describing an event or occurrence; in epidemiology, the proportion of persons with a health problem among a population at risk.

TABLE 8-2
Selected Definitions of Epidemiological Terms

Rate: A rate is a measure of some event, disease, or condition in relation to a unit of population, along with some specification of time.

Infant death: An infant death is the death of a live-born child before his or her first birthday. The age at death may be further classified as neonatal or post-neonatal. Neonatal deaths are those that occur before the 28th day of life; post-neonatal deaths are those that occur between 28 and 365 days of age.

Infant mortality rate: The infant mortality rate is based on period files and is calculated by dividing the number of infant deaths during a calendar year by the number of live births reported in the same year. It is expressed as the number of infant deaths per 1,000 live births. The neonatal mortality rate is the number of deaths of children younger than 28 days of age per 1,000 live births. The post-neonatal mortality rate is the number of deaths of children that occur between 28 days and 365 days after birth, per 1,000 live births.

Incidence: Incidence is the number of cases of disease having their onset during a prescribed period of time. It is often expressed as a rate (e.g., the incidence of measles per 1,000 children 5–15 years of age during a specified year). Measuring incidence may be complicated because the population at risk for the disease may change during the period of interest, for example, due to births, deaths, or migration. In addition, determining whether a case is new—that is, whether its onset occurred during the prescribed period of time—may be difficult. Because of these difficulties in measuring incidence, many health statistics are instead measured in terms of prevalence.

Prevalence: Prevalence is the number of cases of a disease, number of infected persons, or number of persons with some other attribute present during a particular interval of time. It is often expressed as a rate (e.g., the prevalence of diabetes per 1,000 persons during a year).

Source: National Center for Health Statistics (NCHS). (2011). *Health, United States, 2010: With special feature on death and dying.* Hyattsville, MD: Author, pp. 503, 504, 520, 527, 528.

When one wants to compare rates of occurrences between groups, a ratio is usually employed, so there is a common reference point, and there is an easily understood magnitude of difference between the two rates. For example, if City A had a severe depression rate (requiring prolonged hospitalization) in an at-risk population of 125 per 120,602 teenagers that could be converted into a standard rate of "per 100,000 at-risk population," the new standardized rate would be 103 per 100,000. If a City B had a severe depression rate (requiring prolonged hospitalization) in an at-risk population of 492 per 194,301 teenagers, that rate could also be converted into a standard rate of "per 100,000 at-risk population," and City B's new standardized rate would be 253 per 100,000. Reporting these two occurrences with a standard denominator permits some standard quantification.

To further simplify any comparisons between the two cities in regard to these rates, ratios are constructed. This is accomplished by first reducing the number of occurrences of the lower incidence rate to the number 1, and then reducing the higher occurrence rate using the same scale (Smith & Maurer, 2000). Using the severe depression rates among teenagers in City A and City B reported previously, the ratio of these two rates would become approximately 1:2.5, meaning City B has roughly two and a half times the incidence of teenage severe depression than City A. This ratio is arrived at by setting up a simple cross-multiplication of $103/253 = 1/x$; dividing 253 by 103, the result is 2.4563, which can be expressed as a ratio of approximately 1:2.5. Approximately the same results can be arrived at by simply comparing the numerators in the reported rates of 103 and 253; the second number is roughly two and a half times larger than the first.

Accordingly, ratios, proportions, and rates are used in epidemiology to provide a more accurate description of health situations. A **ratio** is the relationship between two numbers expressed as a fraction; the value is obtained by dividing the numerator of the fraction by the denominator. A **proportion** is a specific type of ratio in which the numerator is included in the denominator, and the resultant value is expressed as a percentage (Valanis, 1999). A *rate* is a special form of a proportion that includes a specification of time. It is a statistical measure that can be used to measure and compare the health status in a community. A rate is the proportion of persons with a health problem among a population at risk. The total number of persons in this group serves as the denominator in the proportion; the numerator includes all of the events that are being measured. Rates are used to measure many things, including mortality and morbidity rates.

$$\text{Rate} = \frac{\begin{array}{c}\text{Number of conditions or events that}\\ \text{occur in a specific period of time}\end{array}}{\begin{array}{c}\text{Population at risk during}\\ \text{the same time period}\end{array}} \times \text{base multiple of 10}$$

Common morbidity rates measure the incidence and prevalence of disease risk among populations. **Crude rates** measure the entire population in a designated geographic area in relationship to a condition that is being investigated (Harkness, 1995).

$$\text{Crude death rate} = \frac{\text{Number of deaths in 1 year}}{\text{Average (midyear) population}} \times \text{per 100,000 population}$$

An **incidence** rate measures the number of new cases identified in a measure of time.

Ratio: The relationship between two numbers expressed as a fraction; the value is obtained by dividing the numerator of the fraction by the denominator.

Proportion: A specific type of ratio in which the numerator is included in the denominator, and the resultant value is expressed as a percentage.

Common morbidity rate: A measure of the incidence and prevalence of disease risk among populations.

Crude rate: A measure of the entire population in a designated geographic area in relationship to a condition that is being investigated.

Incidence: The number of new cases identified in a measure of time.

$$\text{Incidence rate} = \frac{\text{Number of new conditions or events that occur in a specific period of time}}{\text{Population at risk during the same period (usually midyear)}} \times \text{base multiple of 10}$$

A **prevalence** rate measures the existing number of cases in a population at a given time or over time.

$$\text{Prevalence rate} = \frac{\text{Number of existing conditions or events occuring within a specific period of time}}{\text{Population at risk during the same time period}} \times \text{base multiple of 10}$$

The **age-specific death rate** is another rate used to index health.

$$\text{Age-specific death rate} = \frac{\text{Number of deaths among persons in a given age group in 1 year}}{\text{Average (midyear) population in a specified age group}} \times \text{per 100,000 population}$$

Prevalence: The existing number of cases in a population at a given time or over time.

Age-specific death rate: The number of people in a defined age group who die each year (or during some other period of time).

Infant mortality rate (IMR): The number of children younger than one year of age who die each year; a statistic used to measure the health of a community or nation.

The Significance of Infant Mortality

The **infant mortality rate (IMR)** is used to measure the health of a community or nation. An infant's mortality can be affected by many external factors. In developing countries, these external factors can include substandard health services and inadequate access to health care, poor water quality, inadequate food sources, and an increased level of infectious disease—in particular, malaria—that contribute to a high IMR. This is the reason why the IMR is considered a good indicator of the overall health of a nation or community.

$$\text{Infant mortality rate} = \frac{\text{Number of deaths in children under 1 year of age during 1 year}}{\text{Number of live births in same year}} \times 1000$$

The worldwide average of IMR is currently about 40 per 1,000 live births (UNICEF, 2012). Health disparities among racial and ethnic groups—in particular, among African Americans in the United States—account for the U.S. ranking of 177th in the world based on IMR; the 2011 IMR was estimated at 6.06 per 1,000 live births in the United States (Central Intelligence Agency [CIA], 2011). This high rate of infant mortality in racial and ethnic groups in the United States is directly related to the high premature birth rate among these subpopulations. In 2010, the March of Dimes indicated that the problem of prematurity had continued to increase since 1981, rising 30% over a 30-year period. More than 543,000 babies (1 in 8) are born prematurely in the United States each year; their care costs 10 times more than the care of healthy babies, totaling as much as $26 billion per year (March of Dimes Foundation, 2012). **Table 8-3** lists the infant

TABLE 8-3
Estimates of Worldwide Highest and Lowest Infant Mortality Rates, 2011, in Rank Order

Rank	Country	Infant Mortality Rate (Deaths/1,000 Live Births), 2011 Estimates
1	Angola	175.90
2	Afghanistan	149.20
3	Niger	112.22
4	Mali	111.35
5	Somalia	105.56
219	Japan	2.78
220	Sweden	2.74
221	Bermuda	2.47
222	Singapore	2.32
223	Monaco	1.79

Source: Central Intelligence Agency (CIA). (2011). *The world factbook 2011.* Retrieved from https://www.cia.gov/library/publications/the-world-factbook/rankorder/2091rank.html#

mortality rate rankings for the countries with the highest and lowest rates. **Table 8-4** documents the causes of infant mortality in the United States for the year 2005.

Types of Epidemiological Investigations

There are three main types of epidemiological investigations: descriptive, analytical, and experimental. These types of investigations use different methodologies and have different purposes for public health. Descriptive investigation is the study of the amount and distribution of disease within a population; analytical investigation attempts to determine why disease is occurring; and experimental investigation tests a hypothesis about a disease or disease treatment in a group of people.

The focus of nurses entering community health practice is to grasp the basics of descriptive epidemiological investigations. The aim of these investigations is to better understand the illness phenomenon. Once it is better understood, information about illness or accidents can be used to identify realistic client health goals to cope with health problems. Understanding of the scope of illness and accidents can be used to develop ways of preventing them. A descriptive epidemiologic study includes an investigation carried out to collect information. Some of the data may be collected by the CHN, while other pieces of information may be collected by a variety of other professionals working for a variety of agencies.

TABLE 8-4
Causes of Infant Mortality in the United States, 2005

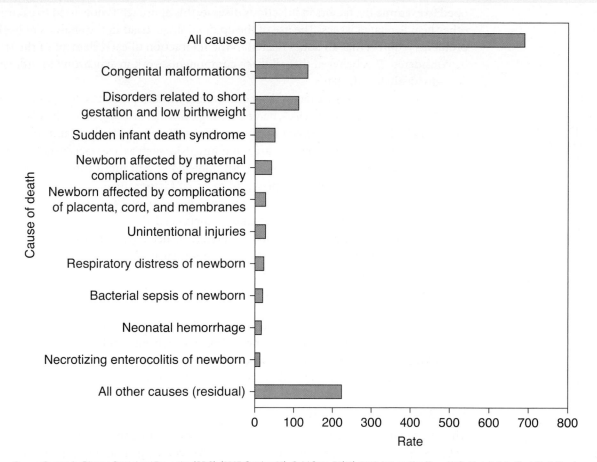

Source: Centers for Disease Control and Prevention (CDC). (2007, October 26). *QuickStats, 56*(42), 1115, in turn citing Kung, H. C., Hoyert, D. L., Xu, J. Q., & Murphy, S. E. (2007). MMWR Quick Stats deaths: Preliminary data for 2005 health E-stats. *Morbidity and Mortality Weekly Report, 56*(42), 1115. Retrieved from http://www.cdc.gov/nchs/data/hestat/prelimdeaths05/preliminarydeaths05_tables.pdf#A

The Natural History of Disease

The goal of public health practice is to provide prevention at every phase of a disease process. Therefore, in addition to looking at prevention as a process that occurs before the onset of disease, CHNs work toward prevention in the phases during and after the onset of the disease process. Various models have been developed to better understand the development of disease; a few of these models are discussed here. To achieve the goal of ensuring prevention at every stage of the disease process, the natural history of disease needs to be understood by the public health nurse, and proper patient education and prevention must occur. The **natural history of disease** is the process by which disease occurs and progresses in humans, involving the interaction of (at least) three different factors: host, agent, and environment.

Natural history of disease:
The process by which disease occurs and progresses in humans, involving the interaction of (at least) three different factors: host, agent, and environment.

Agent (in the disease process): A causative factor that contributes to health problems; it may be chemical, physical, biological, or a deficiency.

Host (in the disease process): A susceptible human (or animal) who harbors and supports a disease-causing agent.

Environment (in the disease process): All external factors surrounding the host that might influence resistance to disease or injury, including biologic, physical, social, cultural, technological, educational, political, legal, demographic, sociological, and economic factors.

Agent–Host–Environment Triad

The notion of the impact of the interaction of the epidemiologic triad—the agent, host, and environment—originated in the work of Leavell and Clark in 1965. Originally developed to examine the factors in infectious disease, this approach is now used to examine other health-related issues. The use of the epidemiologic triad in the analysis of health problems requires that all issues related to the interaction of each element of the triad be considered. It is believed that all three components work in synchrony to influence an individual's health status.

The **agent** is a causative factor that contributes to health problems. It may be chemical, physical, biological (e.g., virus, bacteria, fungi, worms, insects), or a deficiency (e.g., nutritional). The **host** is a susceptible human (or animal) who harbors and supports a disease-causing agent. Host factors are often intrinsic, such as age, race, genetic make-up, lifestyle, exercise level, nutrition, health knowledge, and motivation for achieving wellness. The **environment** comprises all external factors surrounding the host that might influence resistance to disease or injury. Environmental factors include biologic aspects of the environment (e.g., plants and animals needed for food, pathogenic micro-organisms), physical aspects of the environment (e.g., heat, light, atmospheric pressure, radiation, air, water), and social, cultural, technological, educational, political, legal, demographic, sociological, and economic factors.

Changes in one or more of these three variables may allow illness to become manifest. **FIGURE 8-2** represents an intact relationship between the variables, where health status is intact. Changes may occur on any of the three planes of the triangle to maintain health. For example, one can change the pathogen's environment through refrigeration or cooking; hosts can be protected through vaccines or education. These strategies can help prevent diseases from spreading throughout a population.

Chain of Infection

The chain of infection (**FIGURE 8-3**) is a model that describes the infectious process. All of the elements must be present for an infection to occur. If just one element in the chain is broken, then the host cannot become infected. This linkage provides opportunities for intervention and education for the CHN when assisting populations and individuals with disease prevention. For example, proper hand washing can eliminate a mode of transmission, and covering one's mouth when one coughs can eliminate a portal of exit.

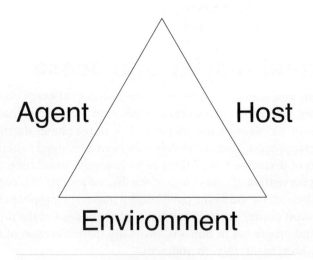

Figure 8-2 The epidemiological triangle.

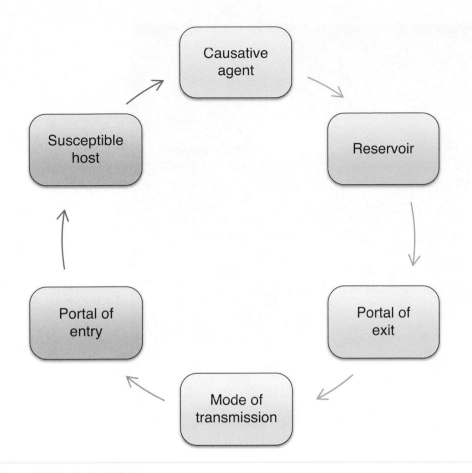

Figure 8-3 The chain of infection.

The Visible Tip of the Iceberg

The iceberg is used as a graphic illustration of colonization versus infection, as it relates to illness. Those patients who are infected with an organism represent just the "tip of the iceberg" of all patients who are colonized or infected (**FIGURE 8-4**). Just because a client is not infected, or showing signs of infection, does not mean that the individual does not carry organisms that could be transferred to another client if proper hand hygiene and other infection control precautions are not taken (Lopez-Moreno et al., 2000).

Web of Causation

Comorbidities do exist, such that some infectious and noninfectious conditions are caused by most of the occurrences at the "right" time, with the right set of circumstances. Two examples are described here: one for infections/communicable disease and the other for a chronic disease heart disease.

The web of causation is extremely helpful in analyzing the origins of an infection or circumstances that have led to a disease's process. The spread of the infectious disease malaria (**FIGURE 8-5**), for example, occurs from multiple causes. An infected human must be bitten by the mosquito, and in turn that mosquito must transmit the multiplying malaria protozoa organisms successfully to the susceptible host, who will develop malaria. Many measures have been put in place to decrease the risk of contracting malaria, such as mosquito netting, draining

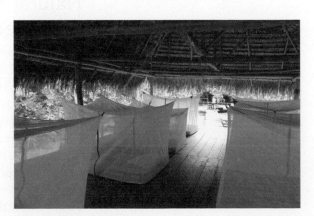

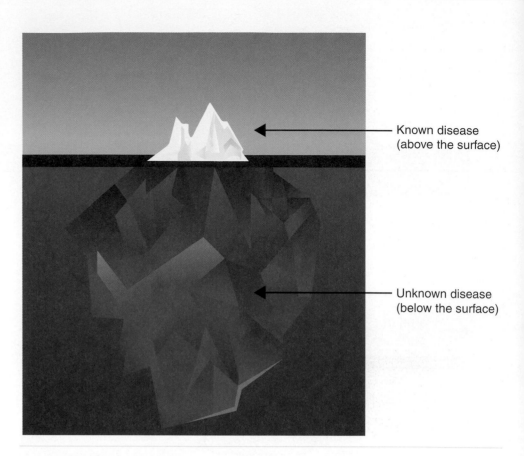

Known disease (above the surface)

Unknown disease (below the surface)

Figure 8-4 The infection iceberg.

standing water, and use of insecticide spray and lotions. In addition, several prophylactic medications can be given to persons who plan to travel into a region where the malaria prevalence is known to be high. Currently, there is no vaccine to prevent malaria, however, and some strains are becoming resistant to the oral antimalaria medications.

In the second example of the web of causation of illness, multiple factors can be seen to relate to infant mortality (**FIGURE 8-6**). In this case, a number of related and seemingly unrelated factors may be critical to the death of infants. A change in various aspects of the interconnected web may change the dynamics of infant mortality, thereby enabling more infants to survive.

Natural History of Disease and Levels of Prevention

The natural history of disease is the basis for intervention. The three levels upon which this prevention is based are aptly named: primary, secondary, and tertiary. Primary prevention aims to prevent the disease from occurring. Secondary prevention is used after the disease has occurred, but often before the person notices that anything is wrong; the goal of this level of prevention is to find the disease early, and treat the disease promptly. Tertiary prevention targets the person who already has the disease, and is related to a rehabilitative stage of recovery (Leavell & Clark, 1965). **Table 8-5** shows the relationship between the progression of an illness and the levels of prevention. Further discussion of the levels of prevention is provided later in this text, using clinical examples that demonstrate how the natural history of disease can be altered.

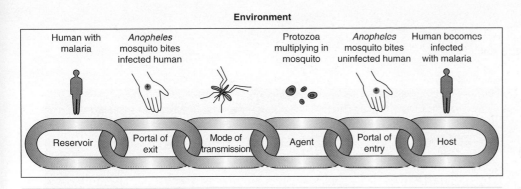

Figure 8-5 Multiple causes of malaria infection.

Source: Adapted from Dever, G. E. (1976). An epidemiological model for health policy analysis. *Social Indicators Research, 2,* 453–466.

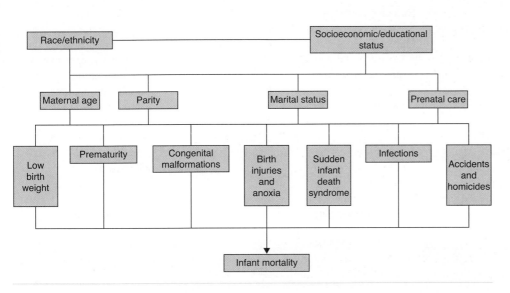

Figure 8-6 Dever's epidemiological model: the web of causation for infant mortality.

Source: Adapted from Dever, G. E. (1976). An epidemiological model for health policy analysis. *Social Indicators Research, 2,* 453–466.

TABLE 8-5
The Natural History of Any Disease in Humans

Interrelations of Agent, Host, and Environmental Factors → Production of Stimulus →		→ Reaction of the Host to the Stimulus → Early → Discernible → Advanced → Convalescence → Pathogenesis Early Lesions Disease		
Prepathogenesis Period		**Period of Pathogenesis**		
Health Promotion	**Specific Protection**	**Early Diagnosis and Prompt Treatment**	**Disability Limitation**	**Rehabilitation**
Health education Good standard of nutrition adjusted to developmental phases of life Attention to personality development Provision of adequate housing, recreation, and agreeable working conditions Marriage counseling and sex education Genetics Periodic selective examinations	Use of specific immunizations Attention to personal hygiene Use of environmental sanitation Protection against occupational hazards Protection from accidents Use of specific nutrients Protection from carcinogens Avoidance of allergens	Case-finding measures, individual and mass Screening surveys Selective examinations Objectives: • To cure and prevent disease processes • To prevent the spread of communicable diseases • To prevent complications and sequelae • To shorten the period of disability	Adequate treatment to arrest the disease process and to prevent further complications and sequelae Provision of facilities to limit disability and to prevent death	Provision of hospital and community facilities for retraining and education for maximum use of remaining capacities Education of the public and industry to utilize the rehabilitated As full employment as possible Selective placement Work therapy in hospitals Use of sheltered colony
Primary Prevention		**Secondary Prevention**		**Tertiary Prevention**
Levels of Application of Preventive Measures				

Source: Adapted from Leavell, H. R., & Clark, E. (1965). *Preventive medicine for the doctor in his community.* New York, NY: McGraw-Hill.

Health Information Systems

The National Electronic Telecommunications System for Surveillance (NETSS) is used by local, county, and state departments of health in the surveillance and reporting of notifiable conditions. This computerized public health data system collects data on notifiable diseases and conditions for the CDC on a weekly basis.

The 8-City Enhanced Terrorism Surveillance Project is a CDC "initiative focused on strengthening key components of traditional public health surveillance in major metropolitan areas" (CDC, 2011, p. 1). Its main focus is ensuring early detection of a terrorist event and maintaining clear lines of communication for urgent disease reporting of outbreaks, terroristic threats, or public health emergencies with the ability to pass the information and consult with leading public health authorities on a 24/7 basis (CDC, 2011).

The National Vital Statistics System (NVSS) at the CDC is the most successful example of intergovernmental data sharing in public health. The National Center for Health Statistics (NCHS) collects and dis-

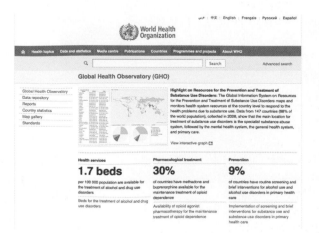

seminates the United States' official vital statistics. The various jurisdictions are legally responsible for collecting the data and registering the life events (e.g., births, deaths, marriages, divorces, and fetal deaths) in the NCHS database.

International vital records are governed by two systems. Most developed countries have a system similar to that used in the United States. Statistical measures as well as principles of registration are similar throughout the world. The World Health Organization and the United Nations in the twentieth century made attempts to standardize vital statistical data collection to evaluate population growth, disease processes, and global health. The Global Health Observatory (GHO) is the WHO's "main record depository making available such data as mortality, the global and regional burden of disease, infectious diseases, risk factors, and health expenditures" (WHO, 2011).

The WHO Statistical Information System (WHOSIS) is a component now incorporated within the GHO. "WHOSIS is an international database containing more than 70 health statistics for 193 World Health Organization member states. Topics include, but are not limited to: perinatal statistics, life expectancy, education, and immunizations" (Harvard School of Public Health, 2009).

Principles of Environmental Health: At Home, Work, School, and Houses of Worship

Environmental health is defined as the freedom from illness or injury related to exposure to toxic agents and other environmental conditions that are potentially detrimental to human health (Institute of Medicine [IOM], 1995). The nursing process regarding environmental health includes all the steps in the nursing process. The environmental health history for the individual has implications for others. If an individual is exposed to a substance at work or home, everyone who enters that workplace or dwelling is potentially exposed to the same substance. Individuals can also carry toxins from one setting to another on clothing, belongings, or themselves. For example, there are documented cases of children who were poisoned by parents who carried lead dust home on their work clothes (Khan, Qayyum, Saleem, Ansari, & Khan, 2010).

More than one-fourth of the global disease burden is attributable to environmental exposures. Given this fact, assessing an individual's environmental exposures is critical in community nursing practice (Barnes, Fisher, Postma, Harnish, Butterfield, & Hill, 2010). Assessment of the environmental health history for the individual also includes the assessment of his or her occupational health history. In addition, it entails an environmental assessment of the home, school, workplace and community of the individual. The nursing plan includes environmental health education for the individual, as well as for families and communities. The education plan should include referral sources for information and further assessment and treatment within the community if indicated, as well as advocacy regarding environmental health safety.

Environmental assessments provide an opportunity for discussion about environmental risk-reduction education and prevention strategies. The implementation of the plan is followed by evaluation of whether the exposure has continued to be avoided or whether prior exposure has subsequently been reduced (Paranzino, Butterfield, Nastoff, & Ranger, 2005). The International Council of Nurses (ICN) describes nurses' environmental and policy-making roles within two policy statements (ICN, 2008, 2011). According to the ICN, nurses should contribute to public policy pertaining to the determinants of health. Included in the nurse's environmental role is patient education on the impact of environmental pollution

Environmental health: The freedom from illness or injury related to exposure to toxic agents and other environmental conditions that are potentially detrimental to human health.

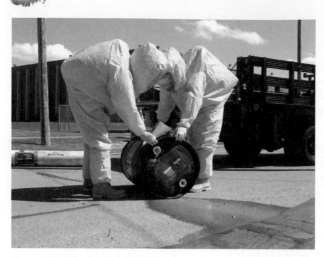

Courtesy of Staff Sgt. Brandie Session/U.S. Air Force.

and the development of coalitions with other professions to lobby for safe waste disposal (Carnegie & Kiger, (2010).

Environmental health threats can be chemical, physical, biological, nuclear, or radioactive. Examples of environmental toxins include pesticides (chemical), industrial waste or by-products (chemical), fire (physical), explosions (physical), injuries from environmental hazards (physical), microbes (biological), poisonous plants or mold spores (biological), and oncological treatments such as implants and seeds (nuclear/radioactive).

Expertise in Occupational Health

In response to the need for nursing expertise in the field of environmental health, the Institute of Medicine, Agency for Toxic Substances and Disease Registry, and National Institute of Nursing Research have designed core competencies for the nursing profession. The IOM competencies focus on four areas: (1) knowledge and concepts; (2) assessment and referral; (3) advocacy, ethics, and risk communication; and (4) legislation and regulation. These competencies establish a baseline of knowledge and awareness necessary for nurses to prevent and minimize health problems associated with exposure to environmental agents (Larsson & Butterfield, 2002).

The American Public Health Association developed environmental health principles for public health nurses in 2006 to standardize practice within the community. These principles, which are found in **Table 8-6**, guide the community health nurse in keeping the workplace, home, school, and house of worship environments safe.

TABLE 8-6
Environmental Health Principles for Public Health Nursing

1. Safe and sustainable environments are essential conditions for the public's health.

2. Environmental health is integral to the role and responsibilities of all public health nurses.

3. All public health nurses should possess environmental health knowledge and skills.

4. Environmental health decisions should be grounded in sound science.

5. The precautionary principle is a fundamental tenet for all environmental health endeavors.

6. Environmental justice is a right of all populations.

7. Public awareness and community involvement are essential in environmental health decision making.

8. Communities have a right to relevant and timely information for decisions on environmental health.

9. Environmental health approaches should respect diverse values, beliefs, cultures, and circumstances.

10. Collaboration is essential to effectively protecting the health of all people from environmental harm.

11. Environmental health advocacy must be rooted in scientific integrity, honesty, respect for all persons, and social justice.

12. Environmental health research addressing the effectiveness and public health impact of nursing interventions should be conducted and disseminated.

Source: American Public Health Association (APHA). (2006). *Environmental health principles and recommendations for public health nursing.* Retrieved from http://www .apha.org/NR/rdonlyres/B4891A3C-F317-468F-8D02-508B82FA729C/0/EHPrinciplesandRecommendationsPHNSection.doc

Educational Changes in the Field of Occupational Health Nursing

Nursing has responded to the new emphasis on environmental health with education of nurses and communities that they serve, inclusion in international policy-making processes, interventions and research regarding environmental health, and the development of environmental health principles for public health nurses. Nurses are increasingly the primary contacts for clients who are concerned about health problems related to their environment. The most recent area of environmental concern is the environment in which people worship. In nursing, the field is referred to as faith community nursing.

Recognized by the American Nurses Association as **faith community nursing practice**, the mission of faith-based, parish, or congregational nursing is "the intentional integration of the practice of faith with the practice of nursing so that people can achieve wholeness in, with, and through the community of faith in which parish nurses work. The focus [of faith community nursing] is on the health and healing needs of the members of a particular faith community and its extended community" (American Nurses Association, 2005, p. 1; Interfaith Health & Wellness Association, 2000).

Both formal and professional development nursing education have been modified to provide nurses working with employee populations with the knowledge base needed to prevent and manage illness and injury and wellness. Nurses who have the appropriate education and experience working within these settings can become certified occupational health nurses (COHN). Achieving such certification requires knowledge of injury prevention; biological, chemical, and physical hazards; disease management; and regulations such as those pertaining to worker's compensation.

In addition to national certification as a COHN, the American Association for Occupational Health Nurses (AAOHN—the professional organization for occupational health nurses) provides a refresher course on occupational health basics. This type of education provides a service to any employee health nurses or occupational health nurses who want to expand their knowledge base regarding injury and illness prevention and management within the worker populations whom they serve ("Use This Checklist," 2008). The National Institute for Occupational Safety and Health (NIOSH) also provides training in the core areas of occupational health nursing at Education and Resource Centers (ERCs) located within universities across the United States (NIOSH, 2011).

Graduate-level occupational health nursing curricula include coursework in toxicology, epidemiology, hazard recognition and control, injury control, safety, the psychosocial covariates with work and health, occupational injury and illness management, and **ergonomics** (the study of body mechanics and movement), in addition to coursework preparing for an advanced practice role (Burgel, 2000). The increasing preparation of nurses to practice in occupational health settings supports better population outcomes in injury prevention and treatment.

Faith community nursing practice: Faith-based, parish, or congregational nursing directed toward "the intentional integration of the practice of faith with the practice of nursing so that people can achieve wholeness in, with, and through the community of faith in which parish nurses work" (American Nurses Association, 2005, p. 1).

Ergonomics: The study of body mechanics and movement.

Understanding Epidemiological Information

The collection of vast and diverse amounts of information is done with the goal of using the information to better prevent disease and accidents in the population. Patterns of data, collected over various periods of time, help the CHN better understand the present condition of a particular population. Comparing past and current data allows the CHN to better understand current therapies, identify resurgent and new problems, and prioritize health-related concerns. A few types of data trends are presented in this section as examples; they include concerns such as life expectancy, response to treatments, changes in how disease is transmitted, and improvements in health status.

Life Expectancy

One concern for most Americans relates to life expectancy. Life expectancy data for men and women between the years of 1900 and 2003 are presented in **Table 8-7**. Analysis of such data over time reveals interesting patterns. For example, life expectancy improved for both men and women over the twentieth century. Women also demonstrate a pattern of living longer than men.

Worldwide, the life expectancy of an individual depends greatly on the country and region of the world in which the person lives, as well as that area's public health infrastructure, diet, health care, and social strife (e.g., war, starvation, and diseases such as malaria and AIDS). In certain African countries, life expectancy has been greatly impacted by the devastating effects of AIDS. For example, the life expectancy in three African countries is extremely short related to the high prevalence of human immunodeficiency virus (HIV) infection:

- Botswana: 31.6 years instead of the 70.7 years that would be expected with HIV
- South Africa: 41.5 years instead of 69.9 years
- Zimbabwe: 31.8 years instead of 70.5 years (United Nations, 2003)

Life expectancy data are used in calculating countries' and regions' Human Development Index (HDI), in addition to the standard of living, adult literacy, and education level. The HDI is used to rank countries as developed (high developed), developing

TABLE 8-7
U.S. Life Expectancy at Birth, by Sex, in Selected Years (in Years)

Years	Total	Males	Females
1900–1902	49.2	47.9	50.7
1909–1911	51.5	49.9	53.2
1919–1921	56.4	55.5	57.4
1929–1931	59.2	57.7	60.9
1939–1941	63.6	61.6	65.9
1949–1951	68.1	65.5	71.0
1959–1961	69.9	66.8	73.2
1969–1971	70.8	67.0	74.6
1979–1981	73.9	70.1	77.6
1989–1991	75.4	71.8	78.8
2002	77.3	74.5	79.9
2003	77.5	74.8	80.1

Notes: Later year estimates are more reliable than those of the early 20th century. The federal civil registration system began in 1900 with the setting up of the Death Registration Area (DRA). States were only admitted as qualification standards were met. Only 10 states and the District of Columbia were in the original DRA of 1900. Statistics prior to 1939–1941 are based on data from the DRA states (which increased in number over time). Alaska and Hawaii are first included in 1959–1961 figures. Also note that data for years 1999–2001 are not reported in this data source.

Source: For data through 2002, the Congressional Research Service (CRS) compilations from National Center for Health Statistics (NCHS), United States Life Tables, 2002, *National Vital Statistics Reports*, vol. 53, no. 6, Nov. 10, 2001. For 2003, NCHS, Deaths: Final Data for 2003, *National Vital Statistics Reports*, vol. 54, no. 13, Apr. 19, 2006.

(middle developed), and underdeveloped (low developed) countries. **FIGURE 8-7** indicates the 2010 HDI rankings.

Response to Medical Advances

Epidemiological data can also demonstrate responses to medical advances. Among the most significant of the major medical breakthroughs were the introduction of vaccines for infantile paralysis/poliomyelitis by Dr. Jonas Salk in 1955 (injectable vaccine) and Dr. Albert Sabin in 1957 (oral vaccine) (McKenzie, 2005; Turnock, 2009). **FIGURE 8-8** demonstrates the effectiveness of both polio vaccines.

Transmission Categories and Morbidity in AIDS

Information on disease and how it spreads, who responds to treatment, and who dies from disease is also collected through epidemiology. Data may be disease specific, as in the following examples of AIDS. **FIGURE 8-9** profiles AIDS diagnoses by transmission category, between 1985 and 2008, for adolescents and adults. Patterns of information become clear as to how transmission categories increase and decrease as they relate to percentage of persons with an AIDS diagnosis. **FIGURE 8-10** compares AIDS diagnoses and deaths for adolescents and adults. Trends for these variables can be monitored between the years of 1985 and 2007.

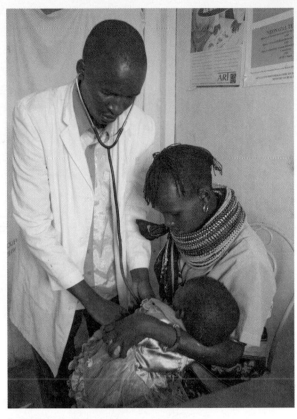

© spirit of america/Shutterstock.com

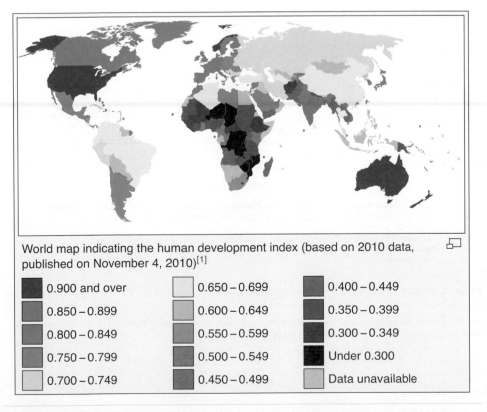

World map indicating the human development index (based on 2010 data, published on November 4, 2010)[1]

0.900 and over	0.650 – 0.699	0.400 – 0.449
0.850 – 0.899	0.600 – 0.649	0.350 – 0.399
0.800 – 0.849	0.550 – 0.599	0.300 – 0.349
0.750 – 0.799	0.500 – 0.549	Under 0.300
0.700 – 0.749	0.450 – 0.499	Data unavailable

Figure 8-7 The Human Development Index.

Source: United Nations. (2010). *UN Development Programme 2010 Human Development Index.* New York, NY: Author. Retrieved from http://hdr.undp.org/en/statistics

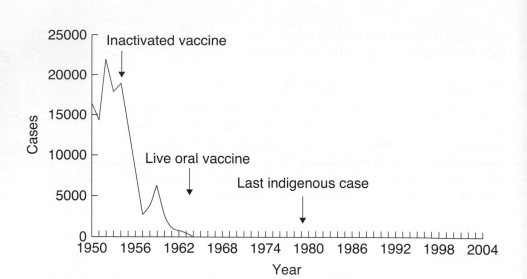

Figure 8-8 Response to poliomyelitis vaccination.

Source: Atkinson, W., Hamborsky, J., McIntyre, L., & Wolfe, S. (Eds.). (2009). Poliomyelitis. In *Epidemiology and prevention of vaccine-preventable diseases (The pink book)* (11th ed., pp. 249–262). Washington, DC: Public Health Foundation.

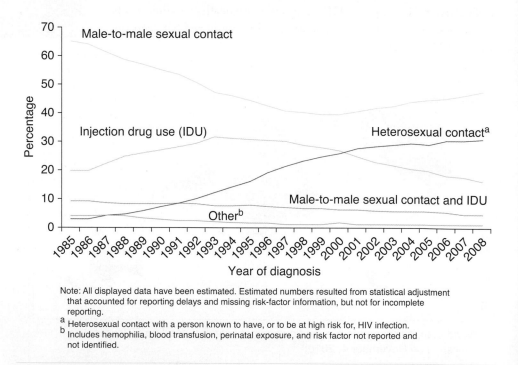

Note: All displayed data have been estimated. Estimated numbers resulted from statistical adjustment
    that accounted for reporting delays and missing risk-factor information, but not for incomplete
    reporting.
a Heterosexual contact with a person known to have, or to be at high risk for, HIV infection.
b Includes hemophilia, blood transfusion, perinatal exposure, and risk factor not reported and
    not identified.

Figure 8-9 AIDS diagnoses among adults and adolescents, by transmission category and year of diagnosis, 1985–2008, United States and dependent areas.

Source: Centers for Disease Control and Prevention (CDC), National Center for Health Statistics (NCHS). (2010). *Health, United States, 2009: With special feature on medical terminology.* Hyattsville, MD: Author.

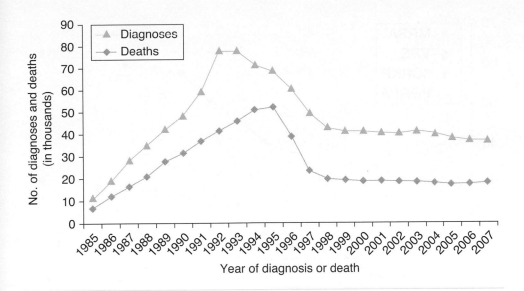

Figure 8-10 AIDS diagnoses and deaths of adults and adolescents with AIDS, 1985–2007, United States and dependent areas.

Source: Centers for Disease Control and Prevention (CDC), National Center for Health Statistics (NCHS). (2010). *Health, United States, 2009: With special feature on medical terminology.* Hyattsville, MD: Author.

The CHN would note that diagnoses of AIDS declined among clients who experienced male-to-male sexual contact to the year 2000, with a slower increase in transmission occurring since that date. AIDS diagnoses among individuals who contracted the disease through injection drug use increased until approximately 1994, then showed a pattern of slow decline. Persons identifying as having both male-to-male sexual contact and injection drug use have experienced little change in their rates of HIV transmission. The largest increase in AIDS diagnoses has occurred among persons who obtain the virus through heterosexual contact. Understanding why these changes have occurred would include understanding the introduction and use of antiviral medications, needle exchange programs, and various safer-sex and possibly sexual abstinence educational programs.

Different data sets provide different information. Figure 8-10, as noted earlier, compares AIDS diagnoses with deaths of adults and adolescents in the United States. Diagnoses peaked in 1992, then demonstrated a steady decline until approximately 1998. Diagnoses leveled off and essentially have not changed since that time. Deaths steadily increased until around 1995, then showed an impressive decline until 1997–1998, with the number of deaths leveling off at approximately 15,000 to 20,000 per year since that time.

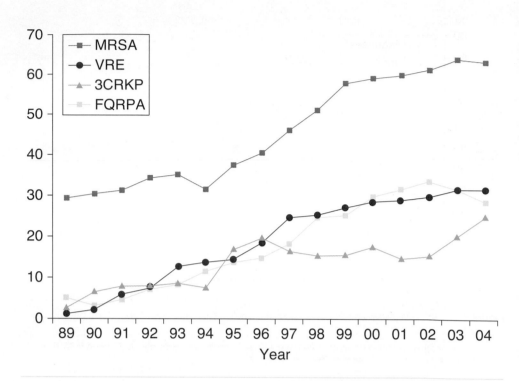

Figure 8-11 The CDC's National Nosocomial Infection Surveillance (NNIS) System, 1989–2004.

Source: Shult, P. A. (2010). MM&I 554: Global emerging and re-emerging infectious disease. University of Wisconsin Course: Infectious Diseases & Bioterrorism.

Nosocomial: Hospital acquired.

Hospital-Acquired Infections

New and emerging problems may also become evident through epidemiological data collection. **FIGURE 8-11** shows the results of monitoring hospital-acquired (**nosocomial**) infections. Such data are useful when comparing how local or regional rates of such infections compare with national trends. As the figure demonstrates, a steady increase in hospital-acquired infections has occurred since data collection began. To fully understand this increase, additional information is necessary related to patterns of hand washing, staffing of units, use and misuse of antibiotics to treat infections, and other possible causes of the spread of infection.

The IOM (1999), in its report *To Err Is Human*, found that 44,000 to 98,000 preventable deaths occur in U.S. hospitals every year and that $17 billion to $29 billion in healthcare dollars is "wasted" because of medical errors. The IOM also discovered that 1.7 million to 2 million nosocomial infections occur annually, resulting in 80,000 to 100,000 deaths each year. Medication errors cause approximately 7,000 deaths per year, and the cost of these errors is estimated at $5 billion to $6 billion per year (IOM, 1999).

Nonfatal Occupational Injuries and Illnesses

Evidence that interventions are working in a population may also be obtained by reviewing data. **FIGURE 8-12** shows a drop in nonfatal occupational injuries and illnesses from 1989 to 2007 in the United States, although the data do not explain why this decline occurred. Once again, additional data are needed to understand the trend of a steady

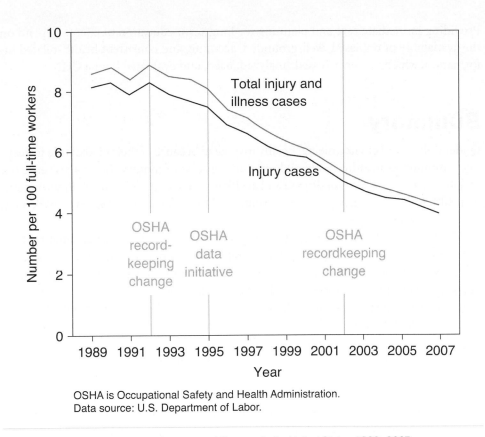

Figure 8-12 Nonfatal occupational injuries and illnesses in the United States, 1989–2007.

Source: Centers for Disease Control and Prevention (CDC), National Center for Health Statistics (NCHS). (2010). *Health, United States, 2009: With special feature on medical terminology.* Hyattsville, MD: Author.

decrease in occupational injuries and illnesses. Occupational injury and illness rates can be affected by many factors, including the "amount and quality of training, employee turnover rates, work experience, extent of mechanization and automation, job-related parameters, and worker gender" (Subramanian, Desia, Prakash, Mital, & Mital, 2006, p. 1). It should be noted that improvements in technology in the workplace as well as employers' and employees' awareness of occupational safety have played a large part in controlling workplace injuries (Subramanian et al.).

Questions that these data raise include the following: Which changes in education have occurred related to injuries and illnesses? Which changes in product safety and management have been occurring, and continue to occur, in the occupational setting? How are occupational injuries and illnesses defined? How have occupational health nursing and industrial hygiene influenced the decline of nonfatal occupational injuries and illness?

Revisiting Validity and Reliability in Epidemiology and Environmental Health

Validity and reliability are key to the work of the CHN in epidemiology and environmental health. The CHN collects information, reporting it according to the relevant protocols, in an attempt to add to the data that reveal patterns of injury and accidents.

Providing immediate care and planning for long-term education of clients depend on the availability of unbiased, well-grounded, accurate, and consistent health-related information, which is then assessed, analyzed, used, and evaluated by the CHN.

Summary

Epidemiology and environmental health are related because of their pivotal role in keeping communities healthy. Epidemiology is the process of inquiry that makes sense out of data related to patterns of disease and accidents, on a population level. Environmental health focuses on local patterns of health and disease where people live, work, play, learn, and pray.

Identifying patterns of illness in populations involves more than calculating total numbers of sick or injured persons. Ratios, rates, and proportions are three methods to present data in meaningful ways. Incidence rates and prevalence rates provide pictures of changing health- and illness-related statistics. The infant mortality rate is both a statistic and a moral statement; the United States has a higher infant mortality rate than many less affluent nations.

Epidemiological investigations may be descriptive, analytical, or experimental in nature. Nurses educated at the baccalaureate level would most likely be involved in descriptive studies, or data collection activities. These activities help the CHN understand the natural history of disease. The natural history of disease may be described through concepts such as the agent–host–environment triad, the chain of infection, the visible tip of the iceberg, and the web of causation.

Health information systems are critical for the collection, analysis, and dissemination of data related to health and illness patterns. National data systems are in place in the United States, but may be missing or incompatible in other countries. A universal set of data markers that would enable epidemiologists to track illness on a global basis is still in early development.

Growing public discomfort with environmental conditions has supported closer monitoring of the environments in which people work, play, and go to school; such environments are usually public and shared. By comparison, less regulation has been directed at the environments in which people live and pray, because they are perceived as more private environments.

Understanding how to use epidemiological information is a critical skill for the CHN. Various types of information may be reviewed by the CHN, including life expectancy, response to treatments, changes in how disease is transmitted, and improvements in health status. Comparing past and current data allows the CHN to better understand current therapies, identify resurgent and new problems, and prioritize health-related concerns.

REFERENCES

American Nurses Association. (2005). *Faith community nursing: Scope and standards of practice.* Silver Springs, MD: Author.

American Public Health Association (APHA). (2006). *Environmental health principles and recommendations for public health nursing.* Retrieved from http://www.apha.org/NR/rdonlyres /B4891A3C-F317-468F-8D02-508B82FA729C/0/EHPrinciplesandRecommendationsPHN Section.doc

Atkinson, W., Hamborsky, J., McIntyre, L., & Wolfe, S. (Eds.). (2009). Poliomyelitis. In *Epidemiology and prevention of vaccine-preventable diseases (The pink book)* (11th ed., pp. 249–262). Washington, DC: Public Health Foundation.

Barnes, G., Fisher, B., Postma, J., Harnish, K., Butterfield, P., & Hill, W. (2010). Incorporating environmental health into nursing practice: A case study on indoor air quality. *Pediatric Nursing, 36*(1), 33–40. Retrieved from Academic Search Complete database.

Burgel, B. J. (2000). OHNs: A valuable resource in workplace safety leadership. *Safety Management, 447*, 1. Retrieved from http://libproxy.adelphi.edu:2048/login?url=http://search.ebscohost.com/login.aspx?direct=true&db=bth&AN=6300056&site=ehost-live&scope=site

Carnegie, E., & Kiger, A. (2010). Developing the community environmental health role of the nurse. *British Journal of Community Nursing, 15*(6), 298–305. Retrieved from CINAHL Plus with Full Text database.

Centers for Disease Control and Prevention (CDC). (2007, October 26). *QuickStats, 56*(42), 1115, in turn citing Kung, H. C., Hoyert, D. L., Xu, J. Q., & Murphy, S. E. (2007). MMWR Quick Stats deaths: Preliminary data for 2005 health E-stats. *Morbidity and Mortality Weekly Report, 56*(42), 1115. Retrieved from http://www.cdc.gov/nchs/data/hestat/prelimdeaths05/preliminary deaths05_tables.pdf#A

Centers for Disease Control and Prevention (CDC). (2010). Summary of notifiable diseases—United States, 2008. *Morbidity & Mortality Weekly Report, 57*(54), 1–100.

Centers for Disease Control and Prevention (CDC). (2011). *Performance criteria for public health disease reporting systems*. Retrieved from http://www.cdc.gov/osels/ph_surveillance/nndss/files/Performance_Criteria_Public_Health_Disease_Reporting_Systems.doc

Centers for Disease Control and Prevention (CDC), National Center for Health Statistics (NCHS). (2010). *Health, United States, 2009: With special feature on medical terminology*. Hyattsville, MD: Author.

Central Intelligence Agency (CIA). (2011). *The world factbook 2011*. Retrieved from https://www.cia.gov/library/publications/the-world-factbook/rankorder/2091rank.html#

Dever, G. E. (1976). An epidemiological model for health policy analysis. *Social Indicators Research, 2*, 453–466.

Friis, R. H., & Sellers, T. A. (2004). *Epidemiology for public health practice* (3rd ed.). Sudbury, MA: Jones and Bartlett.

Harkness, G. A. (1995). *Epidemiology in nursing practice*. St. Louis, MO: C. V. Mosby.

Harvard School of Public Health. (2009). *WHO Statistical Information System (WHOSIS)*. Retrieved from http://dvn.iq.harvard.edu/dvn/dv/dataconnect/faces/study/StudyPage.xhtml?globalId=hdl:1902.1/12516&studyListingIndex=0_a8e0b2421fa032e26e15e7225e8b

Institute of Medicine (IOM). (1995). *Nursing, health and the environment*. Washington, DC: National Academies Press.

Institute of Medicine (IOM). (1999). *To err is human: Building a safer health system*. Washington, DC: National Academies Press.

Interfaith Health & Wellness Association. (2000). *Faith community nursing*. Retrieved from http://www.ihwassoc.org/nursing.html

International Council of Nurses (ICN). (2008). *Participation of nurses in health services decision making and policy development*. Retrieved from http://www.icn.ch/images/stories/documents/publications/position_statements/D04_Participation_Decision_Making_Policy_Development.pdf

International Council of Nurses (ICN). (2011). *Reducing environmental and lifestyle related health risks*. Retrieved from http://www.icn.ch/images/stories/documents/publications/position_statements/E11_Reducing_Environmental_Health_Risks.pdf

Khan, D., Qayyum, S., Saleem, S., Ansari, W., & Khan, F. (2010). Lead exposure and its adverse health effects among occupational workers' children. *Toxicology & Industrial Health, 26*(8), 497–504. doi: 10.1177/0748233710373085

Larsson, L., & Butterfield, P. (2002). Mapping the future of environmental health and nursing: Strategies for integrating national competencies into nursing practice. *Public Health Nursing, 19*(4), 301–308. doi: 10.1046/j.1525-1446.2002.19410.x

Leavell, H. R., & Clark, E. (1965). *Preventive medicine for the doctor in his community*. New York, NY: McGraw-Hill.

Lopez-Moreno, S., Garrido-Latorre, F., & Hernandez-Avila, M. (2000). Historical development of epidemiology: Its growth as scientific discipline. *Salud Pública de México, 42*(2), 133–143. Retrieved from MEDLINE with Full Text database.

March of Dimes Foundation. (2012). *Prematurity campaign*. Retrieved from http://www.marchofdimes.com/mission/prematurity.html

McKenzie, J. F., Pinger, R. F., & Kotecki, J. E. (2005). *An introduction to community health* (5th ed.). Sudbury, MA: Jones and Bartlett.

Merrill, R. M. (2010). *Introduction to epidemiology* (5th ed.). Sudbury, MA: Jones and Bartlett.

National Center for Health Statistics (NCHS). (2011). *Health, United States, 2010: With special feature on death and dying.* Hyattsville, MD: Author.

National Institute for Occupational Safety and Health (NIOSH). (2011). *Office of Extramural Programs page.* Retrieved from http://www.cdc.gov/niosh/oep/centers.html

Paranzino, G., Butterfield, P., Nastoff, T., & Ranger, C. (2005). Development and clinical utility of an environmental exposure history: Pneumonic. *American Association of Occupational Health Nurses Journal, 53*(1), 37–42.

Polit, D. F., & Beck, C. T. (2012). *Nursing research: Generating and assessing evidence for nursing practice* (9th ed.). Philadelphia, PA: Lippincott Williams & Wilkins.

Shult, P. A. (2010). MM&I 554: Global emerging and re-emerging infectious disease. University of Wisconsin Course: Infectious Diseases & Bioterrorism.

Smith, C. M., & Maurer, F. A. (2000). *Community health nursing: Theory and practice* (2nd ed.). Philadelphia, PA: W. B. Saunders.

Subramanian, A., Desia, A., Prakash, L., Mital, A., & Mital, A. (2006). Changing trends in US injury profiles: Revisiting non-fatal occupational injury statistics. *Journal of Occupational Rehabilitation, 16*(1), 123–155. doi: 10.1007/s10926-005-9012-1

Turnock, B. J. (2009). *Public health: What it is and how it works* (4th ed.). Sudbury, MA: Jones and Bartlett.

UNICEF. (2012). Table 1: Basic indicators. *State of the World's Children 2012.* Retrieved from http://www.unicef.org/sowc2012/pdfs/SOWC-2012-TABLE-1-BASIC-INDICATORS.pdf

United Nations. (2003). *UN world population prospects: The 2002 revision.* New York, NY: Author. Retrieved from http://www.un.org/esa/population/publications/wpp2002/WPP2002-HIGH-LIGHTSrev1.PDF

United Nations. (2010). *UN Development Programme 2010 Human Development Index.* New York, NY: Author. Retrieved from http://hdr.undp.org/en/statistics

Use this checklist for cost/benefit analysis. (2008). *Occupational Health Management, 18*(4), 35–36. Retrieved from http://libproxy.adelphi.edu:2048/login?url=http://search.ebscohost.com/login.aspx?direct=true&db=a9h&AN=31625998&site=ehost-live&scope=site

Valanis, B. (1999). *Epidemiology in nursing and health care* (3rd ed.). Norwalk, CT: Appleton & Lange.

World Health Organization (WHO). (2009). *Pandemic influenza preparedness and response: A WHO guidance document.* Retrieved from http://www.who.int/csr/disease/influenza/pipguidance2009/en/index.html

World Health Organization (WHO). (2011). *Global Health Observatory.* Retrieved from http://www.who.int/gho/en

ADDITIONAL RESOURCES

Allender, J. A., Rector, C., & Warner, K. D. (2010). *Community health nursing: Promoting and protecting the public's health* (7th ed.). New York, NY: Lippincott Williams & Wilkins.

Institute of Medicine (IOM). (2011). *The future of nursing: Leading change, advancing health.* Washington, DC: National Academies Press.

Rosen, G. A. (1958). *A history of public health.* Baltimore, MD: Johns Hopkins University Press.

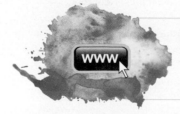

For a full suite of assignments and additional learning activities, use the access code located in the front of your book to visit the exclusive website: http://go.jblearning.com/Holzemer/. If you do not have an access code, you can obtain one at the site.

LEARNING ACTIVITIES

www

1. A nurse defines epidemiology in the following ways. Which statement is correct?

   A. "Epidemiology measures patterns of activity that relate to health, illness, and accidents."

   B. "Epidemiology evaluates the response of vulnerable populations to medical interventions."

   C. "Epidemiology is concerned with how pathogens respond to specific pharmacological agents."

   D. "Epidemiology predicts the need for future health care services using current illness statistics."

2. An ethical implication of how a nation responds to its infant mortality rate (IMR) is reflected in which of the following statements?

   A. An IMR relates to how a nation pays for health care.

   B. An IMR relates to how a nation creates laws to protect the public.

   C. An IMR relates to how a nation values the health and wellness of children.

   D. An IMR relates to how a nation prepares for new epidemics and health problems.

3. A nurse is aware that the major problem with not improving the health of a population with information from epidemiology and environmental health, is related to which of the following concepts?

   A. The staggering cost of healthcare service delivery.

   B. The ability to assist communities to cope with disasters.

   C. The methods of educating healthcare providers.

   D. The loss of human potential for the community.

ADDITIONAL QUESTIONS FOR STUDY

1. Using Table 8-1 as a reference, apply the nursing process to a client who has been diagnosed with hospital-acquired pneumonia, and the epidemiological process to the community in which the client diagnosed with hospital-acquired pneumonia resides. What contrasts and comparisons can you make between these two processes?

2. Using Table 8-2 as a reference, contrast the definitions of incidence and prevalence. Can you list different informational needs in the epidemiological process where one of these measures would answer a question more appropriately than the other?

3. Frequently, there are correlations between other variables (e.g., poverty, economic measures, natural resources) of countries and overall population health measures. Table 8-3 lists the 2011 estimates of worldwide highest and lowest infant mortality rates in rank order. Access the Internet resource for these data (https://www.cia.gov/library/publications/the-world-factbook/rankorder/2091rank.html#) and review other economic indicators listed for countries on this site. Are any economic indicators listed there that you believe would be correlated with infant mortality rates? List these indicators and the reasons you suspect a correlation (positive or negative) would exist.

4. Using Figures 8-2 and 8-3, develop a concept map or nursing care plan for prevention of hospital-acquired urinary tract infections.

CHAPTER OUTLINE

OBJECTIVES

www

1. Explain the differences between primary, secondary, and tertiary levels of prevention.

2. Describe the importance of the three levels of prevention as they relate to problems with individuals, families, other groups, and communities.

3. Define the major areas of *Healthy People 2020* as they relate to health promotion and specific protection of communities.

4. Create a plan to promote primary prevention activities from a nursing perspective.

KEY TERMS

www

Anticipatory guidance

Determinants of health

Health disparity

Health equity

Healthy People 2020

Prepathogenesis

Primary prevention

Secondary prevention

Tertiary prevention

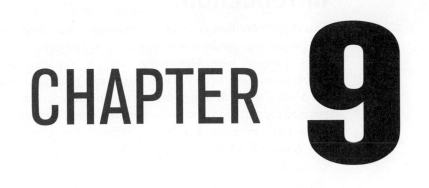

CHAPTER 9

Inquiry and Health Promotion, Health Maintenance, and Health Restoration in the Community

Judith Aponte

Stephen Paul Holzemer

INQUIRY

Action and reaction, ebb and flow, trial and error, change—this is the rhythm of living. Out of our overconfidence, fear; out of our fear, clearer vision, fresh hope. And out of hope, progress.

—Bruce Barton (1886–1969)

Introduction

This chapter examines the concept of inquiry, including how to assist the client in making proper and productive health choices. The community health nurse (CHN) uses skills of inquiry when identifying the appropriate nursing interventions that relate to health promotion, health maintenance, and health restoration. Nursing interventions are derived after a thorough assessment and diagnosis of actual and potential problems, using the nursing process. Following the nursing process, interventions are evaluated by the CHN to ensure that they were effective, or to identify that a change in the plan of care is necessary (American Nurses Association [ANA], 2001, 2010a, 2010b).

The topics of health promotion, health maintenance, and health restoration interventions were introduced earlier in this text, as they relate to primary prevention, secondary prevention, and tertiary prevention activities. Prevention activities aimed initially at preventing the problem from ever occurring are referred to as primary prevention. Preventing problems that do occur from becoming worse or progressing relates to secondary and tertiary prevention. The three levels of prevention are the focus of this chapter.

This chapter begins with a view of health priorities as reflected in *Healthy People 2020*, the United States' national priorities for health. The priorities of *Healthy People 2020* are those that the CHN would expect to be connected to resource allocation. Without the necessary resources, adequate prevention of problems—or a timely resolution of problems once they do occur—is not possible. Examples of how the levels of prevention complement the focus areas of *Healthy People 2020* are discussed in detail in this chapter. Some problems are addressed with a client who is an individual, a family, or another group living in the community. Other problems are addressed at the level of the aggregate or community itself. The chapter ends with a discussion of a multi-problem issue, for which the CHN must decide how to establish priorities with community members to address and intervene with the community in managing their problems.

The Use of Inquiry by the Nurse into the Needs of the Client

Community health nurses focus much of their time and energy on matching the needs of their clients with the resources that are available for those clients' care. The CHN uses inquisitiveness to continuously monitor the changing needs of clients, armed with the changing pool of resources available to them. Inquiry allows the nurse to choose between and among options for care. The national agenda for healthcare delivery known as *Healthy People 2020* provides guidance in how to use inquiry in choosing priorities to resolve client problems or concerns. The process of inquiry is core to effective and appropriate communication, cultural competence, and all levels of client-centered care (The Joint Commission, 2011).

A National Agenda for Healthcare Delivery: *Healthy People 2020*

The *Healthy People 2020* agenda is based on the accomplishments of four previous *Healthy People* initiatives. The national agenda for healthcare delivery has evolved from

Healthy People 2020: The United States' national agenda for healthcare delivery; it strives to improve the health of all groups, with the goals of achieving health equity and eliminating disparities, to allow people to reach their health potential.

nearly 30 years of inquiry, with the latest agenda set to guide care delivery until 2020. The previous programs included the following:

- *Healthy People: The Surgeon General's Report on Health Promotion and Disease Prevention* (1979)
- *Healthy People 1990: Promoting Health/Preventing Disease: Objectives for the Nation*
- *Healthy People 2000: National Health Promotion and Disease Prevention Objectives*
- *Healthy People 2010: Objectives for Improving Health*

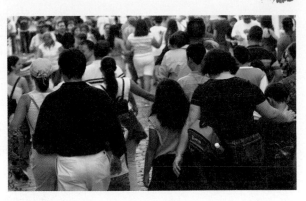

© Joseph/ShutterStock, Inc.

The origins of *Healthy People* focused, in part, on health disparities. Although the term "disparities" often is interpreted to mean racial or ethnic disparities, many dimensions of disparity exist in the United States, particularly in health. If a health outcome is seen in a greater or lesser extent between populations, there is disparity. An African American, a single woman on welfare, an 84 year-old male restricted in movement to a wheelchair, a person identifying as gay or lesbian, or a family in rural Idaho—all may experience disparity that affects their ability to achieve good health outcomes.

Healthy People 2020 strives to improve the health of all groups, with the goals of achieving health equity and eliminating disparities, to allow people to reach their health potential. This agenda defines **health equity** as the attainment of the highest level of health for all people. Achieving health equity requires valuing the health of everyone, and eliminating health and healthcare disparities. *Healthy People 2020* defines a **health disparity** as "a particular type of health difference that is closely linked with social, economic, and/or environmental disadvantage" (U.S. Department of Health and Human Services [DHHS], 2010).

Health disparities adversely affect groups of people who have systematically experienced greater obstacles to health based on variables such as race or ethnicity, religion, gender, and age. Other pertinent variables include socioeconomic status, mental health, physical or emotional disability, sexual orientation or gender identity, and geographic location (DHHS, 2010).

Powerful and complex relationships exist between health and biology, genetics, and individual behavior, and between health and health services, socioeconomic status, the physical environment, discrimination, racism, literacy levels, and legislative policies. These factors, which collectively influence an individual's or population's health, are known as **determinants of health**.

Throughout the next decade, *Healthy People 2020* will assess health disparities in the U.S. population by tracking rates of illness, death, chronic conditions, behaviors, and other types of outcomes in relation to demographic factors. Among the categories in which data are to be collected are the following (DHHS, 2010):

- Race and ethnicity
- Gender
- Sexual identity and orientation
- Disability status or special healthcare needs
- Geographic location (rural and urban)

A renewed focus on identifying, measuring, tracking, and reducing health disparities through a determinants of health approach is the focus of *Healthy People 2020*. Nurses familiar with the *Healthy People* program are aware that new topic areas of concern surface with every 10-year cycle. The new topic areas for *Healthy People 2020* are profiled in **Table 9-1**. **Table 9-2** lists all topic areas for 2020.

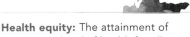

Health equity: The attainment of the highest level of health for all people.

Health disparity: "A particular type of health difference that is closely linked with social, economic, and/or environmental disadvantage" (DHHS, 2010).

Determinants of health: Factors that collectively influence an individual's or population's health, such as biology, genetics, individual behavior, socioeconomic status, the physical environment, discrimination, racism, literacy levels, and legislative policies.

TABLE 9-1
The New Topic Areas for *Healthy People 2020*

- Adolescent Health
- Blood Disorders and Blood Safety
- Dementias, Including Alzheimer's Disease
- Early and Middle Childhood
- Genomics
- Global Health
- Healthcare-Associated Infections
- Health-Related Quality of Life and Well-Being
- Lesbian, Gay, Bisexual, and Transgender Health
- Older Adults
- Preparedness
- Sleep Health
- Social Determinants of Health

Using *Healthy People* Topic Areas to Complement Levels of Prevention

For the novice CHN, making a connection between the focus areas of the *Healthy People* project and levels of prevention can assist in "preplanning" those nursing actions that may be necessary to move the client to a higher or more functional level of health. The term **anticipatory guidance** describes the process of predicting which services may be needed for the client, and guiding the client in the use of those services. As always, clients need a detailed personal assessment that matches their specific needs, with the nurse avoiding the temptation to cluster groups of clients together according to variables that may not be appropriate.

Nursing actions can be effective before a disease occurs (primary prevention), in the earliest stages of disease (secondary prevention), or when residual consequences of disease linger (tertiary prevention). These levels of prevention are derived from the classic work of Leavell and Clark (1965). The CHN may use multiple interventions, from any or all of the three levels of prevention, to address the health needs of the client. Of great importance is the recognition of the role of the client in participating by choosing the level of prevention activity, under the guidance of the CHN.

The levels of prevention are discussed in this section with clinical examples of how the CHN uses inquiry to decide which interventions have the best chance of fostering healthy behaviors. Levels of prevention can be viewed as going beyond the care of individuals. Families, other groups, and communities may all potentially be the recipients of interventions reflecting levels of prevention. The idea of levels of prevention is closely related to the agent–host–environment model, introduced earlier in this text. Manipula-

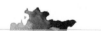

Anticipatory guidance: The process of predicting which services may be needed for the client, and guiding the client in the use of those services.

TABLE 9-2
Healthy People 2020 Topic Areas

• Access to Health Services	• HIV
• Adolescent Health	• Immunization and Infectious Diseases
• Arthritis, Osteoporosis, and Chronic Back Conditions	• Injury and Violence Prevention
• Blood Disorders and Blood Safety	• Lesbian, Gay, Bisexual, and Transgender Health
• Cancer	• Maternal, Infant, and Child Health
• Chronic Kidney Disease	• Medical Product Safety
• Dementias, Including Alzheimer's Disease	• Mental Health and Mental Disorders
• Diabetes	• Nutrition and Weight Status
• Disability and Health	• Occupational Safety and Health
• Early and Middle Childhood	• Older Adults
• Educational and Community-Based Programs	• Oral Health
• Environmental Health	• Physical Activity
• Family Planning	• Preparedness
• Food Safety	• Public Health Infrastructure
• Genomics	• Respiratory Diseases
• Global Health	• Sexually Transmitted Diseases
• Health Communication and Health Information Technology	• Sleep Health
• Healthcare-Associated Infections	• Social Determinants of Health
• Health-Related Quality of Life and Well-Being	• Substance Abuse
• Hearing and Other Sensory or Communication Disorders	• Tobacco Use
• Heart Disease and Stroke	• Vision

tion of any one of these variables may move the person (family, group, or community) closer to or farther away from a preferred state of health.

Primary Prevention

Primary prevention includes interventions implemented before disease occurs, during the prepathogenic stage of an illness. Every disease process is divided into two phases—the prepathogenic stage and the pathogenic stage; **prepathogenesis** is the period prior to illness. Primary prevention efforts undertaken during this period include both health promotion behaviors and specific protection behaviors. Examples of health promotion activities include fostering healthy behaviors in all of the basic human needs, such as human interaction and nutrition. An example of specific protection is providing many, but not all, forms of immunization.

Primary prevention: Interventions implemented before disease occurs, during the prepathogenic stage of an illness; they include both health promotion behaviors and specific protection behaviors.

Prepathogenesis: The period prior to illness.

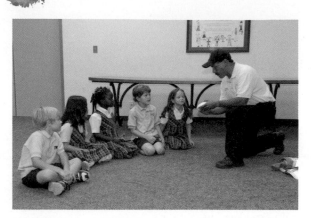

© Jones & Bartlett Learning. Photographed by Glen E. Ellman.

The CHN often works independently in providing primary prevention services that relate to counseling and teaching. When primary prevention activities involve the administration of immunologic agents, for example, physicians direct the intervention. The CHN works with the community health team and the client in anticipating the needs of the community as they relate to primary prevention activities, and provides care to prevent physical disease (e.g., influenza) and diseases of society (e.g., violence) from occurring.

Secondary Prevention

Secondary prevention interventions are used during early pathogenesis; they include early diagnosis, prompt treatment, and the limitation of disability (because of quick action). Examples of secondary prevention include case finding, screening, and other methods that prevent the spread of disease and injury. First-response therapies to treat the disease and prevent further complications are also components of secondary prevention. An acute, emergency hospitalization for a specific disease or condition is part of secondary prevention.

The CHN works closely with acute care specialists when secondary prevention activities are implemented. For example, home care nurses visit clients at their homes after they are discharged following hospitalization, and may perform high-technology care (e.g., use of a vacuum-assisted closure [VAC] pump for wound care) in the home as part of a subacute plan of care, directed by a physician. The CHN uses anticipatory guidance in this level of prevention by assisting the client, for example, with coping with the demands of high-technology care in the home.

Tertiary Prevention

Tertiary prevention is also related to a period of pathogenesis—specifically, the period of convalescence and rehabilitation. Examples of tertiary prevention include reeducation for the client (secondary to physical therapy or occupational therapy) and education of the public (to increase employment opportunities for persons with a disability). As indicated, tertiary prevention activities are often provided under the direction of an occupational therapist or physical therapist. The CHN needs to be clear about the proper role of the nurse when supporting the work of other disciplines. A review of agency protocols, or development of protocols when necessary, assists with this process.

Secondary prevention: Interventions are used during early pathogenesis—that is, after illness has occurred; they include early diagnosis, prompt treatment, and the limitation of disability.

Tertiary prevention: Interventions used during later pathogenesis—specifically, the period of convalescence and rehabilitation; they include reeducation for the client and education of the public.

Applying the Principles of Levels of Prevention to Individuals, Families, and Other Groups

The principles of the three levels of prevention can be applied to individuals, families, and other groups in the community. A thorough assessment is needed before a diagnosis and intervention plan is created. The following examples are used as a basis for discussing the concepts of various clients' needs that are identified with the *Healthy People* priorities, and the levels of prevention related to those priorities. The idea of levels of prevention emerged in response to individuals experiencing disease and disability. Extending these concepts to relate to social and community-based problems requires some creativity.

Any activity could conceivably be used in primary, secondary, or tertiary prevention. To match the activity with the level of prevention, the CHN must ask, "Why am I using this particular intervention?" The various methods used to teach health-related activities will reflect the specific level of prevention that the caregiver aims to provide. If teaching on the topic of nutrition is aimed to prevent a problem from occurring, for example, it is considered primary prevention. By comparison, teaching the protocol for using the 911 emergency system can be considered secondary prevention. Finally, if teaching is intended to foster forgiveness in a client in spiritual distress, it could be linked to tertiary prevention, as a form of rehabilitation.

An Individual and Levels of Prevention

A client, Mr. Jones, is maintained at home on a respirator, and receives 24-hour home health aide services through Medicare. The client has one regular visitor, a friend, although the client's family (mother and two brothers) live only 40 miles away. The client does not want to communicate with the family, and states to a nurse, "Do not let them visit; I don't want to see any of them." After a thorough assessment, the CHN makes nursing diagnoses that relate to the topic areas from *Healthy People 2020*.

The CHN supervising the home care services initially respects the client's choice to live in isolation, but wants to learn more about how to assist the client in experiencing a better quality of life, if the client agrees. The CHN examines the *Healthy People 2020* material, focusing on mental health and mental disorders (communication with family/isolation) as well as medical product safety (use of respirator). In practice, the CHN would fully review the *Healthy People* objectives and activities for these areas. **Table 9-3** provides an example of how the nurse used *Healthy People 2020* and the levels of prevention to assist in planning care for this individual client.

TABLE 9-3
An Individual Client and the Levels of Prevention

Priority *Healthy People 2020* Focus Areas		
Mental Health and Mental Disorders		Medical Product Safety
Primary Prevention Nursing Interventions	Secondary Prevention Nursing Interventions	Tertiary Prevention Nursing Interventions
Discuss, with the appropriate source, the need to secure a secondary generator for electricity (the respirator), and to follow the manufacturer's plan for maintenance of equipment. Refer to the client to a social worker to explore the notification of the electric company concerning the noninterruption of electrical service.	Make a referral to the clinical nurse specialist in mental health to identify the potential for improving family communication. Screen the visitor for caretaker fatigue. Investigate other community resources that may be assistive in maintaining the client's level of health.	Re-institute the plan for physical therapy exercises to decrease contractures and review with home health aide.

Two Families and Levels of Prevention

The Alpha Family

The Alpha Family is made up of a 45-year-old mother and her adopted 20-year-old daughter. The family is preoccupied with dieting. The mother weighs 230 pounds (104.55 kg), and the daughter weighs 120 pounds (54.55 kg). The daughter states, "The best thing for weight loss is actually using cocaine … but I have been 'clean and sober' for 4 years."

The CHN who is providing care treats the family as the client. The CHN examines the *Healthy People 2020* material, focusing on nutrition and overweight, along with substance abuse, as areas of concern. **Table 9-4** provides an example of how the nurse used *Healthy People* and levels of prevention to assist in planning care for this family as client. The interventions identified are examples of the activities that may be appropriate in this situation. An actual plan of care would include more detail, and would require input from other providers as necessary.

The Beta Family

The Beta Family consists of a 70-year-old male and his 66-year-old "live-in girlfriend." The girlfriend says to a nurse, "The old man is good to me. He smokes too much, but the violent threats have stopped. I guess we are fine. Neither of us has seen a doctor in years!" The CHN discovers that the male has a 30-year history of tobacco use. The CHN focuses on mental health and mental disorders (violent threats) and access to health services, using the *Healthy People 2020* guidelines. **Table 9-5** represents possible interventions with the Beta Family and levels of prevention.

The CHN considered "tobacco use" as a *Healthy People 2020* focus area, but chose to initially focus on "access to health care" instead. As a family, both members of this pair have not seen a healthcare provider for some time. Making connections with healthcare services for the pair may be more productive than breaking a 30-year cycle of smoking behavior. The CHN plans to discuss smoking and second-hand smoke with the family after the first two priorities are addressed. One idea would be to explore the possibility of a harm-reduction approach to the smoking situation for the family.

TABLE 9-4
The Alpha Family and Levels of Prevention

Priority *Healthy People 2020* Focus Areas		
Nutrition and Overweight		**Substance Abuse**
Primary Prevention Nursing Interventions	**Secondary Prevention Nursing Interventions**	**Tertiary Prevention Nursing Interventions**
Discuss nutrition as a family concern, focusing on exercise and activity for the daughter.	Make a referral to the nutritionist for development of a plan of nutrition maintenance for the mother (and daughter). Monitor the mother using the agency's protocol for assessment of hypertensive and diabetic conditions. Identify social activities that the mother and daughter might share and do together.	Evaluate the daughter's definition of "clean and sober." Explore the daughter's use of 12-step recovery programs, or other support programs for maintenance of sobriety.

TABLE 9-5
The Beta Family and Levels of Prevention

Priority *Healthy People 2020* Focus Areas		
Mental Health and Mental Disorders		Access to Health Services
Primary Prevention Nursing Interventions	Secondary Prevention Nursing Interventions	Tertiary Prevention Nursing Interventions
Discuss the progression of verbal violence to physical violence. Create a plan for leaving escalating violent situations.	Develop a health screening plan for diseases and conditions of older adults. Identify emergency care and urgent care contacts.	Explore support group options for coping with emotional trauma.

A Group and Levels of Prevention

A 50-year-old client with a history of heart disease is working at a job where lifting heavy boxes is part of his responsibilities. The client states, "My back is always hurting, but I bend my legs like a nurse told me once." The client works for minimum wages and has limited health insurance. He states, "There are about 10 of us employees here in a similar situation." The CHN takes the members of this employee group up on an offer to meet monthly on resolving health concerns as a group.

The CHN collaborates with the occupational health nurse (another CHN) working at the facility to develop a plan of care for the group and to explore the possibility of implementing a program for the whole company in the future. The occupational health nurse looks forward to working with the other CHN, because current work responsibilities prevent the occupational health nurse from running the group that is needed. The group begins with the suggested activities shown in **Table 9-6**.

TABLE 9-6
A Group and Levels of Prevention

Priority *Healthy People 2020* Focus Areas		
Access to Quality Health Services		Occupational Safety and Health
Primary Prevention Nursing Interventions	Secondary Prevention Nursing Interventions	Tertiary Prevention Nursing Interventions
Identify methods of completing job tasks using proper body mechanics. Survey like-businesses in the area for their participation in employee health activities.	List the city resources for health screening that complement the concerns about limited health insurance. Plan to participate in screening activities with work peers for support.	Make a referral to physical therapy for relearning core body strengthening exercises for persons with stress injuries (after proper medical diagnosis), as a part of rehabilitation.

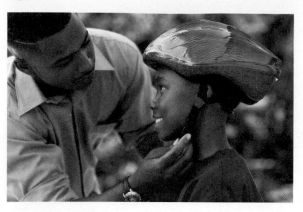

© Creatas/Jupiterimages

Applying the Principles of Levels of Prevention to Aggregates and Communities

Some health-related problems require nursing interventions at the aggregate or community level. Five examples of aggregate or community-level problems needing CHN intervention are (1) accidents in children, (2) homicides, (3) other forms of abuse and violence, (4) cancer, and (5) persons who are overweight. These larger, community-wide problems were identified after the CHN initiated an exploration of the epidemiological trends in the community that include a large percentage of people needing nursing services in the community. As always, the CHN is not working in isolation on aggregate or communitywide programs. Instead, the coordination of many providers, organizations, and people from the community is necessary for this level of intervention.

Accidents in Children

The CHN becomes aware that accidents are the major cause of mortality among children. In particular, accidents pose the greatest threat to children and adolescents ages 10–24 (**FIGURE 9-1**). Additional data are evaluated to identify the percentages of children and adolescents who die from accidents from birth to 19 years of age (**FIGURE 9-2**). Together, these data document the need for aggregate and community intervention. Instead of looking at individuals, families, and other groups, the CHN and the community health team, which includes members of other healthcare disciplines, examine the

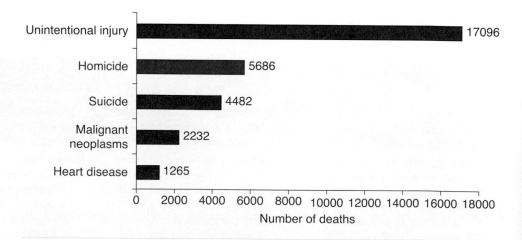

Figure 9-1 Five leading causes of deaths among persons ages 10 to 24 years, United States, 2005.
Source: CDC.

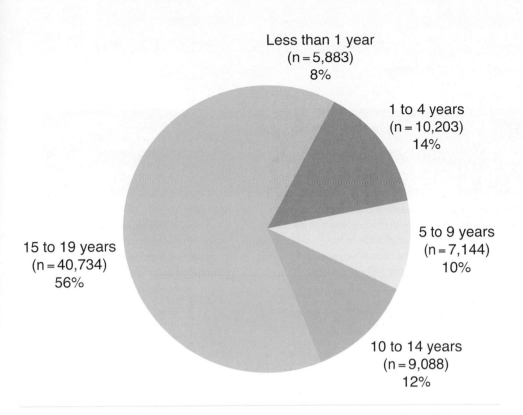

Less than 1 year
(n = 5,883)
8%

1 to 4 years
(n = 10,203)
14%

5 to 9 years
(n = 7,144)
10%

15 to 19 years
(n = 40,734)
56%

10 to 14 years
(n = 9,088)
12%

Figure 9-2 Percentage of injury deaths among children 0 to 19 years, by age group, United States, 2000–2005.

Source: CDC/NCHS, National Vital Statistics System.

best intervention strategies for the community as a whole. **Table 9-7** provides possible examples of levels of prevention related to accidents in children.

Intervention strategies for the aggregate or community include making communitywide changes in areas that relate to, for example, education in all schools in the community, close supervision of public recreation areas, and use of the media to educate parents and others about the general safety concerns for all children and adolescents. Additional data that are made available to the CHN and the community health team identify motor vehicle accidents as a primary cause for concern (**FIGURE 9-3**). With this information in hand, the team can use the same strategies, albeit with an emphasis on the proper use of car seats, analysis of traffic patterns, and police surveillance of drivers who speed while driving.

Homicides

Figure 9-1 identified homicide as the second leading cause of death among persons 10 to 24 years of age. Further investigation reveals that while the rate remains high, there has been a decrease in homicide in the United States from 1991 to 2005 (**FIGURE 9-4**). The CHN takes no comfort in this decline, because the nurse believes that this rate should

TABLE 9-7
Accidents in Children and Levels of Prevention

Priority *Healthy People 2020* Focus Areas		
Maternal, Infant, and Child Health		**Injury and Violence Prevention**
Primary Prevention Nursing Interventions	**Secondary Prevention Nursing Interventions**	**Tertiary Prevention Nursing Interventions**
Secure funding for media and a communitywide safety program. Negotiate with local media (television/radio/Internet) for a 6- to 18-month safety plan of public announcements and teaching activities to apply in schools, houses of worship, and recreational facilities.	Create a plan to assess for (screening) ways to avoid accidents in the home, school, houses of worship, and recreational facilities.	Evaluate records of the safety of public and private spaces for rehabilitation (road repair, asbestos removal, recall of unsafe equipment).

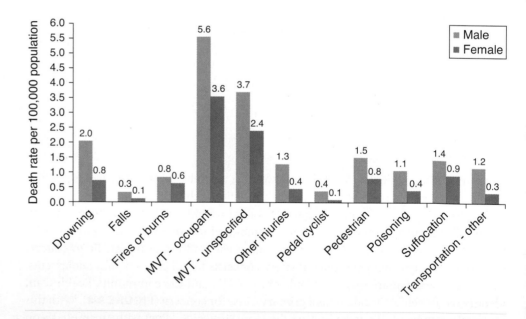

Figure 9-3 Unintentional injury death rates among children 0 to 19 years, by sex and cause, United States, 2000–2005.

Source: CDC/NCHS, National Vital Statistics System.

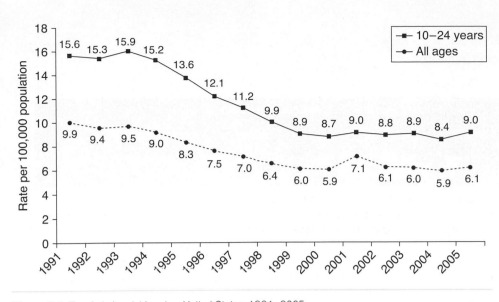

Figure 9-4 Trends in homicide rates, United States, 1991–2005.
Source: CDC.

not exist at all in a civil society. Communitywide intervention strategies directed at eliminating homicides could include teaching conflict management in schools, monitoring the laws concerning the sale and ownership of weapons, and meeting the basic human needs that might make the community less violent in nature. **Table 9-8** relates the concept of homicide with levels of prevention.

Abuse and Violence

Examining the need for a community response to homicide allowed the CHN to become informed about the larger concern of physical and sexual violence in the community. The assessment of the CHN identified the prevalence and incidence of violence among vulnerable segments of the population. The Duluth model (Domestic Abuse Intervention Project, 2011), which articulates the causes and methods of physical and sexual violence, is considered a standard means of assessing violence for many in the field of abuse. Shown in **FIGURE 9-5**, it identifies ways that an abuser maintains power and control.

After further examination, the CHN determines that the Duluth model addresses male-perpetrated violence taking place within a traditional male–female relationship. Thus the model would be helpful to guide discussions of abuse for only part of the problem of abuse. To apply the model to women who abuse others or to same-sex (i.e., gay and lesbian) relationships, the model would need to be refined. An additional review of the literature reveals that a different focus may better describe the concerns of abuse for all persons. A model that focuses on equality in relationships may be better suited for understanding perpetrators of violence (**FIGURE 9-6**). **Table 9-9** relates abuse and violence with levels of prevention.

TABLE 9-8
Homicides and Levels of Prevention

Priority *Healthy People 2020* Focus Areas		
Mental Health and Mental Disorders		**Injury and Violence Prevention**
Primary Prevention Nursing Interventions	**Secondary Prevention Nursing Interventions**	**Tertiary Prevention Nursing Interventions**
Implement cooperation and civil play activities for children. Provide programs that emphasize respect for others, and foster conflict management skills to children in schools.	Screen for impulsive action, anger levels, and sense of hopelessness in older children. Develop a peer crisis team to meet with family and peers in the emergency department after a violent episode.	Create anger management programs to follow students into adulthood. Allow persons involved in perpetrating violence to educate others as to the consequences of action (if and when appropriate). Develop grief resolution groups for adolescents and adults experiencing violent deaths in others in the community.

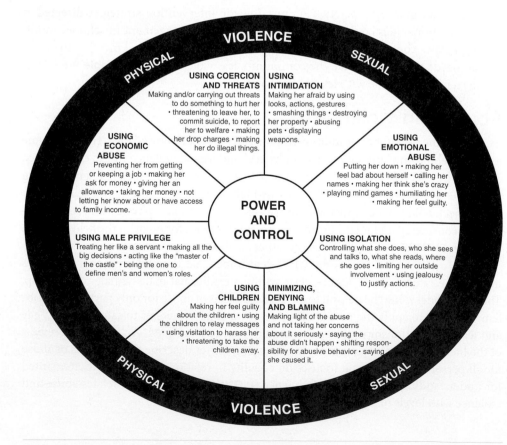

Figure 9-5 The Duluth model for physical and sexual violence.

Source: © 2011 Domestic Abuse Intervention Programs. Used with permission.

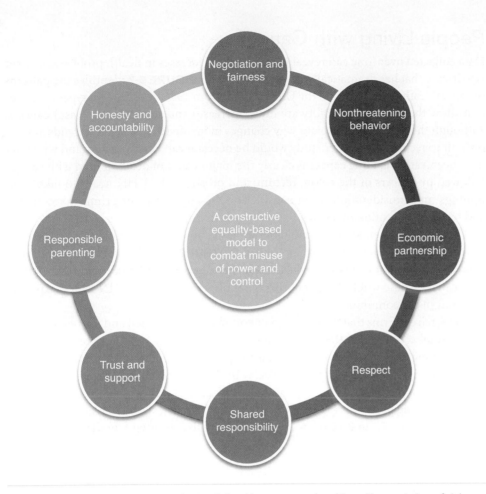

Figure 9-6 A model focusing on equality in relationships as a way of working with perpetrators of violence related to power and control.

TABLE 9-9

Abuse and Violence and Levels of Prevention

Priority *Healthy People 2020* Focus Areas		
Mental Health and Mental Disorders		**Injury and Violence Prevention**
Primary Prevention Nursing Interventions	**Secondary Prevention Nursing Interventions**	**Tertiary Prevention Nursing Interventions**
Implement cooperation and civil play activities for children. Provide programs that emphasize respect for others and conflict management skills to children in schools.	Assess for abuse and violence at any age. Provide short-term counseling for students for personal problems and in response to disturbing local, national, and international events.	Initiate long-term counseling for clients experiencing abuse and violence (rehabilitation).

People Living with Cancer

Data collected over time can reveal increases and decreases in health problems. Cancer is a disease that has dramatically changed over time. **FIGURE 9-7** identifies the patterns of cancer death rates in men in the United States from 1930 to 2002. Two types of cancer that show the greatest variability are lung (increase) and stomach (decrease) cancers. Although the data cannot explain why changes in incidence occur, such trends are important to recognize. Further study would be necessary to better understand why rates have been variable. Lung cancer is clearly the major cause of death of men with cancer, followed by cancers of the colon, rectum, and prostate. The CHN needs to take these findings into consideration when considering the application of primary, secondary, and tertiary prevention measures.

Cancer in women shows some different and some similar findings. Cancer rates for women for the same years are presented in **FIGURE 9-8**. The major ongoing threat is breast cancer, but the cancer whose incidence has grown steadily since the 1960s is lung cancer. These would represent two types of cancer that the CHN would expect to confront in the community.

Research confirms that the common denominator among men and women with lung cancer is tobacco use. **FIGURE 9-9** reveals the relationship between cigarette consumption and lung cancer deaths. Of interest is the pattern of decreased deaths that mirror a decrease in cigarette consumption. The delay in cigarette use and death rates is related to time—a factor necessary to develop the fatal disease. The CHN would identify the necessity of providing programs to target this disease on primary, secondary, and tertiary levels of prevention. **Table 9-10** relates people living with cancer with levels of prevention.

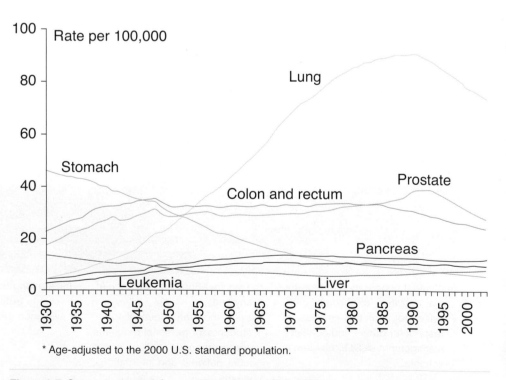

* Age-adjusted to the 2000 U.S. standard population.

Figure 9-7 Cancer death rates*, for men, United States, 1930–2002.

Source: U.S. Mortality Public Use Data Tapes 1960–2002, U.S. Mortality Volumes 1930–1959, National Center for Health Statistics, Centers for Disease Control and Prevention, 2005.

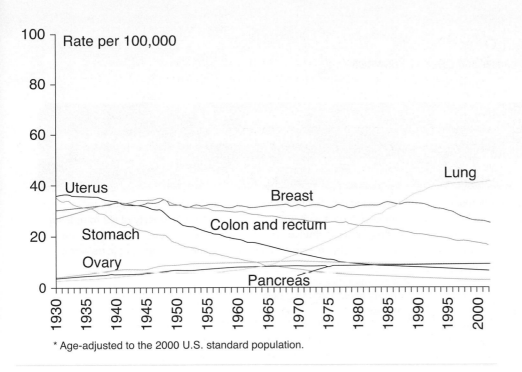

* Age-adjusted to the 2000 U.S. standard population.

Figure 9-8 Cancer death rates*, for women, United States, 1930–2002.

Source: U.S. Mortality Public Use Data Tapes 1960–2002, U.S. Mortality Volumes 1930–1959, National Center for Health Statistics, Centers for Disease Control and Prevention, 2005.

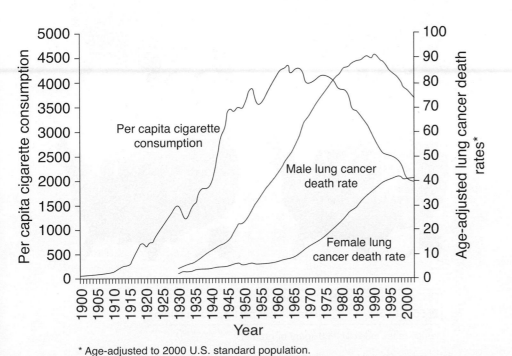

* Age-adjusted to 2000 U.S. standard population.

Figure 9-9 Tobacco use in the United States, 1990–2002.

Source: Death rates: U.S. Mortality Public Use Tapes, 1960–2002, U.S. Mortality Volumes, 1930–1959, National Center for Health Statistics, Centers for Disease Control and Prevention, 2005. Cigarette consumption: U.S. Department of Agriculture, 1900–2002.

TABLE 9-10
People Living with Cancer and Levels of Prevention

Priority *Healthy People 2020* Focus Areas		
Cancer		**Health-Related Quality of Life and Well-being**
Primary Prevention Nursing Interventions	**Secondary Prevention Nursing Interventions**	**Tertiary Prevention Nursing Interventions**
Review aspects of nutrition and exercise as core to healthy living. Promote taking responsibility for risk behaviors (i.e., use of tobacco). Encourage risk-minimizing activities (self-examination of skin, testicular self-examination, breast self-examination).	Screening and case finding for various cancers with age-appropriate groups (i.e., men older than 50 years and prostate cancer). Create peer crisis counselors for people newly diagnosed with cancer.	Introduction of activities to improve quality of life to recover from treatment, or accept the limits of treatment in palliative care.

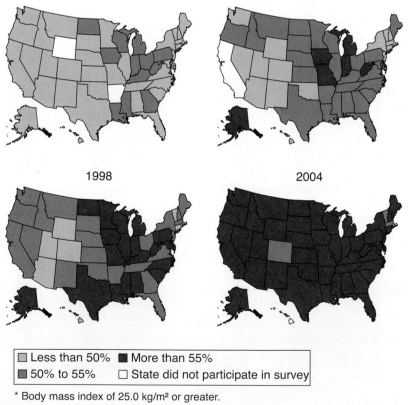

Figure 9-10 Trends in overweight* prevalence (percent), adults 18 and older, United States, 1992–2004.

Source: Behavioral Risk Factor Surveillance System, CD-ROM (1984–1995, 1998) and Public Use Data Tape (2004), National Center for Chronic Disease Prevention and Health Promotion, Centers for Disease Control and Prevention, 1997, 2000, 2005.

Overweight Persons

The number of adults who were overweight in the United States increased sharply between the years 1992 and 2004. In 1992, very few states reported people 18 years and older (adults) as being overweight. At that time, the majority of states had less than 50% of their adult population reported as overweight. Only 12 years later, however, all but two states reported that more than 55% of adults were overweight. **FIGURE 9-10** provides this information in graphic form. The CHN would consider the impact of diet and exercise, for example, in children to prevent the overweight problem, as well as the impact of diet and exercise in the adult population to move toward normalizing weight in the population.

Additional data are necessary to better understand the problem of overweight people in the population. The CHN considers reviewing data concerning children to elucidate the relationship between exercise and weight control. **FIGURE 9-11** reveals the prevalence of high school students (grades 9–12) attending physical education (PE) class daily between the years 1991 and 2003. Two pieces of information from this figure might be significant. First, exercise prevalence initially declined for a few years, but then a somewhat steady rate of student participation in PE classes occurred. Second, the older the students became, the less they participated in daily PE class. **Table 9-11** reviews interventions for overweight persons related to levels of prevention

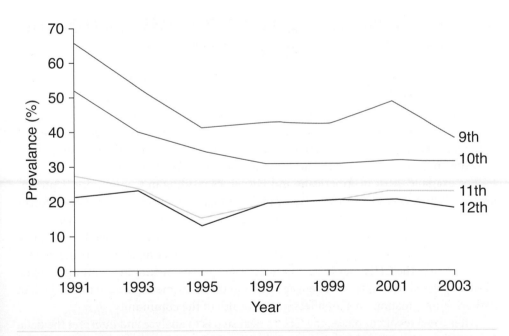

Figure 9-11 Trends in prevalence of high school students attending physical education class daily, by grade, United States, 1991–2003.

Source: Youth Risk Behavior Surveillance System, 1991–2003, National Center for Chronic Disease Prevention and Health Promotion, Centers for Disease Control and Prevention, 2004.

TABLE 9-11
Overweight Persons and Levels of Prevention

Priority *Healthy People 2020* Focus Areas		
Nutrition and Weight Status		Health-Related Quality of Life and Well-being
Primary Prevention Nursing Interventions	Secondary Prevention Nursing Interventions	Tertiary Prevention Nursing Interventions
Review aspects of nutrition and exercise as core to healthy living. Promote taking responsibility for risk behaviors (over-eating).	Use body mass index (BMI) to better understand the meaning of overweight status. Provide food preparation and cooking classes to people who self-identify as overweight (with other family members).	Involve people who have been successful with weight loss to work with others new to improving their health.

The CHN Working with a Multi-problem Concern in the Community

To assist the community in developing appropriate primary, secondary, and tertiary prevention activities, the CHN needs to first assess the health of the community. As part of this assessment, the CHN needs to examine the distribution (i.e., risk) and determinants of health of the particular community. During this phase, the CHN collects demographic data (e.g., age, ethnicity, income, educational level) and examines them to determine how they may be influencing the health outcomes of the community.

For example, African Americans and Hispanics residing in Community "Uptown" are three times more likely to have type 2 diabetes than residents of Community "Downtown." In this situation, the CHN would need to assess the distribution of type 2 diabetes in both communities, along with the possible determinants of health (why these particular ethnic groups are affected by type 2 diabetes) affecting those persons in both communities. The CHN may reach out to key stakeholders within the community (e.g., pastors, priests) in an attempt to engage them in the assessment phase, with the goal of gathering information on gaps affecting the health of the community.

After the assessment phase, the CHN's next step is to analyze and interpret the data. During this phase, the CHN examines all of the data collected (e.g., demographic and health data) for this community to assist the community in developing and planning prevention activities. For example, in the "Uptown" and "Downtown" communities, the data collected during the assessment phase would be analyzed, particularly data on those residents affected with type 2 diabetes, to develop and plan activities such as diabetes awareness initiatives and educational programs.

Throughout this entire process, the community members and CHN need to be partners and stakeholders in identifying, analyzing, planning, and developing an appropriate community health plan, such as prevention activities. As part of this partnership, it is essential that both the community members and the nurse trust each other. Also, it is important that the CHN be receptive to the input of the community members so as to address and accurately identify the health needs of the community.

When developing and planning any community program, a partnership between both entities (e.g., community members and the CHN) is essential. Review the following vignette, "A Multi-problem Concern in an Urban Community."

Although the community's obvious health concerns for adults and children are asthma, diabetes, and obesity, the *primary health concern* has become bullying. The CHN treats the school(s) with bullying as the client. The CHN reviews two *Healthy People 2020* objectives, dealing with mental health and educational and community-based programs. **Table 9-12** provides an example of the *Healthy People 2020* agenda items and levels of prevention used by the CHN to assist in planning care for the schools.

Essential Questions for Setting Priorities

What is important for the community at this current time?

Based on the demographic data collected, asthma, diabetes, and obesity would seem to be the primary health priorities of this urban community. In reality, given the current situation occurring in the schools, the priorities of this community have changed. Now the primary health priority has become bullying.

What is the distribution (i.e., risk) and determinants of health for the health priority identified in this particular community?

Based on the assessment phase, the CHN needs to gather data on the number of people who are admitted to the hospital for bullying. Also the CHN would collect any data available regarding the rates of bullying in this community; any

TABLE 9-12
The CHN Working with a Multi-problem Concern in an Urban Community

Priority *Healthy People 2020* Focus Areas		
Mental Health	**Educational and Community-Based Programs**	
Primary Prevention Nursing Interventions	**Secondary Prevention Nursing Interventions**	**Tertiary Prevention Nursing Interventions**
Discuss bullying as a community concern, focusing on educating the community (including the hospital and schools) on mental and behavioral health. Speak to the teachers and principals of those schools who do not identify bullying as a health concern to create awareness of bullying.	Invite and involve the hospital administrators to meetings with the teachers and principals of the schools and school board in discussions on how to handle behaviors related to bullying in children and adolescents. Create meetings between parents, teachers and healthcare providers (e.g., CHN, social worker) to discuss how to handle behaviors related to bullying of the children and adolescents. Create new initiatives and programs for parents, teachers, and principals on bullying and methods of managing and handling such behavior.	Maintain continuous meetings with parents, teachers and healthcare providers (e.g., CHN, social worker) to provide education on ways to manage behaviors related to bullying of the child or adolescent. Explore developing a parents support program for the parents of those children and adolescents who are admitted to the hospital for behaviors related to bullying. Maintain school board meetings to report feedback on initiatives and programs developed and implemented on bullying, and provide evaluative outcomes.

A Multi-problem Concern in an Urban Community

An urban community of more than 200,000 people comprises an ethnically diverse population. Although the primary health concerns in adults and children living in this community are asthma, diabetes, and obesity, a different health concern affects all residents in the community. Additional investigation suggests that this newly emerging problem will need to be resolved before the community can hope to make any progress in the other health concern areas.

In a large tertiary hospital in this urban community, there has been an alarming rise in the number of admissions in the children's emergency room (ER). This increase is derived from 911 calls placed primarily by public schools in the neighborhood. During the assessment phase, the CHN speaks to the teachers and principals at these schools and learns that 911 is called to deal with children's and adolescents' behaviors. The CHN is informed that the children and adolescents are physically or verbally "misbehaving" or "out of control" in the classroom, and sometimes even violent with other students and teachers.

The teachers and principals describe the students' behavior as "bullying." The teachers and principals state, "We attempt to call the parents and either the telephone numbers are nonworking numbers (e.g., disconnected) or the parents do not answer their phones." They further state, "We have spoken to the parents and understand that the students behave similarly at home, but the parents don't know what to do and feel they have no control." School officials add that they have persistent difficulties with many of the same students and regularly call 911 for them, resulting in the students ending up in the ER.

The statements and issues identified concern the CHN, and the nurse realizes this is a health concern affecting the whole community (e.g., schools, hospital, parents, and all students attending these schools including those with the "bullying" behaviors). Hence, a new priority health concern is identified by the CHN. The CHN is aware that it will take a coordinated effort by many community health providers to address the problem in a meaningful way.

demographic data (e.g., age, gender, ethnicity) on those admitted for bullying; and any reasons, events, or factors that contribute to bullying.

Why is it important to involve other disciplines in the primary, secondary, and tertiary prevention activities in this community?

Given that bullying is the current health priority in this community, representatives from multiple disciplines (e.g., social workers, mental health providers, nurses, and physicians) are important members of the healthcare team. Different members of the healthcare team are essential in assessing this health priority, which affects the teachers, principals, other staff of the schools, families of those with children who are bullying and those who are bullied, and students who witness bullying at the school. Along with community members, these disciplines are important partners in developing, planning, and implementing preventive activities and initiatives in this community.

Summary

This chapter examined the concept of inquiry, focusing on how to assist the client in making proper and productive health choices. The CHN uses skills of inquiry when identifying the appropriate nursing interventions that relate to health promotion, health maintenance, and health restoration. Potential prevention activities may initially attempt to prevent the problem (primary prevention), and then seek to prevent problems (that do occur) from becoming worse or progressing (secondary and tertiary prevention).

Healthy People 2020 represents an attempt to define health priorities within the United States on a national level. Without national guidance, resources may not be allocated appropriately to allow for adequate prevention of problems. Problems may be addressed with a client who is an individual, family, or other group, as well as at the level of the aggregate or community. In the last case, community members are central and essential to making any progress in community health interventions.

REFERENCES

American Nurses Association (ANA). (2001). *Code of ethics for nurses with interpretive statements.* Silver Spring, MD: Author.

American Nurses Association (ANA). (2010a). *Nursing: Scope and standards of practice* (3rd ed.). Silver Spring, MD: Author.

American Nurses Association (ANA). (2010b). *Nursing's social policy statement: The essence of the profession.* Silver Spring, MD: Author.

Centers for Disease Control and Prevention, National Center for Health Statistics (2010). *Health, United States, 2009: With special feature on medical terminology.* Hyattsville, MD: Author.

Domestic Abuse Intervention Project. (n.d.). *Duluth model for physical and sexual violence.* Retrieved from http://www.batteredmen.com/duluwomn2.htm

The Joint Commission. (2011). *Facts about advancing communication, cultural competence, and patient-and-family centered care.* Retrieved from http://www.jointcommission.org/assets/1/18/Advancing_Effective_Comm.pdf

Leavell, H. R., & Clark, E. (1965). Levels of application of preventive measures in the natural history of disease. In H. R. Leavell & E. Clark, *Preventive medicine for the doctor in his community.* New York, NY: McGraw-Hill.

U.S. Department of Health and Human Services (DHHS). (2010, November). *Healthy people 2020.* ODPHP Publication No. B0132. Retrieved from www.healthypeople.gov

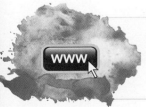

For a full suite of assignments and additional learning activities, use the access code located in the front of your book to visit the exclusive website: http://go.jblearning.com/Holzemer/. If you do not have an access code, you can obtain one at the site.

LEARNING ACTIVITIES

1. Having a conversation with a group of neighbors about exploring chemical analysis of a waste site near their homes is an example of which of the following terms?

   A. Primary prevention
   B. Secondary prevention
   C. Tertiary prevention
   D. Nonprevention fact finding

2. Levels of prevention refer to the stages in which of the following concepts?

   A. Surveillance process
   B. Epidemiological triangle
   C. Natural history of disease
   D. Web of causation

3. The community health nurse encourages a family of survivors of a terror attack to attend a support group, one month after the event. This intervention represents which of the following terms?

   A. Primary prevention
   B. Secondary prevention
   C. Tertiary prevention
   D. Specific protection

ADDITIONAL QUESTIONS FOR STUDY

A nurse is a member of a planning group, whose members are interested in promoting prevention-based behaviors in a community that reflect all levels of prevention. For each of the services, identify the appropriate level of prevention. Choose A, B, or C, where A = primary prevention, B = secondary prevention, and C = tertiary prevention.

1. _____ Volunteering to help others to develop a personal sense of responsibility.

2. _____ Attending long-term grief counseling after the death of a parent.

3. _____ Establishing a study group immediately after failing an examination.

4. _____ Learning about other cultures in an effort to improve understanding and decrease problems from occurring.

5. _____ Administering annual influenza vaccine to children in a school.

6. _____ Anger and frustration assessment in children.

7. _____ Learning responsible parenting, after suspected abuse.

8. _____ Scoliosis identification in primary school.

9. According to the data provided in this chapter, the smallest change in morbidity rates from 1950 and 2003 was found in the area of cancer deaths, when compared to other causes of death. (See Figures 9-7 and 9-8.) What influence do you think that primary, secondary, and tertiary prevention activities have had in preventing deaths from other causes? Why do you think the impact on cancer deaths has been less?

10. Identify a communitywide intervention for primary, secondary, and tertiary prevention, for each of the listed causes of death in Figure 9-1.

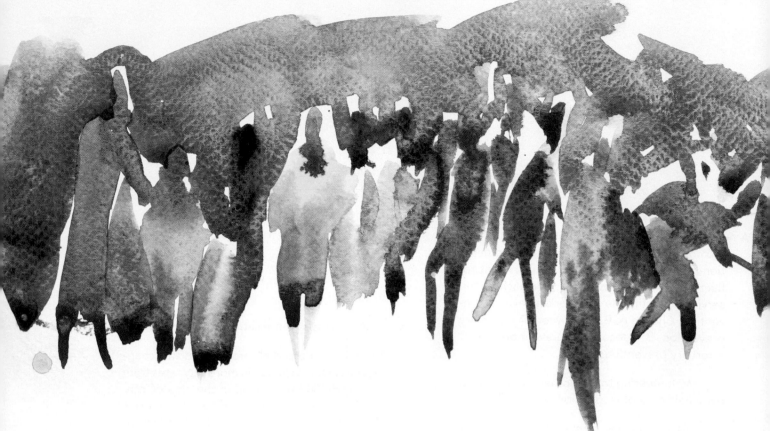

Assessment and Diagnosis Related to the Systems of Care Management and Resource Allocation

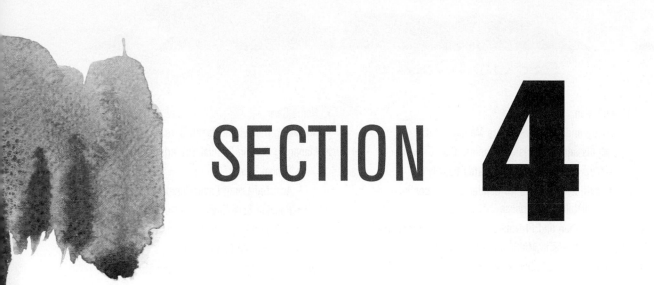

SECTION 4

CHAPTER OUTLINE

- ▸ Introduction
- ▸ Flexibility and Systems of Care Management
- ▸ The Myths and Realities of Seamless Care Delivery
  - • Myth 1: All Clients Are Treated Equally
  - • Myth 2: There Are No Gender Differences in Availability of Services
- ▸ Communication and Providing Care in Various Settings
- ▸ Staffing Patterns in Multiple Levels of Care
- ▸ Managing Care in Public Health in Rural and Urban Settings
- ▸ Managing Care in Acute Primary Care Settings
  - • Emergency Care and Ambulatory Care in Hospitals
  - • Independent Emergency Care Resources

- ▸ Home Care
- ▸ Managing Behavioral Health Care
- ▸ Managing Care in Special Settings
  - • School Health
  - • Assisted-Living Environments
  - • Hospice Care Environments
  - • Community-Based Organizations
  - • Faith-Based Communities
- ▸ Two Personal Stories About Moving Through the Healthcare Delivery System
  - • Eloisa's Story
  - • Jane's Story
- ▸ Summary

OBJECTIVES

1. Explain the need for flexibility in developing and implementing various systems of care delivery.

2. Identify the similarities and differences in meeting the needs of clients in rural and urban settings.

3. Define the nursing role in various settings for clients of various ages.

4. Discuss the potential tension between providing comprehensive care to all clients when the care provider is working from a special interest perspective, like parish nursing, or other faith-based perspective.

KEY TERMS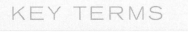

Community-based organization (CBO)

Faith-based community (FBC)

Health ministry

Hospice

School nursing

CHAPTER 10

Flexibility and Systems of Care Management for Providing Care in the Community

Helen Christina Ballestas

Stephen Paul Holzemer

Introduction

This chapter examines the various systems of care management in the community. Clients move through several levels of care to obtain needed health care services. The intent of different levels of care is to provide care to clients by using material and human resources efficiently and effectively. This chapter examines the myth that the current care delivery system is seamless and meeting the needs of the American public.

The role of the community health nurse (CHN) in managing care is explored in rural and urban public health settings, acute primary care (ambulatory and home care) settings, behavioral health care settings, special settings (school health, assisted-living, and hospice care), and community-based organizations and faith-based communities. This chapter also gives voice to clients by including two individuals' personal stories of moving through the healthcare delivery system.

Flexibility and Systems of Care Management

Flexibility is critical in bringing together the various public and private, religious and secular, free and at-cost components of the healthcare delivery system. The CHN has a role in helping manage the services that are available to meet the needs of clients seeking care in the community. One issue of concern is that the CHN, as the provider on the "front lines" of care delivery, or the point of service, is not able to make independent decisions about care management. Instead, the highly complex systems of care management are increasingly being directed by business and fiscal decision makers, far from the client in need of care. Definitions of selected care management settings, as developed by the National Center for Health Statistics (2011), appear in **Table 10-1**.

One concern with managing care relates to the myth that needed services are present and available to clients in a seamless way.

The Myths and Realities of Seamless Care Delivery

Seamless health care is an idealistic notion. Health care itself is a complex entity that involves the cooperative efforts of multiple agencies, professionals, and other institutions that direct and govern how healthcare practice is delivered. Many aspects of health care must be considered—such as the diversity of clients and their needs, the expertise of health professionals, the availability of clinical specialties, and the cost of care—that influence the care that people actually receive. These aspects make the idea of a seamless healthcare delivery experience for clients an impossible notion, at least not without a complex system of care management and great inter-agency and interdisciplinary co-operation. Two myths are discussed in this section that document the need for systems of care that work together effectively to meet the needs of the public.

Myth 1: All Clients Are Treated Equally

While U.S. law requires all healthcare institutions to provide emergency medical services regardless of clients' ability to pay for those services, the reality is that clients with minimal or no insurance coverage may not have access to the services they need. Services that are created for the under-insured and uninsured may not be available because of location, times of operation, or eligibility requirements. The existence of this system

TABLE 10-1
Definitions of Selected Care Management Settings

Health maintenance organization (HMO): An HMO is a healthcare system that assumes or shares both the financial risks and the delivery risks associated with providing comprehensive medical services to a voluntarily enrolled population in a particular geographic area, usually in return for a fixed, prepaid fee. Pure HMO enrollees use only the prepaid, capitated health services of the HMO panel of medical care providers. Open-ended HMO enrollees use the prepaid HMO health services but may also receive medical care from providers who are not part of the HMO panel. There is usually a substantial deductible, copayment, or coinsurance associated with use of nonpanel providers.

Hospital: According to the American Hospital Association (AHA), hospitals are licensed institutions with at least six beds whose primary function is to provide diagnostic and therapeutic patient services for medical conditions; they have an organized physician staff and provide continuous nursing services under the supervision of registered nurses. The World Health Organization (WHO) considers an establishment to be a hospital if it is permanently staffed by at least one physician, can offer inpatient accommodation, and can provide active medical and nursing care. Hospitals may be classified by type of service, ownership, size in terms of number of beds, and length of stay.

Nursing home: A nursing home is a facility that is certified and meets the Centers for Medicare & Medicaid Services' long-term care requirements for Medicare and Medicaid eligibility.

Nursing care home: A nursing care home is a facility that employs one or more full-time registered or licensed practical nurses and provides nursing care to at least half of residents.

Personal care home with nursing: Such a home has fewer than half of residents receiving nursing care. In addition, it employs one or more registered or licensed practical nurses or provides administration of medications and treatments in accordance with physicians' orders, supervision of self-administered medications, or three or more personal services.

Skilled nursing facility: A skilled nursing facility provides the most intensive nursing care available outside a hospital. Facilities certified by Medicare provide posthospital care to eligible Medicare enrollees. Facilities certified by Medicaid as skilled nursing facilities provide skilled nursing services on a daily basis to individuals eligible for Medicaid benefits.

Intermediate care facility: An intermediate care facility is certified by Medicaid to provide health-related services on a regular basis to Medicaid-eligible persons who do not require hospital or skilled nursing facility care but do require institutional care above the level of room and board.

Office visit: In the National Ambulatory Medical Care Survey, a physician's ambulatory practice (office) can be in any location other than in a hospital, nursing home, other extended care facility, patient's home, industrial clinic, college clinic, or family planning clinic. Offices in health maintenance organizations and private offices in hospitals are included.

Outpatient department: According to the National Hospital Ambulatory Medical Care Survey (NHAMCS), an outpatient department (OPD) is a hospital facility where nonurgent ambulatory medical care is provided. The following types of OPDs are excluded from NHAMCS: ambulatory surgical centers, chemotherapy, employee health services, renal dialysis, methadone maintenance, and radiology.

Outpatient surgery: According to the AHA, outpatient surgery is a surgical operation, whether major or minor, performed on patients who do not remain in the hospital overnight. Outpatient surgery may be performed in inpatient operating suites, outpatient surgery suites, or procedure rooms within an outpatient care facility.

Source: National Center for Health Statistics. (2011). *Health, United States, 2010: With special feature on death and dying.* Hyattsville, MD: Author.

suggests that different levels of care are available based on the ability to pay for them. Providers need to stand up to the injustices fostered in a two-tiered healthcare system, and explicate ways that allow all people to get the services they need. The contemporary debate on healthcare reform speaks to the need for making sure that allocated resources are available to those who need them.

Myth 2: There Are No Gender Differences in Availability of Services

Gender neutrality is not apparent, for example, in the assessment, diagnostic, and treatment options available in cardiovascular care. Despite advances in research detailing the differences in gender presentation of cardiovascular disorders such as myocardial infarction (MI), many healthcare providers lack the understanding that MI presents differently in men and women within the clinical setting. Such gender bias may also exist related to diseases that tend to present in females more often than males, such as fibromyalgia. Providers may not consider exploring a disease process that affects one gender more than the other. It requires vigilance and attention to remove bias when treating clients who differ according to gender and other variables such as age, race, and nationality.

Problems with seamless care delivery are becoming more evident and transparent in actual healthcare practices. Today, health care is a business, whose operations are managed by corporations that often do not understand the complexities of client care delivery. All too often, corporate decisions regarding hospital length of stay (LOS) and use of diagnostic testing, laboratory tests, and other services are driven by the financial bottom line. Insurance companies seemingly do not grasp the concept that prevention and screening, in the long run, save money and lives. An investment in primary prevention and early secondary preventive care, considering the health epidemics of diabetes mellitus, obesity, hypertension, hyperlipidemia, and cancer, for example, would have a profound effect on the future financing of health care for all clients in the United States.

Communication and Providing Care in Various Settings

Moving clients through healthcare systems is a daunting task; it is completed for the most part, effectively, on a daily basis. With the advent of continuously changing healthcare technology and the growth of the knowledge base for all health-related professions, however, problems with providing care in a seamless fashion continue to increase. A "disconnect" in how to identify, treat, and evaluate the needs of clients still occurs. Although many issues contribute to this disconnect, one of the biggest challenges is communication (The Joint Commission, 2011).

Communication among healthcare providers is hampered for many reasons, ranging from lack of collaboration between professionals (nurses, physicians, and others) to time constraints in providing care to more acutely ill clients. Unfortunately, the outcome in such cases is often a decrease in effective client management. Conversely, effective communication can improve client management. Theoretically, healthcare technology has been implemented and incorporated, in part, to ease the communication process. Such technology is intended to get information to providers who need the information to make critical decisions and to decrease error rates.

Of course, healthcare technology is only effective when it is used properly. In real-world settings, computers crash; files are erased, lost, and misplaced; differences in nomenclature exist; and providers vary in computer literacy. All of these problems, in turn, contribute to the technology–communication problem. Ultimately, healthcare delivery approaches are limited unless they are supported by effective communication.

Staffing Patterns in Multiple Levels of Care

Research has demonstrated that effective nursing care, with positive care outcomes, is directly correlated to adequate staffing patterns and other safety concerns (Hughes, 2008). Adequate numbers of CHNs are needed to manage care in the many care settings found in the community. Favorable client outcomes, with significant reduction in mortality and morbidity, are possible only when adequate staff is available to provide and manage clients' care. Some institutions believe that the best way to cut their financial debt is to decrease the number of CHNs available to provide care to clients. This practice occurs without regard for the direct positive influence nurses have had on the reduction of pressure ulcers, recognition of complications, improvement of nutrition and hydration, and prevention of falls and other accidents (The Joint Commission, 2011).

Managing Care in Public Health in Rural and Urban Settings

Barriers in maintaining the public's health in rural and urban settings may occur, in part, due to the unique concerns related to geographic location. Large urban hospitals have extensive networking associations that are able to assist in moving clients from one specialty to another specialty, as necessary. The healthcare consumer, in larger urban hospital networks, has ready access to healthcare services due to this connection. Specific public health services, such as immunizations, clean water monitoring, and food production safety concerns, may also be provided and available from multiple providers.

Rural communities have special needs, and CHNs working in those areas can seek support from the National Rural Health Association (ruralhealthweb.org) and the Rural Nurse Organization (rno.org). The special needs of nurses in rural practice center on meeting the three core functions of public health—namely, assessment, health policy, and assurance (Bigbee, Otterness, & Gehrke, 2010). Nurses in rural communities need to be included in the nationwide debate in how the health needs of the public should be met (Association of State and Territorial Directors of Nursing, 2000).

Compared to their urban counterparts, rural clinics and smaller hospitals may not necessarily have as much access to networking with other institutions so as to provide needed care. They often rely on larger urban institutions for complex care, such as advanced trauma care, for clients needing this level of care. Clients may be forced to travel long distances from their homes to receive the level of care they need. In such a case, time becomes a central concern in providing care. The time it takes to transport a critically ill client to a larger city, or the time it takes to assess multiple farms in a suspected *Salmonella* outbreak, has an impact on the health of the public.

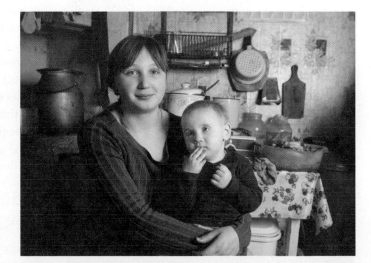
© iStockphoto.com/Moodboard_Images

The unique concerns of rural parts of the country need to be considered in a national response to healthcare needs.

Managing Care in Acute Primary Care Settings

Acute primary care is delivered in emergency departments, in ambulatory care clinics, and in the home via home care services. These levels of care are provided after or in lieu of an acute in-client hospitalization.

Emergency Care and Ambulatory Care in Hospitals

The ongoing healthcare crisis is affecting all aspects of how health services are delivered. Hospital emergency departments and emergent/urgent care clinics are experiencing a major influx of clients, though many of those clients do not actually need emergency care, but rather routine care. Often, clients resort to emergency care for otherwise routine services when they are unable to get timely appointments with their healthcare providers. Accessing the emergency department occurs when seemingly no other choice is left to the client, due to lack of medical insurance, immigrant status, poverty, or the severity of illness related to the unmanaged comorbidities of physical and social diseases such as diabetes, hypertension, and various forms of violence in the community.

Healthcare resources seem to be viewed as infinite by some consumers (and providers). The guarantee of treatment in an emergency department is misused by some

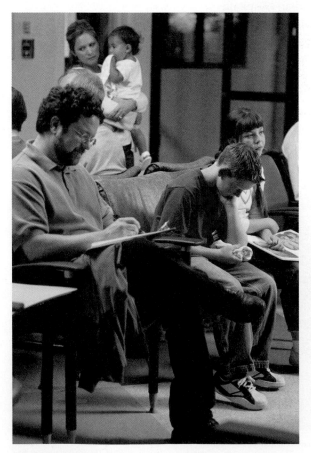

© Ryan McVay/Lifesize/Thinkstock

clients. The majority of clients in this situation are being blamed for misusing resources, when, in fact, there are few other options available to them. Some institutions have responded to this pattern by referring nonemergent clients to a clinic system for care and follow-up. Other institutions move these clients to fast-track services, often managed by nurse practitioners and physician assistants to help scale back costs, while delivering quality care under the supervision of a physician, as necessary.

The major problem that arises when nonemergent clients resort to the emergency department for routine care will not change until adequate care alternatives are developed. A full-scale program of desirable ambulatory care services needs to be developed, outside of a 9:00 A.M. to 5:00 P.M. schedule, to meet the needs of clients who are unable to seek out services during those times (owing to work or childcare issues). Additionally, clustering of ambulatory care services needs to be developed so adults and children can receive comprehensive care in a timely manner. The development of more comprehensive services at the places where people live, work, and go to school is one answer to the question of how to provide services where and when they need healthcare services.

Independent Emergency Care Resources

Independent emergency centers, or urgent care centers, have developed to augment the care people need outside of the hospital environment. "Doc in the box" facilities, where focused yet minimal care is delivered, are examples of community-based organizations that are gaining popularity in today's competitive healthcare environment. These free-standing businesses see clients with basic health issues ranging from lack of immunizations, need for physical examinations and routine blood work, blood pressure management, and other minor emergent problems.

Staffing these facilities are physicians, physician assistants, nurse practitioners, and others working to treat immediate problems. Of major concern is the need to refer clients back to their primary care provider or a designated ambulatory care facility to receive follow-up care. These facilities may also be limited by their inability to perform more sophisticated testing, such as magnetic resonance imaging (MRI), computed tomography (CT) scans, and ultrasound evaluation, that may assist with making a more accurate diagnosis. It is imperative that systems be developed to help the client secure a regular primary care provider, with an accurate record of the many sporadic, episodic care interventions that occur with clients using these facilities.

Home Care

Home care services have increased, in part, due to the shift in healthcare services to include earlier discharges to save healthcare dollars. Clients are followed home by CHNs (and other providers) who provide skilled care that is perceived to be more cost-effective in terms of staffing, infection control, and safety than the option of a longer hospitalization. The perceived advantages of home care include providing care in the client's preferred environment, where easy family access is available.

The disadvantages of home care include the limitations of lay caregivers' interest and ability to provide care that often involves the use of high technology. Caregiver burnout was not anticipated to be such a problem in home care, although the family or support system was often expected to provide care on a round-the-clock basis, without financial compensation. Home care clients are often at the mercy of their insurance carriers when they seek to secure additional skilled or semi-skilled care as part of the goal of making the home a safe place to provide and receive care.

The intent of home care is that professionals, including CHNs, make visits to monitor and provide care related to problems including nutrition and hydration status, medications administration, fall reduction, and improved communication between the client, family, and various providers. The CHN evaluates the client's response to therapy, the need for assistance with activities of daily living, and evidence of social isolation (which may contribute significantly to client depression and anxiety). The CHN advocates for the client, seeking change in the home care environment, when a more assistive or skilled setting is needed for safe care delivery.

Managing Behavioral Health Care

Clients with mental illness and behavioral problems also receive care in the community. Of particular concern is the possibility that their fragile emotional or mental status may make personal, independent decisions difficult. The ability of these clients to make well-reasoned decisions about their care may be further hampered by medication regimens that may compromise their independence for a short or longer period of time. Managing behavioral or mental health care takes time—there are no quick fixes for people in emotional distress.

Although many clients with mental illness and behavioral problems have their care managed without difficulty, problems with routine care and crisis management may

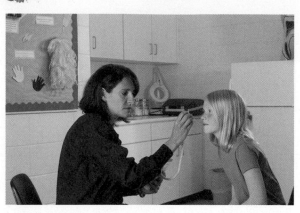

© Brian Eichhorn/ShutterStock, Inc.

result in some clients "falling through the cracks" of the system, and ending up on the streets without support. The growing population of homeless mentally challenged persons is a national problem, and reflects the results of poorly managed behavioral health care. Nurse practitioners and others educated in advanced practice serve as case managers for fragile clients such as the homeless, and other individuals experiencing various mental health crises.

Some clients in the community have dual or triple diagnoses. The client diagnosed with diabetes mellitus, for example, may be schizophrenic as well as addicted to methamphetamine. The client living with HIV/AIDS and alcoholism may also be clinically depressed. It is within the role of the CHN to identify the interlocking medical, psychological, and nursing diagnoses to assist the client in navigating the healthcare delivery system to obtain the needed services. The time the CHN spends with clients gives them special insight into how problems may be solved in the community.

Managing Care in Special Settings

Health care is also managed in special settings. Some of these settings, as discussed in this section, are school health, assisted-living environments, and hospice care environments. Care is also managed in community-based organizations (CBOs) and faith-based communities (FBCs).

School Health

For many of American children, the school nurse may be the only healthcare provider whom they see. The school nurse plays an all-important role in managing care and screening children for a variety of conditions and illnesses. Assessment of vision and hearing, and medication administration following a plan of care (e.g., inhaler use, blood glucose testing, and administration of antibiotics and other medications), are examples of some school nurse responsibilities. The school nurse may also play a pivotal role in discussing and supporting reproductive healthcare choices. Discussions concerning pregnancy and safer sexual practices, including abstinence, are part of this nursing role. School nursing provides children with an advocate for supporting their health care and educational challenges (Vessey & McGowan, 2006; Wolfe, 2012). The National Association of School Nurses (NASN) has clarified the nursing role in educational facilities.

School nursing: A specialized practice of professional nursing that advances the well-being, academic success, and lifelong achievement and health of students.

Definition of School Nursing

The National Association of School Nurses defines **school nursing** as a specialized practice of professional nursing that advances the well-being, academic success, and lifelong achievement and health of students. To that end, school nurses facilitate normal development and positive student response to interventions; promote health and safety, including a healthy environment; intervene with actual and potential health problems; provide case management services; and actively collaborate with others to build student and family capacity for adaptation, self-management, self-advocacy, and learning (NASN, 2010).

Across the United States, violence, weapon possession, drug sale and use, and behavioral problems such as bullying are becoming more pervasive in our schools. School nurses must be at the ready to care for children who are hurt on school grounds, with injuries ranging from minor cuts or scrapes to more serious physical and emotional wounds. Providing education to parents, teachers, administration, and children is the main role of the school nurse. The nurse professional must become fluent in physical aspects of health such as reproductive health and the law, as well as psychological aspects of health such as violence prevention and coping with the possibility of disasters.

The National Health Education Standards (NHES) are written expectations for what students should know and be able to do by grades 2, 5, 8, and 12 to promote personal, family, and community health (**Table 10-2**). The school health nurse, working with teachers and other school officials, assists students in meeting their health goals.

To meet national standards, the role of the school nurse has evolved from provider of first aid services to health professional who is most responsible for the health of children and adolescents. As part of this role, the nurse must assist students with a bundle of complex physical and emotional barriers to learning.

Assisted-Living Environments

As the population of the United States ages, increasing numbers of clients need assistance with activities of daily living. Assisted-living facilities provide a level of supervision that allows the older person to live as independently as possible, albeit in a supervised environment.

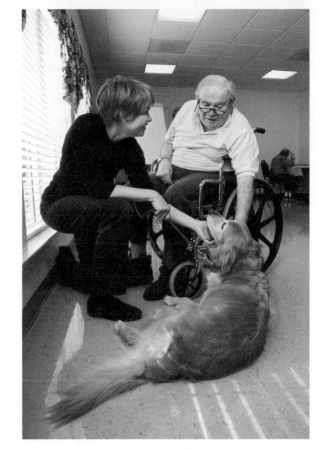
© iofoto/ShutterStock, Inc.

TABLE 10-2
National Health Education Standards

Standard 1: Students will comprehend concepts related to health promotion and disease prevention to enhance health.

Standard 2: Students will analyze the influence of family, peers, culture, media, technology, and other factors on health behaviors.

Standard 3: Students will demonstrate the ability to access valid information, products, and services to enhance health.

Standard 4: Students will demonstrate the ability to use interpersonal communication skills to enhance health and avoid or reduce health risks.

Standard 5: Students will demonstrate the ability to use decision-making skills to enhance health.

Standard 6: Students will demonstrate the ability to use goal-setting skills to enhance health.

Standard 7: Students will demonstrate the ability to practice health-enhancing behaviors and avoid or reduce health risks.

Standard 8: Students will demonstrate the ability to advocate for personal, family, and community health.

Source: Joint Committee on National Health Education Standards. (2007). *National health education standards: Achieving excellence* (2nd ed.). Atlanta, GA: American Cancer Society.

The supervision may be as minimal as occasional discussions with staff, while the client (resident) is living in a private apartment, to placement in a structured housing unit for clients living with dementia or Alzheimer's disease. Frequently, assisted-living facilities have a semi-skilled and skilled nursing care unit for residents needing extended (including 24-hour) supportive care.

Although these facilities have their own nursing staff, the CHN may visit residents who are more independent in their living, or who come to the facility to complete special educational programming. The CHN could focus on groups of older persons to identify and meet their educational needs. The CHN may also be involved in special programs that bring young children into the facility to talk to and interact with the residents. "Foster grandparent" programs are provided to enrich the experience of the children as well as the older person. In addition, the CHN may assist residents with interacting with others outside of the assisted-living environment.

Hospice Care Environments

Hospice: Care of the dying person; more formally, care of a person who has received a medical diagnosis and has an anticipated prognosis of less than six months to live.

Care of the dying person is a responsibility of all healthcare providers and institutions. When the medical diagnosis is made and the client has an anticipated prognosis of less than six months to live, then a referral to **hospice** may be made. Whether the care is delivered as an outpatient or an inpatient, never has the need for a seamless transition been so important. Given the multiplicity of emotions felt by patients and their families, moving through the death and dying process should be a smooth transition, supported by an environment that respects the unique needs of the dying person.

Nevertheless, ideas about death and dying and the possibility of a "good death" experience are not universally agreed upon. Many individuals think that people have a right to a "good death"; death, like birth, is a part of life. The process of death and the ways in which laypeople and professionals think about death vary. This variation is evident in how one answers even the most basic questions: How does the practitioner feel about death? Are the client and family ready for death? How does the concept of fear play into the dying process?

Hospice plays an integral role in assisting clients and families during this stressful time. Hospice provides needed care of the dying patient both in and out of the hospital, meeting the client's needs via pain management, sedation, comfort measures, wound care, ventilator support, psychological care, and other basic needs as the individual moves through the death and dying process. Hospice also tends to the family members who are looking for solace and comfort during a difficult time. The needs of clients and families are reflected in the hospice philosophy statement of the National Hospice and Palliative Care Organization (NHPCO).

> Hospice provides support and care for persons in the last phases of an incurable disease so that they may live as fully and as comfortably as possible. Hospice recognizes that the dying process is a part of the normal process of living and focuses on enhancing the quality of remaining life. Hospice programs provide state-of-the-art palliative care and supportive services to individuals at the end of their lives, their family members and significant others, 24 hours a day, seven days a week, in both the home and facility-based care settings. Physical, social, spiritual, and emotional care are provided by a clinically-directed interdisciplinary team consisting of patients and their families, professionals, and volunteers during the last stages of an illness, the dying process, and the bereavement period. (NHPCO, 2007)

Within the hospital unit, hospice care includes assuring patient and family privacy, facilitation of communication between healthcare providers and patient and family, safe and supportive nursing care, and comfort and palliative care. Home hospice offers the patient and family a high degree of privacy, a familiar environment, and material possessions that are comforting to the patient, such as a favorite quilt or blanket, pets, pictures, and younger family members at the bedside (NHPCO, 2007).

Community-Based Organizations

Community-based organizations often are developed to augment care that is needed by the community in an other-than-hospital type of setting. Free-standing organizations may provide education, support, and often a level of direct care. A community may support a CBO related to cancer care, for example, that provides education about cancer, screens for commonly occurring neoplasms, and provides support groups for cancer survivors. In another example, a CBO for women's health care may provide specific reproductive counseling that is not offered by a hospital or medical center with strong religious ties that do not support full-choice options for women. A CBO may be developed for a particular genetic disorder, sponsored by a special interest group. A CBO with a focus on alcohol and other drug rehabilitation may develop in an area because of a lack of other services for persons in the community with substance abuse issues.

An overarching concern with the development and maintenance of CBOs relates to the "fit" of these organizations with the overall health services needs of the community. Services for the whole community, whether hospital based, CBO based, or home based, should be coordinated and available to the public as needed. The shape of service delivery models is not as important as the fact that clients can get the services they need from qualified professionals.

Faith-Based Communities

Faith community nursing is a part of a broader outreach—namely, health ministry. A **health ministry** focuses on the health and healing needs of the members of a particular faith community and its extended community. In **faith-based communities**, people find continuing connectedness, encouragement, hope, and love. Health ministries continue this tradition by centering on personal presence, listening, and teaching. Examples of health ministries include programs directed toward visiting the homebound or sick; encouraging healthy lifestyles; providing support—either individually or in groups; presenting information on health promotion and disease prevention; monitoring individual concerns and needs; connecting through written or telephone communications; and other activities (American Nurses Association [ANA] & Health Ministries Association [HMA], 2005; Hickman, 2005).

The vision of the Health Ministries Association, an association for faith community nurses, is to engage, educate, and empower people of faith to be passionate and effective leaders for creating healthier communities. This organization's mission is to encourage, support, and empower leaders in the integration of faith and health in their local communities.

Faith community nurses, or parish or congregation nurses, have a variety of roles in the community (ANA & HMA, 2005; Hickman, 2005). The CHN in this field would, for example, have the opportunity to participate in the roles identified in **Table 10-3**. A special sensitivity is needed in caring for clients who may self-identify as atheist, agnostic, or non-religious. Faith community nurses are aware that clients should not be made to feel uncomfortable if they have non-faith-based beliefs.

Community-based organization (CBO): In health care, a local organization developed to augment care that is needed by the community in an other-than-hospital type of setting; such free-standing organizations may provide education, support, and a level of direct care.

Health ministry: A type of outreach that focuses on the health and healing needs of the members of a particular faith community and its extended community.

Faith-based community (FBC): A group of people who find continuing connectedness, encouragement, hope, and love through a shared sense of faith.

TABLE 10-3
Roles of the Parish Nurse

Health Educator: Focusing on a variety of educational activities for all ages that explore the relationship between values, attitudes, lifestyle, faith, and health.

Personal Health Counselor: Assisting individuals to deal with health issues and problems; may include hospital, home, nursing home, and other visits.

Referral Agent: Providing congregational and community resources for healing and wellness.

Health Advocate: Encouraging all systems (congregant, faith community, primary health resources) to find the best solution for healing and wholeness—body, mind, and spirit.

Facilitator of Volunteers: Recruiting and coordinating resources within the faith community to serve in its various health ministries.

Developer of Support Groups: Facilitating the development of support groups to meet member needs and those of the external community.

Integrator of Faith and Health: Seeking, in all activities and contacts, to promote the understanding of the relationship between faith and health.

Two Personal Stories About Moving Through the Healthcare Delivery System

Care settings have become so specialized that it could be expected that any person needing care might interact with more than one setting. An adolescent may receive emergency care at a hospital, to be followed with supervision of the recovery process by a school nurse. A person at the end of life may receive care at home, yet need a transfer to an in-hospital hospice due to some complication. A severely ill neonate nay need intensive care, while the single mother receives support from a CBO specializing in mental health.

The two personal stories presented here relate to problems with clients moving through the healthcare delivery system. The first story is about Eloisa, who disappeared in the healthcare system for three days. The second story is about Jane, who, after being in an accident, was suddenly expected to cope with a six-week hospital and rehabilitation experience. These stories are followed by essential questions that the CHN must ask when caring for clients in any journey through the healthcare delivery system.

Eloisa's Story

Introduction

Eloisa is a 98-year-old Hispanic female living in a large metropolitan city. A fiercely independent woman, she lives in an apartment by herself, despite the concerns of her family. Eloisa disappeared for three days within the healthcare system of this large city. Her family and local law enforcement checked every hospital, clinic, emergency room, restaurant, diner, supermarket, bodega, bus terminal, surrounding building, basement, and friend's house, and along the river walk, for 3 frantic days. The story of how healthcare institutions contributed to, and aided in, the recovery of Eloisa is an example of the good, the bad, and the ugly of today's healthcare system expectation of a seamless transition.

Eloisa has glaucoma, macular degeneration, mild Alzheimer's dementia, and diminishing hearing. She also has a history of multiple cerebral infarcts. Yet she maintains the ability to meet her activities of daily living, as her physical ability, gait, and balance are not disturbed. On one of her daily outings, she becomes confused. She cannot remember where she is, who she is, and what she is doing. Frantically, she attempts to find something within her environment that is recognizable, something signaling that she is near her home, but nothing seems familiar. In her confusion, she falls and hits her head on the pavement in front of a local theater company.

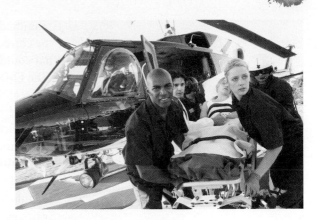

© Monkey Business Images/ShutterStock, Inc.

Emergency Medical Services

The theater company calls the emergency medical services (EMS) system when employees find an elderly female lying on the ground in front of their theater. When EMS caregivers arrive, Eloisa is aroused and able to give her name correctly. She is taken to the local emergency department (ED) for care. Eloisa is frightened by her new environment and becomes combative. Factors that lead to the combative behavior are the awareness that she is not home, a lack of familiar faces in the ED, and the absence of someone who speaks her language. While the ED providers do everything possible to make this patient comfortable, Eloisa is in a crisis state of mind.

Hospitalization

Upon admission, Eloisa is asked her name again, and this time she gives an entirely different name. The name given by the client the second time is not verified with the name given to the EMS staff originally. Meanwhile, Eloisa's family is calling every hospital within 50 miles of her home. Each call to the various EDs leads to the same result: "No one was admitted to the ED with that name." The family contacts local authorities and after the first 24 hours of disappearance, the case is assigned to the detective unit.

Diligently, the detectives work out the details of the person, the last known site seen, the clothing that she was wearing, identifiable information that she might have on her person, frequent spots visited, and addresses of other family members in the vicinity. After an exhaustive search, the detectives make a discovery. They check local EMS records from the day of disappearance to find that an ambulance picked up an elderly woman. But where did it take her? EMS records are reviewed and the hospital is identified. Upon checking the hospital, the detectives find that Eloisa was never admitted. How is this possible? Again, the name given by the client was not verified with the name given to the EMS staff. Armed with a picture of Eloisa, the detectives visit each hospital again. They finally make a startling discovery: Eloisa was indeed admitted to a nearby hospital, as verified by photography. The family is elated to find their family member and is eternally grateful to the detectives for their diligent search.

Essential Questions

What could have been done differently from the perspective of the hospital?

Hospitals need to check the accuracy of their admission records, especially in a case involving an acutely confused client. The hospital needs to provide a way for staff providing care and working in admitting offices to list clients who are admitted with confusion, and to verify demographic information that may not be correct.

What could have been done differently from the perspective of EMS?

The EMS staff need to acknowledge the level of confusion exhibited by some clients, and identify their history as possibly inaccurate. An immediate social services referral could be made to cluster information on confused clients for easier identification. A clearinghouse for client identification could be developed in all communities as the population ages.

What could have been done differently by the client and family?

Special identification cards could be carried by mobile clients who are at risk for confusion and wandering, depending on their level of cooperation. Families could work with local institutions to establish policies and procedures to assist with the proper identification of clients. Navigating the waters of health care is far from easy. An effort to work with the special needs of clients and their families, including the special needs of the elderly, should be a priority, because of the cognitive changes that are a part of long-term care.

Jane's Story

Introduction

My name is Jane and I am 54 years old. I work in the financial industry as an executive assistant, and I am an actor as well. I do various projects and plays throughout the year at an Off-Off Broadway theater. I lead a very active, engaging life. I am lucky enough to have good health insurance through my day job.

On February 3, I was walking to the subway to come to work at 8:30 A.M. It was a particularly icy and slippery day. I was just starting to cross the street and, as I stepped off the curb, I twisted my ankle. I felt a snap. As I went down, I heard someone screaming and realized it was me. The pain was instantaneous and far greater than I had ever felt before.

Emergency Medical Services

Within a very short time, people on the street had called for emergency medical technicians (EMTs), and they were on their way. Looking at my foot was upsetting to me as my leg was going one direction and my foot another and there was a large lump forming on the inside of my ankle. When the EMTs arrived, they were very careful with me—they got me onto the stretcher and into the van without hurting my ankle any further. To move it in any way was excruciatingly painful. The two men worked very well as a team. Once I was in the van, they asked if I could please not scream as it was a very small space. We laughed, and they tried to calm me down.

The EMTs took me to the closest emergency department, a satellite of a large metropolitan hospital. On the way there, they told me that they thought it was probably just a bad dislocation and that I would be in and out soon. They reassured me the team there was great at the ED, so I was in good shape. All in all, they were very supportive and efficient. They promised to look in on me throughout the day. That was very comforting. Knowing that they were concerned about me and my injury helped me face the unknown that was coming.

Hospitalization

My accident happened at 8:30 A.M. By 9:45 A.M., I was in a bed in the ED. Some of the timing in the ED is a bit fuzzy for me after this, as I was drifting in and out of consciousness because of the pain medication I received. I could not eat all day either, as the providers were not certain if I was going to have surgery. Extreme pain takes you a bit out of yourself, and the pain medications remove you a bit further. They had to set my ankle three times, as my break was pretty severe. The pain medication they gave me relieved the pain quickly, but unfortunately, the pain came back quickly as well. During the first part of the day, the staff was pretty attentive to my medication needs; that changed as the day continued.

It did seem that as the day wore on, I was given less priority. Although I became more and more hungry and exhausted, I was less a priority. I think they got used to me! A case came in late in the day that was pretty serious. At that point, I really was no longer a priority for the staff. Luckily I was waiting on a bed to be transferred to the parent hospital.

One of the biggest drawbacks of being in the hospital for a patient is the fact that you live in public. I had no control over who entered my room or at what time, what the noise level was around me, or when I would do whatever activity I had that any number of people had scheduled for that day. It was very difficult. The nurses are a patient's link to the hospital. If anyone knows what is going on with a patient, it is the nurse. I cannot tell you how important that relationship is. And even though the nurses are there 12 hours a day, they do get to go home and leave the environment of the hospital. As a patient, you do not. You have to stay there—in a crisis environment—until someone else decides you are well enough to go home.

All that being said, I thought the care I received was excellent. The majority of the nurses I had were so very conscientious and hard working. The more specific and focused the nurse was, the better I felt about the care I was receiving. My favorite nurse was one who at the beginning of every shift would come in with my chart and review everything and address any needs that had arisen. It did not matter if he had seen me the day before; he took the time to carefully review everything and touch base to see how it all was going. I never felt like an imposition; he really did know what my condition was, and what my needs were on a daily basis. The doctors would come by once a day; they would quickly review my case and then off they would go. They kept track of the general overview, but the day-to-day specifics of my case were in the hands of the nurses. The care I received from the nurses was pivotal in my recovery.

While I was in the hospital, after my first surgery, my mother passed away. She had been sick, but we expected her to live a bit longer. So here I was, in the hospital recovering from surgery and having to deal with the death of my mother. Luckily, for the most part, around this time the staff who took care of me remained constant, so they were aware of my emotional fragility. They were supportive and understanding. That was the case for the first few days after her death. It was very helpful. As time went on and I was shifted from room to room, that was not the case.

In the hospital, they treated me with respect and courtesy. Then, once I began to be able to move around, the level of debilitation I had sunk to proved shocking. To walk 10 feet was a huge effort. Partly because of my limitations and the sudden nature of the injury and the length of stay I had in the hospital, I was desperate to get out—to get back into the real world, as it was. I felt so isolated and cut off from my life and any semblance of a reality that I enjoyed and felt I could participate in. So, as soon as possible, I left for rehab. I was in the hospital for 4 weeks and 1 day.

Subacute Rehabilitation

I went to subacute rehab because I did not have the strength for acute rehab. Unfortunately for me, the rehab center I went to was populated mostly by elderly people. I was the youngest person there by 15 to 20 years. My situation was opposite to the situation in the center in so many ways! I wanted to stay there for 1 to 2 weeks. The standard of care shifted dramatically from the hospital to the nursing facility. There were more patients per nurse there, and the nurses seemed to run constantly. The care of the patients was left primarily to the aides, and that was not to the benefit of the patients. The response time between when the bell was rung and when someone would arrive doubled. I was on complete non-weight-bearing status and could not walk more than 20 feet when I got there. I was still in a highly dependent state.

I would see the nurse once a day—usually at the beginning of his or her shift. The nurses would hurriedly go through the medication and any notes they had, and do the wound care necessary for my injury. That would be it for the day, unless I requested medication, in which case there would be a hurried visit. Any of my other needs were attended to by the aides. It was as if their work was never done, so they just "gave up" on getting it done. I would ring the bell for assistance and often wait 25 to 30 minutes for help. I believe that this attitude came partly from dealing with elderly patients. The aides seemed to think that I did not know what was best for me and that they had a clearer picture of what was in my best interest.

Their attitude was verging on condescending. To get anything done in a timely manner, you had to play nice with them—to please them so they would not get angry and leave you alone to stew in whatever mess you were in. There was an undercurrent in the place that was very unhealthy. It took the staff 4 to 5 days to grasp my situation—that is, what my needs were and what I hoped to accomplish. By that time, I was so frustrated and fed up, I left by day 7. They suggested I stay another week to get stronger, and I was approved by my insurance to do so, but I was fed up with having to fight for everything I needed. I had to state my needs over and over before anyone would pay attention.

I was discharged home, with many limitations, to the care of a network of friends and occasional visits by the Visiting Nurse Service. I left the rehabilitation facility as soon as I could, preferring to be housebound and looked after by my friends rather than in such a noncaring environment. I had hesitated to go home, as I live alone, and would have to rely on friends to take care of me instead of professionals. After the stress of having to state and state again my goals and needs, being at home was so much more attractive, even with the stress of having to rely on my friends, with minimal professional supervision.

Throughout my stay in the hospital, I was keeping my friends updated as to my situation on Facebook. Two different friends suggested a website to me, LotsaHelpingHands, as a place to go to organize the volunteers whom I needed to take care of me. When I left rehab, I still needed care on a 24/7 basis. This website let me create my own calendar and requests for help. With any friends who volunteered, I made them a member of the group and could send emails to them and give them access to the calendar to see with what and when they could help. This worked amazingly well for me. I had more than 50 friends sign up to help.

For the first week, I had someone with me around the clock. The next week I dropped the overnight caregivers, as I was comfortable enough to be on my own to sleep. A week or so later, I cut the shifts down to center on the meals only, and in a few more weeks it was even less time. The website proved to be so helpful, not only for scheduling people, but also for letting people know what was going on. I knew that I was contacting people who wanted to be actively involved in my recovery.

Essential Questions

What could have been done differently from the perspective of the hospital and the skilled rehabilitation facility?

Hospitals and other healthcare facilities need to monitor their "on-time" delivery of services. The emotional state of clients should not be considered adequate for them to be expected to negotiate with so many different people to meet their needs. Client ambassadors or patient care advocates need to monitor the day-to-day operations of care, rather than waiting for a crisis to occur. More attention needs to be given to prepare clients for a change in care that occurs when moving from one level of care (and facility) to another.

What could have been done differently by the client and family?

Clients and identified family members or significant others need to have the opportunity to prepare themselves for differing systems of care delivery, and the level of care each system provides. More attention should be given to the special needs of clients when transfer to another facility is planned. Although the transfer from one facility to another is often driven by finances, transferring clients to a facility on a weekend, when services are not available, should be avoided.

Summary

A variety of systems of care management are present in the community, and clients often move through various levels of care to obtain needed healthcare services. The intent of different levels of care is to provide services to clients while using material and human resources efficiently and effectively. This chapter examined the myth that the current care delivery system is seamless and meeting the needs of the American public. The role of the CHN in assisting with care management may take place in rural and urban public health settings, acute primary care (ambulatory and home care) settings, behavioral health care settings, special settings (school health, assisted living and hospice care) settings, community-based organizations, and faith-based communities.

REFERENCES

American Nurses Association (ANA) & Health Ministries Association (HMA). (2005). *Faith community nursing: Scope and standards of practice.* Silver Springs, MD: Authors.

Association of State and Territorial Directors of Nursing. (2000). *Public health nursing: A partner for healthy populations.* Washington, DC: American Nurses Association.

Bigbee, J. L., Otterness, N., & Gehrke, P. (2010). Public health nursing competency in a rural/frontier state. *Public Health Nursing, 27*(3), 270–276.

Hickman, J. S. (2005). *Faith community nursing.* Philadelphia, PA: Lippincott Williams & Wilkins.

Hughes, R. G. (Ed.). (2008). *Patient safety and quality: An evidence-based handbook for nurses.* Rockville, MD: Agency for Healthcare Research and Quality.

The Joint Commission. (2011). *Facts about advancing communication, cultural competence, and patient- and family-centered care.* Retrieved from http://www.jointcommission.org/assets/1/18/Advancing_Effective_Comm.pdf

Joint Committee on National Health Education Standards. (2007). *National health education standards: Achieving excellence* (2nd ed.). Atlanta, GA: American Cancer Society.

National Association of School Nurses (NASN). (2010). *Definition of school nursing.* Retrieved from http://www.nasn.org/Default.aspx?tabid=57

National Center for Health Statistics. (2011). *Health, United States, 2010: With special feature on death and dying.* Hyattsville, MD: Author.

National Hospice and Palliative Care Organization (NHPCO). (2007). *Hospice philosophy statement.* Alexandria, VA: Author.

Vessey, J., & McGowan, K. (2006). A successful public health experiment: school nursing. *Pediatric Nursing, 32*(3), 255–256.

Wolfe, L. C. (2012). The profession of school nursing. In J. Selekman, *School nursing: A comprehensive text.* Philadelphia, PA: F. A. Davis.

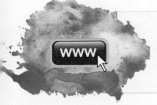

LEARNING ACTIVITIES www.

1. To which of the following care settings would a CHN refer, or arrange to immediately transfer, a client with unpredicted behavior and fluctuating vital signs?

   A. A hospital
   B. An assisted-living facility
   C. A skilled nursing facility
   D. A hospice program

2. To which of the following care settings would a CHN refer, or arrange to immediately transfer, a client with a need for assistance with one or two activities of daily living?

   A. A hospital
   B. An assisted-living facility
   C. A skilled nursing facility
   D. A hospice program

3. To which of the following care settings would a CHN refer, or arrange to immediately transfer, a client without an acute problem, but with an inability to participate in self-care?

   A. A hospital
   B. An assisted-living facility
   C. A skilled nursing facility
   D. A hospice program

ADDITIONAL QUESTIONS FOR STUDY

1. Thinking about the "Eloisa's Story," what essential information should older persons (or potentially disoriented or confused clients) carry on their person?

2. How should the person carry the information so a healthcare provider could find it?

3. How would electronic medical records assist in improving care for clients moving from one care setting to another?

CHAPTER OUTLINE

- ▶ Introduction
- ▶ Justice and Resource Allocation
- ▶ The Myths and Realities of Resource Allocations
  - Myth 1: My personal health insurance will cover everything I need for my family and myself.
  - Myth 2: All people need the same services because morbidity and mortality rates are essentially the same for everyone.
  - Myth 3: The care of children is the number one priority in American health care. All healthcare services for pregnant women and child care are equal.
- ▶ Federal, State, and Local Government Funding for Health Care
  - Medicare
  - Medicaid
- ▶ Third-Party Reimbursement
- ▶ Philanthropy
- ▶ Service Learning and Volunteerism
- ▶ The Limits of Futile Care and Outspending Healthcare Resources
- ▶ Resource Allocation as a Global Concern
- ▶ Summary

OBJECTIVES

www

1. Explain the meaning between the myths and realities of healthcare financing.

2. Identify groups or populations that may not be able to negotiate for the resources they need in health care.

3. Explore the concept of resource allocation from the local, national, and international or global perspectives.

4. Link the reality of resource allocation with the values and beliefs of the people who secure resources for themselves and others.

KEY TERMS

www

"Doughnut hole" (in Medicare)

Formulary

Futile care

Global health

Medicaid

Medicare

Not-for-profit (non-profit) organization

Resource allocation

Secondary insurance

Third-party reimbursement

CHAPTER 11

Justice and Resource Allocation for the Family and Community

Maureen C. Roller

Introduction

This chapter examines the way healthcare resources are allocated. It begins with a discussion of three myths and realities of resource allocation. Next, it examines the official role of federal, state, and local governments in funding healthcare services. This chapter also reviews private efforts directed toward funding health care, such as philanthropy, service learning, and volunteerism. The limits of "futile care" are also examined in terms of this issue's impact on healthcare expenditures. Resource allocation is a primary concern of the community health nurse (CHN) as programs are developed to meet the needs of clients in the community. Responsible resource allocation allows for meeting the needs of clients needing services both today and in the future.

Justice and Resource Allocation

Resource allocation is the way a community distributes its available funds among competing groups and programs. Decision making about resource allocation in the community includes a balancing act of healthcare needs versus social needs. The resources could be allocated for groups, programs, and individual needs. The ethical principle of justice is a key concern for resource allocation. As noted earlier in this text, justice is an ethical concept that suggests that there is a fair way to allocate resources (Rawls, 1971). Justice requires the existence of a transparent way of meeting the needs of persons with various threats to their health in the community, by distributing healthcare resources fairly.

Resource allocation can be considered just when it meets the needs of families and groups in the community. Examples of just resource allocation may include providing a senior citizen services center, a teen work/study center, needed medical equipment, or a meeting space for health teaching. Other programs could include providing health fairs, cancer screening, and exercise programs to promote a healthy lifestyle changes in the community. The mix of services needs to closely correspond to the mix of client needs.

Individual needs, for example, might be addressed with justice through resource allocation to indigent clients (or other vulnerable clients) seeking health care in the community or hospital. Americans must decide how to allocate the resources that best suit their individual community, thereby promoting a just society ("Resource Allocations," 2010). Vulnerable clients need to be given a voice, and they need to be able to participate in the discussion about how resources should be allocated (de Chesnay & Anderson, 2008).

The Myths and Realities of Resource Allocations

Numerous myths have emerged in conjunction with healthcare delivery, often related to the way resources are allocated to meet the needs of the community. Three such myths are identified here, along with the complementary realities of healthcare delivery.

Myth 1: My personal health insurance will cover everything I need for my family and myself.

The U.S. healthcare system continues to change; most Americans contribute to their healthcare costs. Demands on resource allocations for health care are increasing due to skyrocketing healthcare costs. Due to population shifts owing to an aging population and the high cost of health care, the existing healthcare system is evolving into a managed care system that places a greater emphasis on prevention, health promotion, and

Resource allocation: The way a community distributes its available funds among competing groups and programs.

wellness (de Tornyay, 1992; Malloch & Porter-O'Grady, 2010). Allocation of resources depends on the various levels of government funding, and other resources available for the community that needs them.

Public hospitals subsidize approximately 70% of inpatient care and approximately 50% of outpatient and ambulatory services. The coverage of patients' health benefits depends on the insurance provider—specifically, whether it is a private company or the government health insurance system. Before World War II, most individuals directly paid the physician for services rendered. An analysis comparing hospital care to home care costs on an international basis revealed that costs were lower for clients who received care in the community setting; this meta-analysis included 10 studies from Australia, Italy, the United Kingdom, and New Zealand of stroke victims' care (Shepperd et al., 2009).

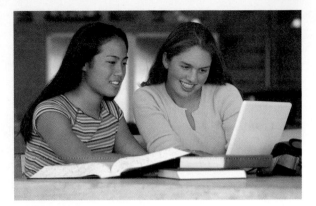

© LiquidLibrary

The values and beliefs of a community will dictate which resources are allocated and to whom. Diversity within cultures and between groups in the community will influence how resources are utilized as well. Community health nurses need to evaluate the health needs of the populations whom they serve to encourage appropriate healthcare services allocations. Community-based organizations are especially widely used health-related facilities in the United States, as the country does not have an integrated national, state, and local health system guaranteed to its citizens (Institute of Medicine, 2011).

The number of uninsured adults in the United States increased 60% from 2003 to 2007, when this population reached an estimated 25 million. The uninsured group includes both individuals below the poverty level and middle-income Americans who cannot afford health insurance. "More than half of the underinsured (53%), and two-thirds of the uninsured (68%) went without needed [health] care—including not seeing a doctor when sick, not filling prescriptions, and not following-up on recommended tests or treatments. Only 31 percent of insured adults went without such limited care" (Schoen, Collins, Kriss, & Doty, 2008, p. 1). Underinsured and uninsured Americans typically lack the ability to access health care due to the increasing cost of insurance. How does this situation affect the health of the public? Lack of vaccinations, screening tests, and procedures surely leads to more expensive treatment of conditions later in life, when they have become more severe.

On March 23, 2010, President Barack Obama signed into law the Affordable Care Act. This law puts into place comprehensive health insurance reforms that are intended to hold insurance companies more accountable and lower healthcare costs, guarantee more healthcare choices, and enhance the quality of health care for all Americans ("Understanding the Affordable Care Act," 2010). It has a goal of improving access to quality health care for all Americans and should help reduce health disparities in the population as a whole ("Health Disparities and the Affordable Care Act," 2010). Changes in the U.S. healthcare system through this federal legislation are due to take effect in most areas by 2014. (The law is currently being reviewed by the U.S. Supreme Court, and the Court's decision on the act's legality will determined whether some, or all, parts of it are ultimately implemented.)

Myth 2: All people need the same services because morbidity and mortality rates are essentially the same for everyone.

To take but one example, rates for new cancer diagnoses (incidence) and deaths vary widely among people of different racial groups (**FIGURE 11-1**). In the United States, rates of new cancer cases and deaths from cancer in 2007 among African Americans and white

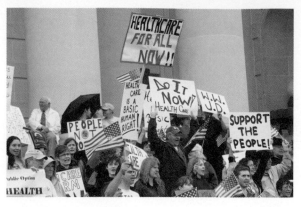

Americans were higher than those among Asian and Pacific Islander Americans. By comparison, lower rates were found among American Indians and Alaskan Natives. Male cancer rates and deaths were higher than the corresponding rates for females across all racial groups (National Cancer Institute, 2010; U.S. Cancer Statistics Working Group, 2010). Resources need to be allocated to affect health outcomes among all populations in need.

Of course, healthcare allocation decisions cannot be made by simply referring to one chart or data set. For discussion purposes, consider that the variability of the rates in Figure 11-1 suggests that further information is needed. Women who are less affected by cancer incidence may be seen as needing fewer resources in cancer care. In fact, this is not the case when data are reviewed related to breast, ovarian, and uterine cancers. Care must be taken to make decisions from oversimplified data.

Myth 3: The care of children is the number one priority in American health care. All healthcare services for pregnant women and child care are equal.

Infant mortality rates (IMRs) vary widely among racial groups. **Table 11-1** compares the IMRs among women of different racial or ethnic backgrounds between 2000 and 2006.

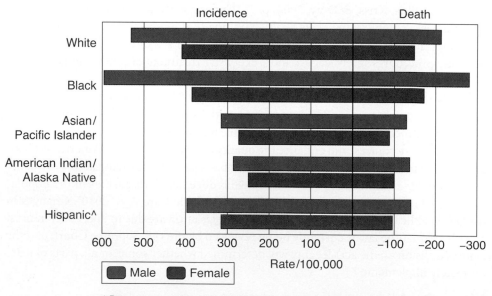

Figure 11-1 Rates* of new cancer cases and deaths by race/ethnicity and sex, United States, 2007.

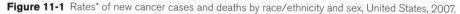

Source: National Cancer Institute. (2010). *Health disparities defined.* Rockville, MD: U.S. Department of Health and Human Services, National Institutes of Health, National Cancer Institute; U.S. Cancer Statistics Working Group. (2010). *United States cancer statistics: 1999–2007 incidence and mortality web-based report.* Atlanta, GA: Department of Health and Human Services, Centers for Disease Control and Prevention and National Cancer Institute. Retrieved from http://www.cdc.gov/uscs

TABLE 11-1

Comparison of Infant Mortality Rates, by Maternal Race, United States, 2000 and 2006

Maternal Race/Ethnicity	2000 Infant Mortality Rate	2006 Infant Mortality Rate	Change in Infant Mortality Rate, 2000–2006 (%)
American Indian/Alaska Native	8.3	8.28	−0.2
Asian/Pacific Islander	4.87	4.55	−3.2
Black, non-Hispanic	13.59	13.35	−1.4
White, non-Hispanic	5.7	5.58	−1.2
Hispanic*	5.59	5.41	−1.8
Total	6.89	6.68	−0.21

Infant mortality rate includes the number of deaths among infants aged less than 1 year per 1,000 live births.

* South or Central American, Cuban, Mexican, Puerto Rican, and other categories of Hispanic origin and Hispanics whose specific category is unknown.

Source: U.S. Department of Health and Human Services, Centers for Disease Control and Prevention (CDC), National Center for Health Statistics. (2010). *Period linked birth–infant death public-use data files* [Downloadable data files]. Hyattsville, MD: Author. Retrieved from http://www.cdc.gov/nchs/data_access/VitalStatsOnline.htm

These rates are declining across all ethnic groups. Among African American infants, the IMR remained high at 13.35%, compared to the much lower IMR of 4.55% among Asian and Pacific Islander American infants (U.S. Department of Health and Human Services [DHHS], CDC, National Center for Health Statistics, 2010). Allocations of resources for American children should reflect the specific community needs to improve health outcomes.

Federal, State, and Local Government Funding for Health Care

Medicare

Definition and Population Served

Medicare is a health insurance program managed by the U.S. federal government for people older than age 65, and younger individuals with disabilities and end-stage renal disease requiring dialysis or transplantation (Centers for Medicare & Medicaid Services [CMS], 2010). The origins of Medicare and its evolution demonstrate changes in federal funding with respect to resource allocation.

History

In 1945, President Harry Truman requested that Congress establish a national health insurance plan. Medicare and its companion program, Medicaid (which insures indigent recipients), were finally signed into law 20 years later, during President Lyndon Johnson's administration, in 1965; the first enrollee in Medicare was ex-President Truman. In 1972, program benefits increased to include coverage for disabled persons younger than age 65 and those with end-stage renal disease. Subsequently, chiropractic services, speech therapy, and physical therapy and payments to health maintenance organizations

Medicare: A health insurance program managed by the U.S. federal government for people older than age 65, and younger individuals with disabilities and end-stage renal disease requiring dialysis or transplantation.

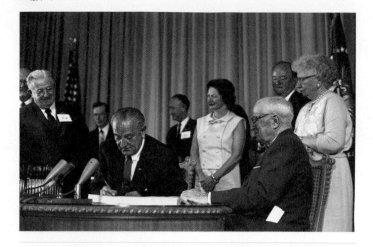

Signing of the Medicare Bill on July 30, 1965: (left to right) President Lyndon B. Johnson, Lady Bird Johnson, President Harry S. Truman, Vice President Hubert Humphrey, Bess Truman.

Courtesy of the Lyndon B. Johnson Presidential Library.

Formulary: A list of drugs reimbursed by a healthcare insurance company.

"Doughnut hole" (in Medicare): A coverage gap under Medicare Part D that occurs after a beneficiary reaches the initial coverage limit for prescription medications and becomes responsible for the total costs of all medications; when the next coverage limit is reached, the beneficiary becomes eligible for catastrophic coverage.

(HMOs) were added to Medicare services. Hospice benefits were added on a temporary basis in 1982; they became permanent in 1986. All federal employees were covered under Medicare in 1984. Fee for service was established as the means of physicians' payment in 1992. Medicare Part B, which covers outpatient and home care services, was established in 2000 ("History of Medicaid," 2010).

President George W. Bush, on December 8, 2003, signed into law a revision of Medicare called the Medicare Modernization Act (MMA). This historic legislation added an outpatient prescription drug benefit to Medicare. The Medicare Part D prescription privileges began January 1, 2006 ("Medicare Services," 2010).

Components

Medicare has four parts: A, B, C, and D. The hospital insurance component (Part A) assists with coverage of inpatient hospital and skilled nursing facilities care, hospice, and home health care. The medical insurance component (Part B) assists with coverage of physician services, outpatient care, home health care, and some preventive services. Part C is an Advantage plan for hospital insurance, similar to that provided by a preferred provider organization (PPO) or HMO; this option is offered by private insurance companies approved by and under contract with Medicare including Part A and Part B, and usually covers prescription drugs. The prescription insurance component (Part D) is a prescription drug option offered by private insurance companies under contract and approved by Medicare and helps cover the cost of prescription drugs (Kaiser Family Foundation, 2010).

The cost of prescription drugs can be an overwhelming expenditure for Medicare clients. Medicare Part D is designed to assist the older adult in dealing with these expenses, but many times the cost of a plan can be deceptive. Supplemental coverage with the lowest premium is not the best option if the insurance company's **formulary** (covered drug list) does not include the medications prescribed for a beneficiary, or if an available pharmacy that a beneficiary uses does not participate in the beneficiary's plan. Changes can also occur in drug prices, so that what appears to be the cheapest drug plan one week is not be the cheapest plan the next week. CMS has even stopped providing information about some plans on its prescription drug plan finder because of discrepancies in information about drug costs.

A beneficiary who reaches the initial coverage limit under Medicare Part D falls into the **"doughnut hole"** (coverage gap) and becomes responsible for the total costs of all medications. The statutory standard initial coverage limit is $2,610 for 2012. A beneficiary who incurs $4,700 in "true out-of-pocket" expenses (TrOOP) in 2012, which include any deductible, copayment, or coinsurance, would reach the other side of the doughnut hole and become eligible for catastrophic coverage (Center for Medicare Advocacy, n.d.).

Individual state programs are instituting supplementary drug programs to assist the older adult. For example:

> Elderly Pharmaceutical Insurance Coverage (EPIC) is a New York State program that helps seniors pay for their prescription drugs. More than a quarter million EPIC enrollees are saving an average of 90 percent of the cost of their medicines. Most enrollees have Medicare Part D or other drug coverage, and use EPIC to lower their drug costs even more by helping them pay the deductibles and co-payments required by their other drug plan. EPIC also helps members pay for Medicare

Part D premiums. Eligibility is you must be a New York State resident 65 or older with an annual income under $35,000 (single) or $50,000 or less (married) to qualify for the program. (EPIC Program, 2010)

Funding

Participants generally pay a set amount for health care (deductible) before Medicare pays its share of the total cost of care. Employers or union coverage may pay the costs not covered by the original Medicare option. Some plan participants choose to buy a Medigap (Medicare Supplement Insurance) policy to assist with uncovered costs. Participants usually pay a monthly premium for Part B services.

Federal law requires doctors, hospitals, skilled nursing facilities, and home health agency providers and suppliers to file Medicare claims for supplies and covered services on behalf of their clients. If the provider accepts Medicare assignment of costs, the out-of-pocket costs will be less for the participant. There is a 60-day benefit period of inpatient hospital deductible for each benefit period. There is no limit to the number of benefit periods. Copayments are due for each service unless the participant has a supplementary insurance plan. Contact for Medicare information is available at 1-800-633-4227 (1-800-MEDICARE) or www.medicare.gov (CMS, 2010).

Medicaid

Definition and Population Served

Medicaid is a state-administered healthcare program funded by federal statutes. It is available to eligible low-income individuals and families recognized by federal and individual state law guidelines (CMS, 2012). Criteria for eligibility include being a U.S. citizen or a lawfully admitted immigrant. A 5-year limit applies to lawful permanent residents for Medicaid. Income regulations vary from state to state, and rules may be different for disabled children and nursing home residents. Medicaid can be purchased by other individuals who may be disabled and whose income is exceeded by their medical expenses (CMS, 2012).

Adult services include physician visits, medication, lab tests, and radiological exams as medically needed. The Medicaid Early and Periodic Screening and Diagnostic Treatment Benefit includes, for children, a comprehensive history and physical exam; lab tests; immunizations; dental, vision, and hearing care; and education services (CMS, 2010).

> **Medicaid:** A state-administered healthcare program funded by federal statutes that is available to eligible low-income individuals and families recognized by federal and individual state law guidelines.

History

President Lyndon Johnson signed the Medicaid program into law in 1965. In 1972, the Supplemental Security Income (SSI) program was established for the elderly and disabled poor. SSI recipients are automatically eligible for Medicaid ("History of Medicaid," 2010).

Funding

Medicaid sends payments directly to healthcare providers. Depending on the individual state's regulations, participants may also be asked to pay a small amount (copayment) for some medical services (CMS, 2010). Medicaid is a state and federal partnership program, with each level of government having a part in designing programs and funding. The federal medical assistance percentage—that is, the share of matching federal funds provided to the states—ranges from a minimum of 50% to a high of 83% depending on the needs of the state ("Federal Medical Assistance Percentage," 2011).

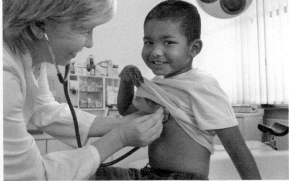
© iStockphoto/Thinkstock

Local Healthcare Funding

Local communities may fund some healthcare services by applying taxes to goods and services sold in the community (Klainberg, Holzemer, Leonard, & Arnold, 1998). For example, a community may fund a senior center or an early childhood daycare program to provide services to its citizens that are not available from national or state government agencies. Local interest groups can influence the community resources offered and their funding mechanisms; politics in the local community may also affect the services provided to the residents. Since 1988, the Robert Wood Johnson Foundation has partnered with local communities to address their unmet healthcare needs; health issues that are unique to individual areas can receive financial support (from grants and philanthropic groups) via local funding partnerships to promote better health care (Robert Wood Johnson Foundation, 2011).

Third-Party Reimbursement

Third-party reimbursement: A healthcare funding mechanism in which the provider bills the insurance company and is paid directly for the services rendered to the client.

Secondary insurance: A type of insurance, from either a public or private source, that covers some costs that are not paid by the primary insurance policy.

Third-party reimbursement influences health care by affecting how the healthcare provider is paid. In this system, the provider bills the insurance company and is paid directly for the services rendered to the client. As a consequence, the client may seek out a provider for services and expect the insurance company to pay the fee submitted by the provider. Due to rising healthcare costs, however, this system has been changed to a managed care component. The future is likely to include a cost-effective health care system managed by private and government insurers to support and encourage services at home and in the community (Klainberg et al., 1998).

Secondary insurance may cover some costs that are not paid by the primary insurance policy. The source of secondary insurance can be either public or private. Terms outlined in the secondary insurance policy provide supplementary coverage and call for it to be coordinated with the primary insurance plan. Secondary coverage may be provided through the primary insurer of a spouse or partner. In addition, individuals with disabilities, low-income families, children, and the elderly have the option of public health secondary insurance. Public policies usually do not require a payment, whereas private secondary insurance may require a monthly or bimonthly premium. Such a policy will often cover hospital costs, copayments, and services that the primary insurance does not cover in full, but only after the primary insurance pays first (Harrison, 2010).

Philanthropy

Philanthropy can fund projects of special interest groups. For example, advocacy groups can empower underfunded causes, such as relief efforts directed toward hurricane and terrorist victims. Celebrities have drawn both attention and funds to certain community causes such as "Farm Aid" through events such as music concerts. Philanthropy organizations may also take advantage of social networking sites to obtain fundraising contact information, such as cell phone numbers and online information.

A number of websites have been specifically developed for fundraising efforts aimed at assisting communities in giving and engendering social action such as Change.org, Changing the Present, Razoo, and Care2 ("Community Philanthropy and Social Media," 2008). Change.org is a platform for online activism that partners with nonprofit organizations. Its supported causes include health, education, environment, poverty, sustainable food, and human rights (Change.org, 2011). Changing the Present (2011) is an organization that helps nonprofit organizations raise money for worthy causes with charitable gifts, fundraising ideas, and guidance.

Many community foundations have taken their own knowledge bases and networks of local information and put them online for their current and prospective donors to use. In 2008, for example, the Columbus Foundation (Ohio) inspired $750,000 worth of giving in less than one hour through a creative campaign it launched to announce its Power Philanthropy program. Based on the Donor Edge platform, Power Philanthropy brings credible, foundation-vetted information on nonprofit organizations to the foundation's donors ("Community Philanthropy and Social Media," 2008, p. 2).

A **not-for-profit (or nonprofit) organization** is an incorporated organization that exists for educational or charitable reasons, and from which its shareholders or trustees do not benefit financially ("Not for Profit Organization Definition," 2010). Any money earned must be retained by the organization and used for its own expenses, operations, and programs. Many nonprofit organizations also seek tax-exempt status, and some may be exempt from local taxes including sales taxes or property taxes. Well-known national nonprofit organizations include Habitat for Humanity, the Red Cross, and United Way. Community-based nonprofit organizations can supplement the residents' resources with services not provided by insurance or the government in times of crisis and need.

Not-for-profit (nonprofit) organization: An incorporated organization that exists for educational or charitable reasons, and from which its shareholders or trustees do not benefit financially.

Service Learning and Volunteerism

Some CHNs have the challenges of managing their clients at home. In many cases, volunteers are needed to support the family and significant partners through supplemental aid networks in the community. Services may include meals on wheels, hospice volunteers, housekeepers, companions, and lay caregivers for assistive roles. People living with terminal illness may require the assistance of group homes or skilled nursing facilities; hospice visiting nurses provide services to this community of clients. All types of support groups for the client and caregivers are important resources for the community (Klainberg et al., 1998).

Service organizations, with the cooperation of the CHN, can foster a safer local environment. Populations at risk need to be identified by the CHN. The availability of Alcoholics Anonymous, Al-Anon, Alateen, Mothers Against Drunk Driving (MAAD), and Students Against Drunk Driving (SAAD) meetings and services can enable the CHN to share information with the community concerning available resources. Health programs can be designed and developed by the CHN in conjunction with the members of the community to engage them in serving their own neighbors.

The Limits of Futile Care and Outspending Healthcare Resources

Nurses manage complicated, technological health care, which poses a dilemma in relation to the difficult decision of resources allocation when benefits may be minimal for the patient. Families may demand

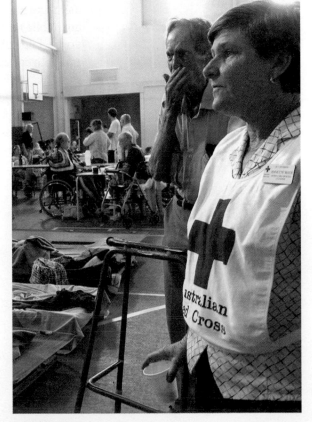

© GYI NSEA/iStockphoto

Futile care: Interventions and treatments that cannot end dependency on intensive care and treatments and medical interventions that have no medical benefit.

Global health: Health concerns of the international community (e.g., malaria eradication, vaccination programs, AIDS treatment) rather than individual nations' health issues.

treatments for the patient that will not change the outcome and add to the ethical issue of futile health care. Interventions and treatments that cannot end dependency on intensive care and treatments and medical interventions that have no medical benefit constitute **futile care**.

A descriptive survey design research was conducted among critical care nurses. The results revealed a significant relationship between nonbeneficial futile care and moral distress. Specifically, futile care had a significant relationship to emotional exhaustion, which is a component of burnout in critical care nurses (Melzer & Huckabay, 2004).

Futile care likely to become even more of an issue as healthcare costs rise further. State governments are attempting to manage and balance budgets to promote fiscal stability. Healthcare resources are being limited, in turn, and reimbursement for providers will be affected. In 2010, for example, providers in 39 states had Medicaid payments reduced or frozen (Hoppel, 2011).

Resource Allocation as a Global Concern

A global community has emerged to improve global health, with international healthcare systems evolving throughout the world. The World Health Organization is the major international agency impacting world health issues (WHO, 2010). **Global health** refers to health concerns of the international community rather than individual nations' health issues; public health issues in the global community include efforts to eradicate malaria, vaccination programs, and AIDS treatment, to name a few (Brown, Cueto, & Fee, 2006).

The European Union (EU) has established healthcare regulations with which new members must comply before admission to the union. "The EU plays its part in improving public health in Europe, and in so doing provides added value to Member State actions while fully respecting the responsibilities of the Member States for the organization and delivery of health services and health care" ("European Union Health Care," 2010, para. 2). "[A European] Community framework for safe, high quality and efficient health services will help to support dynamic and sustainable health systems. Providing clarity regarding application of European Community law to health services and supporting Member States in areas where coordinated action can bring added value to health systems" (Commission of European Communities, 2007, p. 10).

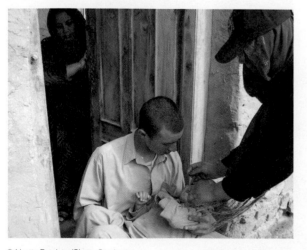

© Lizette Potgieter/ShutterStock.com

The philanthropic efforts of the Bill and Melinda Gates Foundation formed the Global Health Council—the world's largest membership alliance dedicated to saving lives by improving health throughout the world community. Its mission is to disseminate information and resources so as to improve global health. "The diverse membership is comprised of health-care professionals and organizations that include [nongovernmental organizations], foundations, corporations, government agencies and academic institutions that work to ensure global health for all" (Global Health Council, 2010, para. 2).

Adequate healthcare services is just one of the many basic human needs that remains to be addressed on a global level. Promoting and protecting health, and participating in respecting, protecting, and fulfilling human rights, are interconnected, as shown in **FIGURE 11-2**. Ill health can result from violations of human rights as slavery, torture, genital mutilation, and violence. Reducing vulnerability can improve and promote health, whether through provision

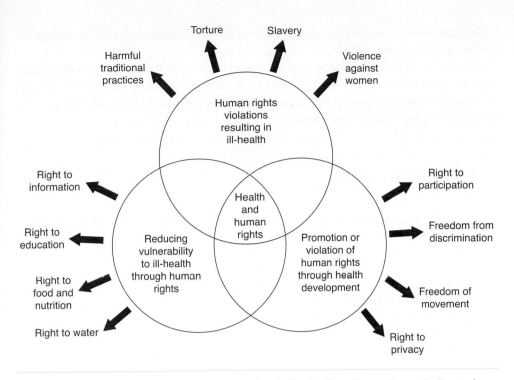

Figure 11-2 The connection between promoting and protecting health and respecting, protecting, and fulfilling human rights.

Source: World Health Organization (WHO). (2012). *Linkages between health and human rights.* Retrieved from http://www.who.int/hhr/HHR%20linkages.pdf

of education, clean water, adequate food, or information. Promotion of human rights through health development includes freedom of movement, freedom from discrimination, and rights to privacy and participation—all factors interconnected for health and human rights.

Summary

This chapter examined the way resources are allocated, including myths and realities of resource allocation. The healthcare system is a complicated infrastructure of hospitals, public health facilities, and community services. In the United States, the population is aging and the reliance on health insurance is increasing. To deal with these pressures, the country is moving toward a new healthcare system with the goal of a more equitable delivery of services to all its citizens. The CHN should be knowledgeable concerning the various types of health insurance utilized and the populations without health insurance in the community served by the nurse.

Federal, state, and local governments all play roles in funding healthcare services. Facilities in the community, whether funded by government, private, not-for-profit, or volunteer organizations are valuable resources that CHNs can use to their advantage in improving the health of their clients. Private efforts directed at funding health care include philanthropy, service learning, and volunteerism. In the future, as in the present, CHNs will be wearing many hats as advocates, educators, care providers, planners, screeners, coordinators of care, supervisors of assistant personnel, and lay caregivers (Institute of Medicine, 2011).

The limits of "futile care" were also examined in terms of their impact on healthcare expenditures. Cost-effective care will be at the forefront of future healthcare debates, and the CHN will continue to provide services in the community as healthcare delivery moves away from high-priced inpatient care.

REFERENCES

Brown, T. M., Cueto, M., & Fee, E. (2006). International to global public health. *Public Health Then and Now, 96*(1), 62–72.

Center for Medicare Advocacy. (n.d.). *Part D: Prescription drug benefits.* Retrieved from http://www.medicareadvocacy.org/medicare-info/medicare-part-d/#standard%20benefit

Centers for Medicare & Medicaid Services (CMS). (2010). Retrieved from http://www.medicare.gov

Centers for Medicare & Medicaid Services (CMS). (2012). Retrieved from http://www.medicaid.gov

Change.org. (2011). Retrieved from http://www.change.org

Changing the Present. (2011). Retrieved http://changingthepresent.org/nonprofits

Community philanthropy and social media: An update. (2008). Retrieved from http://www.communityphilanthropy.org/downloads/CF_FutureMatters_Summer08.pdf

Commission of European Communities. (2007). *Together for Health: A Strategic Approach for the EU 2008–2013* [White paper]. Brussels, Belguim: Author. Retrieved from http://ec.europa.eu/health/strategy/policy/index_en.htm

de Chesnay, M., & Anderson, B. A. (2008). *Caring for the vulnerable: Perspectives in nursing theory, practice, and research* (2nd ed.). Sudbury, MA: Jones and Bartlett.

de Tornyay, R. (1992). Reconsidering nursing education: Pew Health Professions Commission. *Journal of Nursing Education, 31*(7), 296–301.

Elderly Pharmaceutical Insurance Coverage (EPIC) Program. (2010). *New York State Department of Health.* Retrieved from http://www.health.state.ny.us/health_care/epic/medicare.htm

European Union health care. (2010). Retrieved from http://ec.europa.eu/health-eu/health_in _the_eu/policies/index_en.htm

Federal medical assistance percentage. (2011). Retrieved from http://www.hhs.gov/recovery

Global Health Council. (2010). Retrieved from http://www.globalhealth.org/Who_we_are.html

Harrison, H. (2010). What is the definition of secondary health insurance? *E How.* Retrieved from http://www.ehow.com/facts_5679211_definition-secondary-health-insurance_.html

Health disparities and the Affordable Care Act. (2010). Retrieved from http://www.healthcare.gov/law/infocus/disparities/index.html

History of Medicaid. (2010). Retrieved from http://www.seniorjournal.com/medicaid.htm

Hoppel, A. (2011). Dollars and sense countering Medicaid cuts. *Clinical Reviews, 21*(3), 1, 23–34.

Institute of Medicine (IOM). (2011). *The future of nursing: Leading change, advancing health.* Washington, DC: National Academies Press.

Kaiser Family Foundation. (2010, April). *Medicare: A primer.*

Klainberg, M., Holzemer, S., Leonard, M., & Arnold, J. (1998). *Community health nursing: An alliance for health.* New York, NY: McGraw-Hill.

Malloch, K., & Porter-O'Grady, T. (2010). *Introduction to evidence-based practice in nursing and health care* (2nd ed.). Sudbury, MA: Jones and Bartlett.

Medicaid home page. (2010). Retrieved from http://www.cms.gov/home/medicaid.asp

Medicare services. (2010). Retrieved from http://www.hhs.gov

Melzer, L. S., & Huckabay, L. M. (2004). Critical care nurses' perceptions of futile care and its effect on burn out. *American Journal of Critical Care, 13,* 202–208.

National Cancer Institute. (2010). *Health disparities defined.* Rockville, MD: U.S. Department of Health and Human Services, National Institutes of Health, National Cancer Institute.

Not for profit organization definition. (2010). Retrieved from http://www.investorwords.com/3331/non_profit_organization.html

Rawls, J. (1971). *A theory of justice*. Cambridge, MA: Harvard University Press.

Resource allocations. (2010). Retrieved from http://www.ahc.umn.edu/bioethics/prod/groups /ahc/@pub/@ahc/documents/asset/ahc_75702.pdf

Robert Wood Johnson Foundation. (2011). Retrieved from http://www.lifp.org/html/funders /fundingopportunities.html

Schoen, C., Collins, S. R., Kriss, J. L., & Doty, M. M. (2008). How many are underinsured? Trends among U.S. adults 2003 and 2007. *Health Affairs Web Exclusive, 102*, 289–309. Retrieved from http://www.commonwealthfund.org

Shepperd, S., Doll, H., Angus, R., Clarke, M., Ifille, S, … Wilson, A. D. (2009). Avoiding hospital admission through provision of hospital care at home: A systematic review and meta-analysis of individual patient data. *Canadian Medical Association Journal, 180*(2). doi:10.1503/cmaj.081491

Understanding the Affordable Care Act. (2010). Retrieved from http://www.healthcare.gov/law/ introduction

U.S. Cancer Statistics Working Group. (2010). *United States cancer statistics: 1999–2007 incidence and mortality web-based report*. Atlanta, GA: Department of Health and Human Services, Centers for Disease Control and Prevention and National Cancer Institute. Retrieved from http:// www.cdc.gov/uscs

U.S. Department of Health and Human Services, Centers for Disease Control and Prevention (CDC), National Center for Health Statistics. (2010). *Period linked birth–infant death public-use data files* [Downloadable data files]. Hyattsville, MD: Author. Retrieved from http://www.cdc. gov/nchs/data_access/VitalStatsOnline.htm

World Health Organization (WHO). (2010). Retrieved from http://www.un.org/millenniumgoals

World Health Organization (WHO). (2012). Linkages between health and human rights. Retrieved from http://www.who.int/hhr/HHR%20linkages.pdf

ADDITIONAL RESOURCES

American Nurses Association (ANA). (2007). *Public health nursing: Scope and standards of practice*. Silver Spring, MD: Author.

Calculating costs to and through the Part D doughnut hole. (2010). Retrieved from http://www .medicareadvocacy.org/InfoByTopic/PartDandPrescDrugs/PartD_CalculatingCostsThrough DonutHole.htm

Rover, J. (1996). The safety net: What's happening to health care of a last resort? *Advances, 1*(suppl), 1, 4.

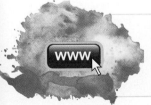

For a full suite of assignments and additional learning activities, use the access code located in the front of your book to visit the exclusive website: http://go.jblearning.com/Holzemer/. If you do not have an access code, you can obtain one at the site.

LEARNING ACTIVITIES   www

1. The community health nurse is servicing a Medicaid-supported client. Which of the following services are available to the client?

   A. Physician visit, immunizations, medications
   B. Physician visit, immunizations, food stamps
   C. Immunizations, medications, 6-year immigrant service limit
   D. Immunizations, food stamps, 5-year immigrant service limit

2. A Medicare client is reviewing the rules of Part D. The CHN explains to the Medicare-supported client which of the following concepts?

   A. Part D covers all medications for all older adults on Medicare.
   B. Part D covers only generic medications for older adults who elect to have this type of Medicare coverage.
   C. Part D covers unlimited medications for older adults who elect to have this type of Medicare coverage.
   D. Part D covers medications for older adults who elect to have this type of Medicare coverage up to a limited amount.

3. The largest increase in the number of health-related facilities is occurring in which of the following types of organizations or facilities?

   A. Community-based organizations
   B. Long-term health facilities
   C. Hospitals or medical centers
   D. Hospice services

4. Community healthcare providers primarily receive compensation for the services rendered to their clients by which of the following mechanisms?

   A. Secondary insurance
   B. Third-party reimbursement
   C. Medicare Part B
   D. Fee for service

ADDITIONAL QUESTIONS FOR STUDY

Ms. Annie Chung is a recent immigrant from China to the northeastern United States. She is married and joins her husband, who is a college student. Ms. Chung has a work visa for 1 year and is a trained nail technician. She works from 9 A.M. to 7 P.M. six days per week in a local community nail salon to help the couple meet their expenses. She has no health insurance. Two months have passed, and Ms. Chung has not experienced her menses. An over-the-counter pregnancy test reveals a positive result.

1. Is there health care available in your (student) local area for an uninsured immigrant woman?

2. Where should Ms. Chung secure information about available healthcare services?

3. What are the options available for prenatal care of the uninsured immigrant?

4. Is there health care available for the infant after birth in the United States?

5. Using the concept of a communication huddle, who needs to be involved in securing resources for Ms. Chung?

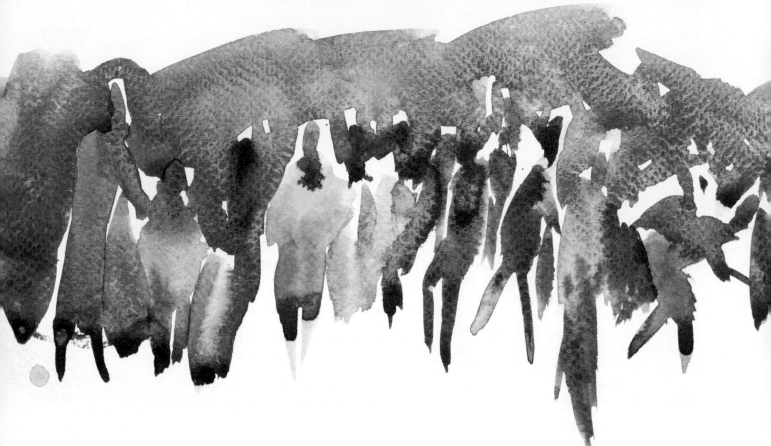

Community Program Development: Program Planning, Program Implementation, Program Evaluation, and Program Termination

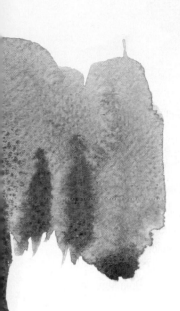

SECTION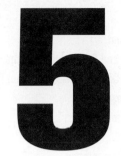

CHAPTER OUTLINE

- ▶ Introduction
- ▶ Precision and Program Development
- ▶ Essential Components of Program Development
  - • Assessment
  - • Diagnosis
  - • Plan
  - • Implementation
  - • Evaluation
  - • Program Termination
- ▶ Three Clinical Examples of Community Program Development
- ▶ Clinical Example 1: Responding to the H1N1 Influenza Pandemic
  - • Introduction
  - • Program Planning
  - • Program Implementation
- • Program Evaluation: Lessons Learned
- • Program Termination
- ▶ Clinical Example 2: Confronting Physical and Emotional Abuse in the Community
  - • Creating a "Safe Space Coalition"
  - • First Attempt at Program Development
  - • Second Attempt at Program Development
  - • Formative (Periodic) and Summative (Final) Evaluation
- ▶ Clinical Example 3: Alcohol and Other Drug Abuse in the Community
  - • The Effect of Addiction on the Community
  - • Role of the Community Health Nurse
  - • Working with People Living with Addiction
  - • Working with People Living with Alcoholism
- ▶ Summary

OBJECTIVES

1. Define the phases of program development in community health nursing.

2. Explain the necessity for a team-approach for all aspects of program development.

3. Articulate the key role of the client in program development, from concept through evaluation.

4. Explore the role of "lessons learned" in potentially improving the process and outcome of program development.

KEY TERMS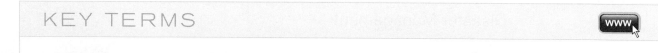

Community
assessment

Community
diagnosis

Formative evaluation

Planned change

Summative
evaluation

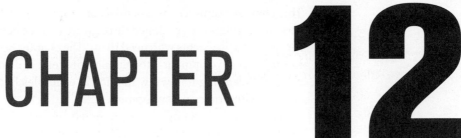

CHAPTER 12

Precision and Principles of Community Program Development

Stephen Paul Holzemer

Marilyn Klainberg

Deborah J. Murphy

Kenneth C. Rondello

Danielle Smith

Introduction

This chapter examines the essentials of program development in the community. Successful programs are developed through an alliance between the professionals providing services and the clients who need them. The chapter begins by examining the major tool in program development—the nursing process. A discussion of specific concerns with program planning follows, with clinical examples highlighting the process, to ensure success with program development.

Three clinical examples are presented in this chapter: (1) responding to a potential H1N1 influenza pandemic, (2) responding to physical and emotional abuse in the community, and (3) coping with addiction in the community. These clinical examples are intended to emphasize the fact that the community health nurse (CHN) needs to be precise in following a comprehensive plan in program development; secure needed resources, often from a variety of sources; and at times allow the client to direct the program development process.

Precision and Program Development

Precision is an interesting concept to use with program development. Programs change frequently and at times drastically, and they must do so with the goal of keeping services to clients ongoing. The problems encountered within the community are diverse and need individual attention to develop appropriate programs for problem resolution. Precision is needed when engaging key people in all aspects of program development and evaluation. It is also needed in selecting appropriate locations and support services to meet program needs. Precision is needed to monitor aspects of project management—including securing and using material and human resources wisely. Finally, precision is needed to take a hard and honest look at lessons learned from a project, through debriefing after the experience, in an effort to improve the chance of success in future programs.

Essential Components of Program Development

Program development for a community begins with assessing community needs. Planning for the development of a program should be determined by many factors in relationship to these needs. The focus when planning and developing programs is on partnering with a community. The CHN uses the nursing process with an emphasis on diagnosing the needs of a population and setting priorities, especially in terms of health education, health promotion activities, and client advocacy. An important first step is in the assessment component of program development, which entails interviewing and speaking with community members. These activities can be carried out by using focus groups—for example, forming an advisory community committee and partnering with members who represent the community.

As previously noted, the notion of caring for the community as a client is often a difficult concept for many nurses to grasp. As the world grows smaller due to increased travel and communication, today's CHN may focus not only on communities consisting of local populations, but also on global societies. The community as a client then may demonstrate a variety of unique concerns that need to be explored to be resolved. An important part of caring for the health needs of a community as client is the creation of programs aimed at prevention as well as crisis intervention, due to a variety of potential health-related crises. Using the nursing process, the CHN completes the following activities:

- Assesses needs and determines the main concerns of a community by talking to people (key informants) in the community
- Explores available resources and the capacity of community members to meet their needs
- Develops a set of realistic diagnoses for problem resolution
- Develops a plan to meet the needs of the community, including the education of stakeholders who will be central in the process of promoting health change
- Works with the community to implement the plan
- Evaluates the success of the plan

Assessment

A **community assessment** is the process of searching for and validating relevant community-based data, according to a specified method, to learn about the interactions among the people, resources, and the environment. This term is used to denote one phase of the nursing process—the assessment phase—applied to the community as a client. Assessment is an extremely important part of planning for any community as a whole, or for a portion of a community. The community may be global, national, or a subsystem of a larger community. Thus the community may be limited to a small subsystem, such as a naturally occurring retirement community (NORC), or it might include members of a large industry or an institution. Regardless of its size, the assessment of the community must be accurate. Errors in assessment are fatal in the sense that they portend inaccurate program development and inadequate program evaluation.

Assessment is how the CHN gets to know the community. It may be done in several ways, such as completing a windshield survey and visiting the community to assess the physical environment of the community, safety, and other critical variables that were previously introduced in the Alliance for Health Model. As part of the assessment, it is also important to learn about the politics of the community, and it is vital to work with leaders or those who represent the community in a variety of situations.

Community assessment: The process of searching for and validating relevant community-based data, according to a specified method, to learn about the interactions among the people, resources, and the environment.

Community diagnosis: A broad statement that represents a major concern in the community, made after the CHN (and other providers) collects and analyzes demographic data and other observed information related to the community, assesses the community's ability to respond to actual and potential threats, and determines how they can be resolved.

Diagnosis

A **community diagnosis** is made after the CHN (and other providers) collects and analyzes demographic data and other observed information related to the community. The CHN needs to assess the community's ability to respond to actual and potential threats, and to determine how they can be resolved. Community diagnoses are broad statements because of the large concerns they represent. In the three clinical situations discussed later in this chapter, they may be worded in the following or similar ways:

- Threat of an influenza pandemic in the community
- Potential ineffective response to preventing abuse in the community
- Inability to cope with endemic addiction in the community

Plan

After the community assessment takes place and one or more nursing diagnoses are formulated, a plan is developed. This plan must include the stakeholders of the community if it is to be successful. The creation of a successful partnership with the community by the CHN or the healthcare team depends on many factors, including the plan's inclusion of factors identified during the assessment: Who are the stakeholders in the community, and who do they represent? Has

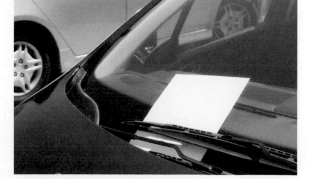
© iStockphoto/Thinkstock

Planned change: A systematic, purposeful, collaborative effort to integrate change for health in a community, through the use of the agreed-upon actions or goals.

Formative evaluation: A prospective assessment that reviews strengths and weaknesses of how a program is unfolding; it is used to help revise project direction and is ongoing.

Summative evaluation: A retrospective assessment that analyzes the outcomes and achievements of the project in a final way, at the end of the program.

the actual need for intervention been validated by validating the diagnosis with the community? Are the stakeholders truly represented by the community leaders who purport to represent them? These questions should be answered in the affirmative, and the resulting plan should include input from groups in the community, especially those who often are underrepresented and do not have a voice, such as the homeless, the poor, and the elderly.

When considering the plan, it is important to remember that the plan will usually require change. **Planned change** is a systematic, purposeful, collaborative effort to integrate change for health in a community, through the use of the agreed-upon actions or goals. The CHN needs to work with others to identify short- and long-term goals that will further guide the use of the nursing process. Working with more experienced CHNs will help identify goals that are realistic for a particular community.

Implementation

Once goals and objections for change have been decided upon by all stakeholders affected by the plan, implementation may occur. Collaboration is the key to success, especially when identifying and linking possible sources of funding for the plan. The most important component of implementation is community ownership and support of the program. If community ownership and support is not considered, the program may fail, despite financial support or the perceived value of the program.

Evaluation

Both qualitative and quantitative approaches are used to measure and evaluate outcomes of interventions, previously identified as short-term and long-term goals of the various interventions. Both formative and summative evaluation methods should be used in the evaluation process. A **formative evaluation** is prospective, and reviews strengths and weaknesses of how a program is unfolding. It is used to help revise project direction and is ongoing. A **summative evaluation** is retrospective, and analyzes the outcomes and achievements of the project in a final way, at the end of the program. It is also important to integrate early evaluation findings into ongoing implementation, and to use outcomes to reassess community-based needs. Evaluation should include recommendations for both ongoing and future assessment strategies, as well as necessary staffing needs and future funding of programs.

One of the most important aspects of the success of community programs is how the community assesses its own needs, and makes resources available to resolve problems identified through this assessment. A close fit between problems and needed resources promotes program success. The variables that need to be evaluated during this process are the same as those needed for assessment, as reflected in the Alliance for Health Model.

Working collaboratively with a team, and with the community stakeholders, to meet the needs of a community is vital. According to John Steen (2009), "Community health planning [including evaluation] is a deliberate effort to involve the members of a geographically defined community in an open public process designed to improve the availability, accessibility, and quality of healthcare services in their community as a means toward improving its health status" (p. 1).

Program Termination

Programs are at times terminated when their short- and long-term goals are met. Sometimes they end when they are no longer working as they should. Programs have a life cycle. To maintain viability, they must change with the needs of the public. If programs do not respond to the need for change, they need to be discontinued, thereby making way for new and more innovative programs.

Three Clinical Examples of Community Program Development

The first clinical example explored in this chapter relates to responding to the H1N1 influenza pandemic. The focus of this example is a discussion of all the steps necessary in program development. The second clinical example relates to confronting physical and emotional abuse in the community by creating a theoretical "Safe Space Coalition." The focus of this example is on the way a variety of agencies or institutions can come together to share resources so as to meet program development needs. The third clinical example, addressing alcohol (and to some extent, other forms of drug) abuse in the community, provides an example of program development that is managed by lay persons, with technical assistance by professionals.

Clinical Example 1: Responding to the H1N1 Influenza Pandemic

Introduction

Some community-based programs are developed with the intent of serving the community for years. Other programs are developed to respond to a time-limited threat or problem that needs immediate resolution. The example presented here relates to the 2009 unfolding of the novel H1N1 influenza pandemic and the subsequent legislation that had the potential to disrupt the statewide learning of many nursing students (and other healthcare providers) who did not comply with mandatory vaccination against seasonal and H1N1 influenza, as required by New York State.

In a response to the growing realization that an influenza pandemic was developing, the New York State Department of Health announced an emergency regulation (which took effect on August 13, 2009) for all direct healthcare providers to be immunized against seasonal and H1N1 influenza by November 30, 2009. After that date, any providers without proof of immunization, including students, would be restricted from direct-care activities. Confusion about the importance of immunization and the actual consequences of not receiving the vaccine compounded the problem of assisting students, faculty, and staff to comply with the immunization requirement.

Soon after the emergency regulation went into effect, a restraining order blocking mandatory immunization was imposed until a New York Supreme Court hearing could review the policy of the Department of Health. In late October, New York's governor, David Paterson, decided that the original requirement for mandatory vaccination was unreasonable due to the lack of vaccine supply; at the same time, President Barack Obama declared a state of national emergency as a result of the influenza pandemic.

Responses to the threat of a combined seasonal and H1N1 influenza epidemic occurred at both the university level and the school of nursing level, each with its own priorities. The university in this example activated its Threat Assessment Team (TAT) to protect the campus in the event of an influenza outbreak. The school of nursing created a

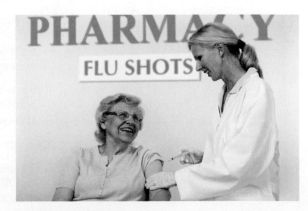

H1N1 Workgroup, with the goal of preparing students and faculty for the initial November vaccination deadline.

Program Planning

The University Threat Assessment Team

Preserving the safety and security of students and employees was a top priority for the university, and one that required vigilance, communication, and coordination. To facilitate collaboration among the many individuals whose work affected the university's collective security, the university established a TAT. This workgroup, coordinated by the Office of Public Safety, was designed to monitor and discuss reported incidents and implement action plans as necessary. In times of nonemergency, group members met semi-monthly to evaluate potential campus threats. However, once the H1N1 pandemic became a concern, the TAT began to meet several times per week to proactively address new developments.

A primary goal of the TAT was to attempt to ensure continuity of university operations in the event of either mass faculty/staff absence due to illness or forced closure mandated by the County Department of Health. To that end, the TAT implemented both preventive and contingency measures, as outlined in **Table 12-1**. The TAT continued to meet on a regular basis to discuss potential changes in protocol and alertness posture until the crisis phase of the pandemic passed. The TAT then returned to the nonemergency schedule of meetings, monitoring the ongoing health and wellness of the campus.

TABLE 12-1
Preventive and Contingency Measures of the Threat Assessment Team

1. Weekly situation status (SitStat) conference calls with the County Department of Health and the other institutions of higher education in the county.

2. Installation of more than 60 touchless antimicrobial gel dispensers in high-traffic academic and residential buildings on campus, including common-use computer labs and shared bathroom dormitories.

3. Distribution of H1N1 awareness/precaution flyers throughout all four campuses.

4. Conduct of public information sessions offering a Q&A forum with local public health experts.

5. Development of a "sick student" plan that would relocate the well roommate, deliver food and other necessities to the isolated student, and conduct periodic assessments of the sick student until he or she is deemed well enough to return to normal activities.

6. Encouragement of faculty to develop both synchronous and asynchronous online distance-learning tools so that they might be able to continue instruction in the event of a campus closure or their own illness.

7. Coordination of a campus vaccination initiative with University Health Services.

8. Provision of regular updates from the County Department of Health, the New York State Department of Health, and the CDC to the university community through campus-wide email alerts.

Preparation of Various Academic Departments

The university also sponsored a university-wide panel consisting of representatives from various academic departments to discuss electronic-based learning activities, which could be used in the event that the university was closed due to an influenza epidemic. The presentation by the school of nursing presented the unique dilemma of clinical programs that could not operate effectively without student and faculty compliance with immunization requirements. Programs in social work, education, and psychological counseling, which had less or little "direct patient contact," were less directly affected by the State Department of Health mandate, and adapted their school response accordingly.

The Creation of the H1N1 Workgroup

Although the requirement for mandatory immunization related to both seasonal and H1N1 influenza, the H1N1 Workgroup was created after a discussion with the undergraduate faculty. It offered the opportunity for the entire faculty to participate in creating proactive strategies in response to the pandemic. All faculty members were encouraged to participate in the H1N1 Workgroup and to work with members of the student council and other interested students to demystify the pandemic and to discuss related concerns.

An immediate (and ongoing) assessment of how other schools of nursing were responding to the state mandate for immunization yielded curious results. Anecdotally, faculty members from other schools reported that their colleagues were not formally responding to the perceived consequences of the mandate. The lack of an organized response appeared to be laissez-faire in character. Few, if any, faculty members had faced such a mandate for immunization during their professional careers. The fact that vaccination against polio and other childhood illnesses was mandated (and had been for many years) did not seem relevant to some faculty members, who questioned (and objected to) the need for a different and new public health requirement.

The work of the H1N1 Workgroup began with distributing information to all students and faculty via electronic mail concerning the state Department of Health mandate and the consequences of noncompliance. Anger and confusion were the immediate responses of many faculty and students. Without proof of immunization, students (and faculty) would not be able to meet the requirements of their clinical courses.

Information about the requirements for immunization and the consequences for noncompliance was sent to students and faculty on a weekly basis. Copies of communications were posted in public areas; additional copies were made available to students in the student lounge and office space of the administrative assistants for the school of nursing. Copies of important announcements were hand-delivered to student government meetings, and made available to students during open general informational meetings, which were scheduled when most classes were not in session.

Problems with Communication

When asked, students were polarized about receiving "too much" or "not enough" information regarding the immunization situation. A pattern of student and faculty members ignoring electronic mail notices fostered misinformation and generated many questions about information that was previously sent to them via electronic mail. The H1N1 Workgroup members experienced frustration with the need to correct misinformation, which was generated by some faculty and students who were not referring to various science-based local and national websites for their information.

The information provided by the Centers for Disease Control and Prevention and by the New York State, New York City, and county health departments did not always appear to be consistent or in agreement. Competing informational websites—some appearing legitimate and others not so legitimate—added to the confusion. Scholarly discussion of the benefits and perceived limitations of mandatory immunization for healthcare workers was, in part, circumvented by the legal requirement for immunization. The public opposition by the New York State Nurses Association to mandatory immunization made discussion of the real consequences of choosing not to be immunized—a decision made by some individuals—unrealistic and unjust.

Providing Support for Students Refusing Vaccination

Most clinical agencies used by the school of nursing were uniform in supporting the mandate for vaccination. Institutions were threatened with financial sanctions as a penalty for noncompliance with the immunization mandate. The temptation to seek out clinical opportunities at federal agencies, which were not bound by the mandate, or small community-based agencies, which might not be as concerned about following the mandate, created a serious ethical dilemma. A number of students who, for a variety of self-identified reasons, refused or wanted to delay immunization could be placed in certain agencies. The H1N1 Workgroup was clear that sending non-immunized and potentially infectious students into a healthcare environment was a clear violation of professional ethics.

Keeping Routine Operations of the School of Nursing on Track

Supporting a strict requirement for student attendance in clinical experiences has always been standard practice. Typical influenza treatment, with its emphasis on a 7- to 10-day period of isolation from others, translated easily into (at least) two clinical absences if students acquired the flu. The H1N1 Workgroup, with the support of the academic dean of the school of nursing, encouraged faculty to develop a number of alternative learning experiences to be used if necessary to keep students on track with their learning goals. Although non-direct-care learning activities were not considered a replacement for clinical learning, strategic alternative learning would be available for emergency use, as necessary.

The unique challenge of developing these activities was that the students would need to be able to complete the assignments independently, and then discuss them with other students and faculty without face-to-face instruction. Asynchronous learning strategies, similar to an online course, would need to be used in many learning situations. Face-to-face learning with other students, faculty, and clients (patients) would have to wait until the emergency threat was lowered or eliminated.

Program Implementation

Influenza clinics were held on campus at times when students could receive the immunizations and pre-immunization counseling that were required. Immunizations were administered at a campus location from the morning through evening hours. Support services were secured for food, emergency services (vaccine reaction), and counseling as necessary. Students, faculty, and staff who could not attend the immunization clinics were allowed to receive immunizations on an individual basis from the University Health Services.

Program Evaluation: Lessons Learned

The anxiety that students experienced related to the pandemic was underestimated. During student involvement in four campus-wide immunization efforts, a number of students demonstrated what some faculty considered to be "unprofessional" behaviors. In one situation, a student argued loudly and in public about her disagreement with the rationing of injected (dead) versus inhaled (attenuated) vaccine. Heath services staff had developed a decision tree about requirements and restrictions of the two vaccine forms. In this instance, the student's behavior increased confusion among vaccine recipients about which form of the vaccine was best for them to receive.

Students had received information about how vaccine development (nasal versus injectable) varied and which form of the vaccine was best for recipients to receive. The student who raised public objections to the plan (and others) had not completely worked through her feelings of safety, powerlessness, and threat to her continued studies in nursing. Some students reported that their fear-based feelings overshadowed their understanding that the immunizations were required by law.

Students were directed toward activities to decrease their anxiety and increase their insight in how to participate in the immunization program, becoming aware of the consequences of their actions. Students were encouraged to share their concerns with other students, faculty, and the university counseling center as necessary. The concerns of a number of students were incorporated into an anonymous written article published in the undergraduate communication forum, a monthly publication of student issues and concerns.

Program Termination

The program ended with two interesting phenomena occurring. First, there was not a great increase in the incidence and prevalence of H1N1 influenza; and second, the mandate for immunization was lifted, in part due to vaccine shortages. Because the flu is seasonal, the program ended, with planning for the next potential influenza outbreak the next year.

Clinical Example 2: Confronting Physical and Emotional Abuse in the Community

Creating a "Safe Space Coalition"

In a theoretical example, a number of CHNs attending a local conference on community data management identified that there was not a uniform, coordinated plan to work with women and men who are abused in the community. They agreed to discuss the issue with their supervisors—in particular, the possibility of an invitational brainstorming session for care providers, law enforcement officials, and persons who experienced abuse in the past to establish an approach to address the problem.

First Attempt at Program Development

Two CHNs agree to spearhead the project as co-leaders. They decide to invite people from different agencies and from the public to begin to address the problem. They want to "get people on board" who can commit resources for program development. To the surprise and concern of the co-leaders, the response to the program, "A Safe Space Co-alition for People Living with Abuse," was not favorable. Potential participants offered many excuses for being unable to make this project a priority, beyond offering verbal support.

Wisely, the CHNs aborted their plan for a think-tank, and continued to investigate the problem by reading research studies and interviewing specialists in the field of domestic violence and clients who had experienced abuse. Unfortunately, only after the

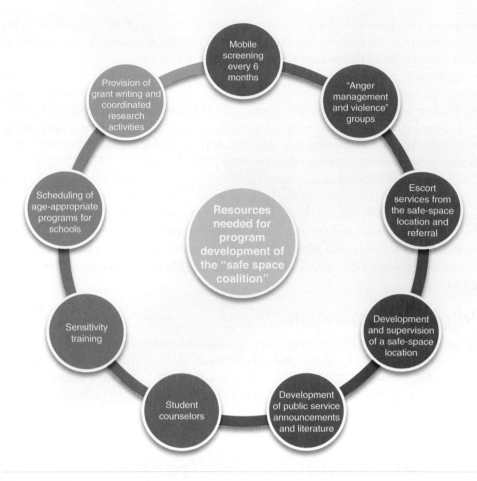

Figure 12-1 Resources needed for program development.

severe beating of a woman and her 6-month-old child in the community, resulting in the death of the infant, did the topic become more important to the community. The community was now motivated to take action.

Second Attempt at Program Development

The nursing co-leaders reintroduced the idea of developing a program for people who are abused and their dependents. Multiple participants from nine agencies or departments agreed to work together and to develop a pilot program to confront abuse. After 6 months of negotiation, several agencies and departments decided to make in-kind (nonmoney) contributions until funding was secured, thereby enabling the coalition to continue its work for one year. **FIGURE 12-1** depicts the various services that were necessary to secure in program development of the project. **Table 12-2** documents the agency in-kind contributions to the coalition related to service delivery. Program planning for the coalition would follow a systematic process.

Formative (Periodic) and Summative (Final) Evaluation

An evaluation of the year-long program on domestic abuse—the Safe Space Coalition—provided evidence that the program was successful. Periodic evaluation meetings were held, and changes in parts of the policies and procedures were developed. For example, the visiting nurse service made sure that a bilingual staff member was available for the program, and the legal court system was added to the list of coordinating agencies. The

TABLE 12-2
Agency In-Kind Contributions to the Safe Space Coalition

Agency	Contribution
City hospital A	Provide mobile screening every six months and provide staff to participate in two community health fairs.
Community hospital B	Manage five "anger management and violence" groups for the teenaged and young-adult persons in the community on weekends, at various locations.
Visiting nurse service agency	Provide escort services from emergency departments to a safe-space facility, and complete social service referrals on a 24-hour, 7-day-per-week basis for abused persons and families.
Assisted-living facility	Develop and supervise a safe-space location at an undisclosed location.
Interfaith network (local Lutheran church, synagogue, and mosque)	Accept responsibility for developing nondenominational, lay, public service announcements (radio and television) as well as literature on abuse for local distribution.
Police department	Sensitivity training for law enforcement staff, and development of a continuing education program for professionals (with hospital A and the assisted-living facility), and K–12 students.
Local university, school of nursing and health science	Provide student counselors as part of a service learning program, and offer a discounted college-credit course for the community on preventing abuse.
Local university, school of business	Provide grant writing and coordinated research activities for the coalition, and host a yearly fundraising event for the community.
Board of education	Schedule age-appropriate programs for K–12 schools on safety in the home and abuse prevention. Provide in situ classes for children of abuse in an undisclosed location (as necessary).

courts provided a liaison to work with the people experiencing abuse. In the last summative evaluation meeting, it was announced that funding was secured to continue the program, and the team decided to add subprograms in the areas of elder abuse and dating violence for future community outreach efforts.

Clinical Example 3: Alcohol and Other Drug Abuse in the Community

Addiction is a progressive and chronic disease affecting millions of people from all ethnic and socioeconomic backgrounds. Many people relate addiction to the use of drugs or alcohol and assume that it can be fixed by simply eliminating the substance. Over the years, a growing body of research has shown that addiction is actually a chronic disorder, such that the ultimate goal of long-term abstinence often requires sustained and repeated treatment (Coombs, 2004). Nearly all addicts believe that they initially have control over their usage, but as the disease progresses, their ability to stop use of the substance without help diminishes. Research has shown that long-term drug usage can significantly alter brain function. Changes in brain chemistry result in behavioral consequences, including the compulsion to use the drug despite negative consequences—the defining characteristic of addiction (Leshner, 1999). Unfortunately, even after abuse has stopped, these changes in the brain may persist.

Addiction is a progressive disease that worsens over time. As the disease progresses, cravings emanating from the primitive reward center create a compulsion despite the knowledge residing in the prefrontal cortex that compulsion leads to adverse effects. Once the cycle of addiction begins, the drug-induced reward system continues to grow, even during a time of abstinence. For this reason, individuals who resume use of alcohol or drug after periods of abstinence progress to full addiction more rapidly with each period of returned use (DuPont, 1997).

Many people have a misconception of addiction and drug use. The stereotype suggests that drugs users choose not to quit and become criminals to support their addiction. It can be wrongfully assumed that drug abusers lack moral principles or willpower; the truth is they are affected by a disease of the brain, much like a person with diabetes suffers a disease of the pancreas. People of all ages, socioeconomic statuses, and ethnical backgrounds are afflicted with addiction. No single factor can predict whether a person will become addicted to drugs of abuse. Although risk for addiction has been shown to be influenced by factors including genetics, social environment, age, stage of development, and personal support systems (National Institutes of Health, 2011), a full understanding of risk for addiction remains elusive.

Genetics plays a large role in addiction. Family history has been shown to affect the presence of addiction much in the same way that family history affects the presence of bipolar disorder or schizophrenia. Moreover, family and peer involvement can affect a person's perception of using drugs and alcohol. Strong social approval or disapproval can greatly alter an individual's viewpoint on the use of drugs and alcohol. Drug or alcohol use in a child's home, or by peers, has been shown to increase the likelihood of substance abuse. Factors such as peer pressure, physical or sexual abuse, stress, and the quality of parenting can greatly influence the occurrence of drug abuse (Coombs, 2004).

The Effect of Addiction on the Community

Addiction affects not only the individual and his or her family and friends, but also the community as a whole. The estimated cost of substance abuse in the United States, including treatment, crime-related cost, and collateral damage, exceeds $600 billion annually. This total includes approximately $181 billion in costs associated with use of illicit drugs, $193 billion associated with use of tobacco, and $235 billion associated with use of alcohol (Coombs, 2004). Although addiction has a drastic impact on the economy, it has an even more drastic effect on public health and safety implications. Situations such as domestic violence, loss of employment, failure in school, child and sexual abuse, homelessness, and other social problems often have a connection to the use of alcohol and other drugs.

Individuals, families, and communities who are affected are considered sick and need medical, psychological, emotional, and spiritual assistance as with other diseases. Although this chapter focuses on chemical addiction, similarities exist between this addiction and addictions related to gambling, sexual behavior, spending money/shopping, eating disorders, and Internet/computer use. Specific education and training are needed for the CHN or other provider to be able to provide comprehensive care to the person experiencing addiction.

Role of the Community Health Nurse

Addictions are not something that can be resolved with a "quick fix" solution; they require lifelong treatment. It is true that addicts will probably always be biochemically programmed to crave the target of their addictions. This fact, however, does not mean that addicts cannot be aware of their compulsions, and change their responses to them. Promoting awareness and providing knowledge about addiction are major goals of the CHN.

The CHN has the ability to be present to all levels of a community, from preschool to assisted living facilities, so as to assist clients addicted to various chemicals (alcohol and other drugs). Most notably, prevention and long-term treatment are key to breaking the cycle of addiction. As with other problems, the first step is to identify the issue of addiction in the community as a problem. By assessing the community, the CHN is able to see the effects of addiction and identify a need for intervention. A thorough assessment will allow the CHN to determine the risk factors present, the type of addiction needing intervention, and target groups at risk. The health planning stage will include plans to implement primary, secondary, and tertiary prevention measures.

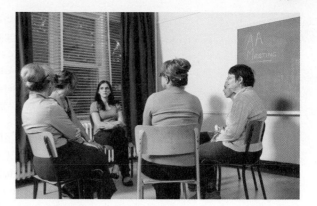

© The Power of Forever Photography/iStockphoto

The goal of care is to determine the effectiveness of the prevention interventions at the primary, secondary, and tertiary levels, as well as the need to avoid any lapses or gaps in prevention and treatment. The CHN should become very familiar with any and all mental health, substance abuse, and addiction centers available in the community, including Alcoholics Anonymous, Narcotics Anonymous, and support groups located at, for example, houses of worship. A relationship should be established with these facilities in an effort to build a partnership and network within the community. The CHN should include these groups in planning and implementation of the health plan for the community; oftentimes these groups are run by community members themselves.

Working with People Living with Addiction

The design of a community health plan to treat and prevent addiction includes primary, secondary, and tertiary prevention measures. **Table 12-3** provides examples of such preventive activities. Acute detoxification from alcohol and other drugs is a medical emergency. The CHN needs to guide clients needing detoxification to supervised medical care services, which may occur in either an outpatient or an inpatient setting. After

TABLE 12-3
Sample Primary, Secondary, and Tertiary Prevention Activities Related to Addiction

Primary Prevention Activities	Secondary Prevention Activities	Tertiary Prevention Activities
Age-appropriate educational programs on substance abuse prevention Self-awareness and self-esteem programs beginning in grade school Rewards program for abstinence programs	Crisis centers and comprehensive treatment centers for the physical/emotional/spiritual components of addiction (pediatric–geriatric) Full-service employee assistance programs Special and specific sensitivity training for athletic coaches, club and activity sponsors, problem identification, and specific counseling/treatment programs	Follow-up and support for rehabilitation programs including, but not limited to, 12-step recovery programs Treatment program relationship with employment support services, food banks, and temporary housing Congregate housing and supervised supportive housing options

initial treatment (secondary prevention), a follow-up program is essential because of the high incidence of relapse (tertiary prevention). Treatment and follow-up programs focus on abstinence or risk reduction, or some combined approach to care. The focus of this discussion is on 12-step recovery programs, which emphasize abstinence from alcohol (or other substances) for life. Rehabilitation from addiction is based on a philosophy of ongoing recovery—one day at a time.

Alcoholics Anonymous is the prototype for a number of other 12-step programs directed at addictions or compulsions. Some examples include Adult Children of Alcoholics (ACOA), Al-Anon, Codependents Anonymous, Crystal Meth Anonymous, Narcotics Anonymous, and Workaholics Anonymous. A more comprehensive list of resources can be found at http://www.12step.org/12-Step-Groups.

Working with People Living with Alcoholism

Alcoholics who are seeking sobriety should be encouraged to participate in a support program/network such as Alcoholics Anonymous (AA). The CHN will find that a unique aspect of AA and other 12-step programs is that they are managed by alcoholics or people with other addictions. The AA program is a spiritual (not religious) program in which participants work with other alcoholics to find support and fellowship. Members of AA are encouraged to complete 12 steps or activities to move them toward a sober life. The 12 steps of the Alcoholics Anonymous program can be found online at http://www.aa.org/en_pdfs/smf-121_en.pdf. In recognition of the fact that some alcoholics may experience a "dual diagnosis" with an emotional or mental illness, Dual Recovery Anonymous offers the similar steps of a dual recovery program at http://www.draonline.org/dra_steps.html.

The role of the CHN may be indirect in caring for the client involved in a 12-step recovery program such as AA. As previously stated, the meetings and fellowship activities undertaken by these programs are directed by other alcoholics. The CHN may choose to attend an AA meeting to better understand the dynamics of the program, but should be careful to attend an "open meeting" during which guests are encouraged. Closed meetings are only for people who self-identify as having an alcohol problem and do not wish to interact with guests, usually for the purpose of anonymity. Local AA offices provide lists of meetings that are clearly identified as "open" or "closed."

One means by which the CHN may support the alcoholic is to encourage the client to follow the suggestions of his or her sponsor. A **sponsor** is a fellow alcoholic who volunteers to assist the person with his or her recovery. A sponsor does not act as a therapist or healthcare provider. The CHN should encourage the person living with alcoholism to seek medical, emotional, psychiatric, or spiritual care from a licensed provider with those skills.

Sometimes the CHN can support alcoholic individuals with their work with other therapists by discussing their progress or the meaning of their recovery. **FIGURE 12-2** provides one example of an art therapy project used to assist a client living with alcoholism to identify the positive attributes of recovery, by labeling the ingredients of a "recovery sandwich." Part of the role of the CHN in working with clients experiencing addiction is to reinforce the positive attributes of recovery, because the disease of addiction often includes relapse. Working closely with other providers skilled in care of addicted persons allows the CHN to prepare individuals living with alcoholism (or other addiction) to cement their recovery by allowing them to work with other persons seeking recovery.

In the three clinical examples, the CHN is often the central person in ensuring that the comprehensive needs of the client are met. The CHN has the responsibility to work with other team members, assist with securing the various resources needed for program success, and allow the client to manage his or her care, with assistance, when appropriate.

Sponsor: In Alcoholics Anonymous or similar programs, a fellow alcoholic or drug abuser who volunteers to assist the person with his or her recovery.

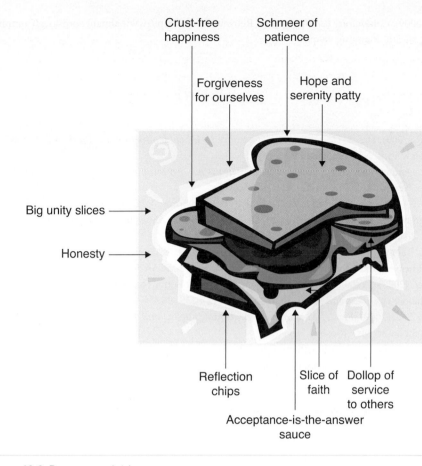

Crust-free happiness

Schmeer of patience

Forgiveness for ourselves

Hope and serenity patty

Big unity slices

Honesty

Reflection chips

Slice of faith

Dollop of service to others

Acceptance-is-the-answer sauce

Figure 12-2 Recovery sandwich.

Summary

This chapter examined the essentials of program development in the community. Successful programs are developed through a partnership between the professionals providing services and the clients who need them. The major tool in program development is the nursing process. Clinical examples of program development in the community presented in this chapter included (1) responding to a potential H1N1 influenza pandemic, (2) responding to physical and emotional abuse in the community, and (3) coping with addiction in the community.

REFERENCES

Coombs, R. H. (2004). *Handbook of addictive disorders: A practical guide to diagnosis and treatment.* Hoboken. NJ: John Wiley & Sons.

DuPont, R. L. (1997). *The selfish brain: Learning from addiction.* Washington, DC: American Psychiatric Press.

Leshner, A. (1999). *Principles of drug addiction treatment: A research-based guide.* Bethesda, MD: National Institute on Drug Abuse.

National Institutes of Health. (2011). *NIDA InfoFacts: Understanding drug abuse and addiction.* Retrieved from http://www.drugabuse.gov/publications/drugfacts/understanding-drug-abuse-addiction

Steen, J. (2009). *Community health planning*. Retrieved from http://www.ahpanet.org/files/Community_Health_Planning_09.pdf

ADDITIONAL RESOURCES

Alcabes, P. (2009). *Dread: How fear and fantasy have fueled epidemics from the Black Death to avian flu*. New York, NY: Public Affairs.

Alcoholics Anonymous World Services. (2011). *This is AA: An introduction to the AA recovery program*. New York, NY: Author.

Bostick, N. A., Subbarao, I., Burkle, F. M., Hsu, E. B., Armstrong, J. H., & James, J. J. (2008). Disaster triage systems for large-scale catastrophic events. *Disaster Medicine and Public Health Preparedness, 2*(suppl 1), S35–S39.

Hsu, E. B., Thomas, T. L., Bass, E. B., Whyne, D., Kelen, G. D., & Green, G. B. (2006, March 20). Healthcare worker competencies for disaster training. *BMCMedical Education, 6*, 19.

Kapucu, N. (2008). Collaborative emergency management: Better community organizing, better public preparedness and response. *Disasters, 32*(2), 239–262.

Veenema, T. G. (2009). *ReadyRN: Handbook for disaster nursing and emergency preparedness* (2nd ed.). St. Louis, MO: Mosby Elsevier.

Weiss, W. M., Winch, P. J., & Burnham, G. (2009). Factors associated with missed vaccination during mass immunization campaigns. *Journal of Health, Population, and Nutrition, 27*(3), 358–367.

Wineman, N. V., Braun, B. I., Barbera, J. A., & Loeb, J. M. (2007). Assessing the integration of health center and community emergency preparedness and response planning. *Disaster Medicine and Public Health Preparedness, 1*(2), 96–105.

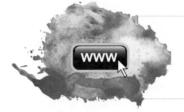

For a full suite of assignments and additional learning activities, use the access code located in the front of your book to visit the exclusive website: http://go.jblearning.com/Holzemer/. If you do not have an access code, you can obtain one at the site.

LEARNING ACTIVITIES

WWW

1. A CHN is concerned about flooding in a particular region of the community because of a history of flooding there. When should the CHN begin to address concerns about flooding with the residents of the community?

   A. Immediately, as soon as a meeting can be arranged

   B. As soon as the community has had the opportunity to understand the significance of the problem

   C. Six months after radio programs and newspaper articles can be distributed

   D. After the nursing department has the opportunity to budget a comprehensive flood prevention program

2. What is the greatest cost to a community working with a group of adolescents addicted to methamphetamine?

   A. The cost of incarceration of those individuals

   B. The loss of human potential in the group

   C. The loss of businesses that do not want to locate near the problem

   D. The cost of ongoing psychiatric counseling

3. Where should the focus be of prevention activities related to a potential epidemic such as influenza?

   A. Primary prevention

   B. Secondary prevention

   C. Tertiary prevention

   D. Combination prevention

4. Which of the following is a potential "key informant" or an important person in a community who can promote change? Choose all that apply.

   A. A visitor attending college for two years with plans to leave after graduation

   B. A grandmother who volunteers at two local soup kitchens

   C. A recluse male who never leaves his home and is under psychiatric care

   D. A CHN who directs programs for women and children in the school district

   E. An elected official who is serving a third term as mayor

5. What are the major resources needed for successful program development and management?

   A. Stable staff, interest in program planning, and sound evaluation

   B. Leaders, followers, and evaluators

   C. Financial support, people, and time

   D. Reimbursement, additional personnel, and administrative support

ADDITIONAL QUESTIONS FOR STUDY

1. Identify (through the local department of health) the five major causes of morbidity and the five major causes of mortality in the community. Meet with classmates to prioritize both lists. Choose a topic from each list. Brainstorm on developing two programs focusing on client education that you think would be appropriate for the community. Identify how you could share resources in program development.

OBJECTIVES

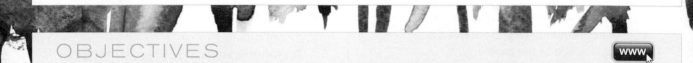

1. Identify the roles of key players in the project management process.

2. Define the role of the community health nurse in the project management team.

3. Discuss the way that the coordination of the resources of time, material, and personnel are central to the success of project management.

4. Describe the method for terminating health-related projects that no longer serve the needs of the client.

KEY TERMS

Execution risk	Integration risk	Project	Scope creep
Gantt chart	Process	Project management	Stakeholder

CHAPTER 13

Using Project Management for Successful and Viable Community Program Change

Christine Coughlin

I'm always making a conscious effort to be viable and accessible.

—Richard Thompson (1949–)

Introduction

Using project management to coordinate community program development represents an attempt to foster a lasting change that is viable—that will survive. Project management gives life to ideas, nurturing and developing them until they can become part of standard operating procedures. This chapter examines the usefulness of project management as a tool for viable change in community program development. It explores both the components of project management and the four phases of the process—concept development, planning, execution, and closing.

This chapter also emphasizes the importance of developing a plan for quality, use of resources, and communication. These plans are critical to the success of the project manager as well as to the project itself. The construction and work of the project management team are essential to ensuring the viability of the project and implementing the process of lasting change. Nurses working in the community are potentially key players in the process of project management because of their special relationship as advocates for their clients in the community.

Viability and Project Management

The concept of viability is important as it relates to project management. The community health nurse (CHN) uses scarce resources to develop needed programs. Viability of programs is central to the core functions of public health—in particular, the function of assurance. The community that is served by programs adequate to meet its health-related needs grows in confidence that future services, when needed, will be made available by a competent healthcare delivery system.

Project Management

What Is a Project?

Project: A task that requires strategizing to get the work accomplished and is not part of the normal work day.

Project is a term used to describe something that is not part of the normal work day. It can be initiating a new charting system, switching from paper records to electronic records, setting up a community health education program, developing a smoking cessation program for new immigrants, or something as small as painting the oncology day infusion center. Projects can be short term with a quick turnaround, such as planning a celebration for Nurses Week, or longer and larger, such as moving a homeless shelter to a new location. A project can affect just a few departments or the entire organization and the community.

Building a community day care center is an example of a huge project that would need support and input from both the healthcare organization and the community. It is called a project because it will require strategizing to get the work accomplished and it is not a part of the daily routine. A project has a well-defined beginning and end. In health care, there is always a need to change and improve services. Projects, both large and small, are part of the ongoing change that keeps health care fluid and not static. Health care is part of the community, and as such, healthcare projects need to meet public scrutiny.

Although projects may have different goals and outcomes, they share a specific framework. Projects are temporary; they have a beginning and an end; they are assigned a specific budget. The budget includes the fiscal cost, time cost, and project scope. A project usually involves the work of multiple disciplines, and frequently multiple projects are underway at the same time.

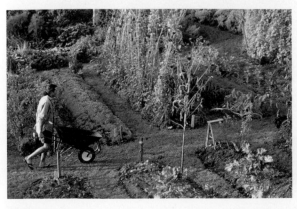

© Photodisc

In contrast to a project, a **process** is continuing ongoing activity. Many changes in health care do not end; these processes are referred to as the daily operations of the organization. The process activity needs to be managed, and its budget is part of the ongoing operational budget. When a project finishes, it ends and daily operations begin. An example would be implementing new critical guidelines for patients on home dialysis. After the guidelines are implemented, the use of the guidelines becomes part of the organization's daily operations—that is, the process of delivering care. The caregivers take responsibility to manage the ongoing process, and the project team disbands.

Another example demonstrating the difference between a project and a process is development of an educational program for new immigrants to promote smoking cessation. The project would include establishing the need for this population, establishing deliverables, researching the best methods to target the population, and designing the program and the outcome evaluation methods. After the program is implemented, however, it is turned over to the manager who will be responsible for the operation of this new program (i.e., the process).

Process: Continuing ongoing activity.

Project management: The concept of managing a one-time activity that has a well-defined set of outcomes, comprising the application of skills, knowledge, tools, and techniques to meet the requirements of a project.

What Is Project Management?

Project management is the concept of managing a one-time activity that has a well-defined set of outcomes. It entails the application of skills, knowledge, tools, and techniques to meet the requirements of a project. Using a consistent methodology to manage projects ensures success (Houston & Bove, 2007). Well-defined steps for project management have been summarized in the classic six-stage project management model (Elbeik & Thomas, 1998): define, plan, team building, control, communications, and review and exit. The Project Management Institute (www.pmi.org) identifies five phases of a project: initiating, planning, executing, controlling, and closing. Still other experts have identified four phases of a project: defining and organizing, planning, managing the project, and closing (Harvard Business Essentials, 2004). Wysocki (2006) defines five phases as part of traditional project management: scope project, develop project plan, launch plan, monitor/control, and close out project.

These models are all similar and identify a project life cycle. Utilizing a specific model with defined steps can eliminate mistakes, save money, and keep the project moving toward its end goal efficiently. The phased approach to project management is not unlike the steps in the nursing process: assessment, diagnosis, planning, implementation. and evaluation (Overgaard, 2010). **FIGURE 13-1** provides a visual representation of the steps in project management.

Managing a Project

Managing a project comprises leading a team, whose members may have never worked together before, to accomplish a task that has never been done before within a given amount of time and within a specific budget. Every project includes three basic elements: the task, the resources, and time. Resources include people, material, and money. Most projects have a sense of time urgency.

Phases of Project Management

Development of a Concept

The first phase in project management is the initial development of the concept. A project is usually initiated by a leader in the institution that sees the need for change or the opportunity to grow and improve the business. However, the initial idea can come

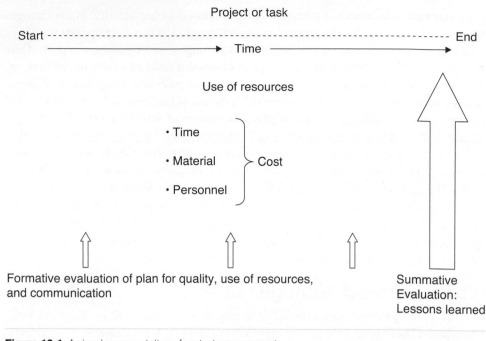

Figure 13-1 A visual representation of project management.

from anyone in the organization if the organization remains open and encourages and rewards creativity. The idea for change is usually driven by an organizational need to remain competitive, to be fiscally responsible, or to meet the demands of regulatory agencies. In health care, the idea of improving the business is synonymous with improving client outcomes.

It is usual for an organization leader to become a key stakeholder or sponsor of the project. This leader may have either initiated or championed the project. Every project needs a champion at a high level in the organization; without a champion, projects usually fail. Other stakeholders also need to be identified before initiating a project; a **stakeholder** is anyone who will be affected by the project. Stakeholders may include the project team, individuals or groups affected by the project (clients/families), the community, organizations that might be affected by the change, professional bodies, employees, and unions in a community (Martin, 2002). In a major community project such as initiating a physical activity plan for women, the stakeholders might include neighborhood social organizations and religious groups. Stakeholders need to be kept informed throughout the duration of the project.

After concept development and approval of the concept, the project moves into the planning phase.

Stakeholder: Anyone who will be affected by a project.

The Planning Phase

The key stakeholders of the project and the leadership team put together a project team. In some large healthcare institutions, there may be employees whose sole responsibility is project management. Such individuals will either lead or act as consultants to all major project teams. In smaller operations and for smaller projects, a member of the healthcare team will be selected to handle project management. Whether you are a team leader or a member of the team, knowledge of project management is essential for success.

During the planning phase, the reason for the project should become very clear. This phase is the time to ask key questions: Why are we doing this? What are the deliverables? Is the project in alignment with the goals and mission of the institution? Who are the stakeholders? A well-intentioned project can fail because the appropriate people were not included in the process. For this reason, it is important to get a sign-off from the key stakeholders and the project sponsor very early in the planning phase. Projects can affect many departments that are not directly involved in the change but will be impacted by it. The sign-off should include a confirmed agreement and understanding about the project's scope, deliverables, and budget.

As an example, a project to put hand sanitizers outside every patient door for the use of visitors almost failed at one extended-care facility because the project manager failed to include the head of housekeeping as a stakeholder. The housekeeping department would ultimately be responsible for maintaining the hand sanitizing equipment. You can imagine the housekeeping department head's surprise when the project team's recommendations were presented at a leadership meeting; a possible supporter was turned into a possible saboteur. Another example in which omission of key stakeholders in planning could wreck the outcome would be when developing a physical activity plan for neighborhood women without including the local child care center (see the case study at the end of the chapter).

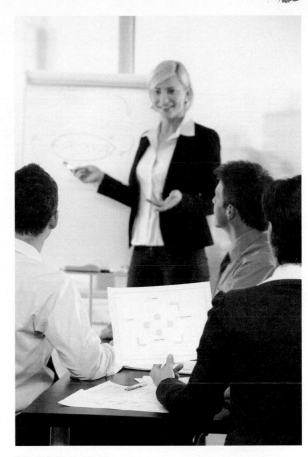

© StockLite/ShutterStock, Inc.

From Plan to Reality

The planning phase is the time to evaluate the project's chances of success. For some projects, it is valuable to mark a decision point at which time it will be decided if the project will be aborted or will continue; this decision is based on specific criteria. For other projects, unforeseen problems may arise that have implications for the decision to continue. For instance, if in the initial team meeting it is discovered that a valuable assessment tool used by caregivers will be eliminated by the project, the goal of the project needs to be revaluated. Stopping at the appropriate moment to reconsider the worthiness of the project can save the project from failure further down the line.

Building the Plan

In building the plan, the project scope should be validated. To do so, it is helpful to review the current state and the idealized future state. In this way, the deliverables become clear to team members. The work involved needs to be broken down into manageable segments so that the needed resources can be determined. As mentioned earlier, resources include people, time, facilities, and money. The work needs to be estimated: What will be the effort and duration? When this information is available, a schedule can be built.

It is helpful to use a **Gantt chart** to build your schedule and develop a work flow. A Gantt chart is the equivalent of a horizontal "to do" list (**Table 13-1**). To use this tool, you establish a deadline for completion of the project and then work backward to see if the time estimate is feasible. By laying out the work plan, you can see which parts of the work have to occur in sequence and which parts of the work can be done concurrently.

Gantt chart: A tool used to build a project schedule and develop a work flow.

TABLE 13-1
Gantt Chart

Team project — December

Number	Task	Start	End	Duration	% complete	5	6	7	8	9	10	11	12	13	14	15	16	17	18	19	20	21	22	23	24	25	26	27	28	29	30	31
1	Assemble team	12/5/12	12/8/12	4		█	█	█	█																							
2	Define project scope	12/5/12	12/8/12	4		█	█	█	█																							
3	Meet with stakeholders	12/5/12	12/15/12	11		█	█	█	█	█	█	█	█	█	█	█																
4	Kick-off meeting	12/16/12	12/16/12	1													█															
5	Decide on software product	12/16/12	12/30/12	15													█	█	█	█	█	█	█	█	█	█	█	█	█	█		
6	Delivery of software	1/12/13	1/13/13	2																												
7	Redesign process and plan launching	1/2/13	1/10/13	9																												
8	Educate staff	1/2/13	2/1/13	28																												
9	Execute	1/25/13	2/9/13	13																												
10	Provide support and evaluate	2/9/13	3/1/13	21																												
11	Close project and celebrate	3/1/13	3/1/13	5																												

Team project — January

Number	Task	Start	End	Duration	% complete	1	2	3	4	5	6	7	8	9	10	11	12	13	14	15	16	17	18	19	20	21	22	23	24	25	26	27	18	19	30	31
1	Assemble team	12/5/12	12/8/12	4																																
2	Define project scope	12/5/12	12/8/12	4																															
3	Meet with stakeholders	12/5/12	12/15/12	11																															
4	Kick-off meeting	12/16/12	12/16/12	1																															
5	Decide on software product	12/16/12	12/30/12	15																															
6	Delivery of software	1/12/13	1/13/13	2													█	█																	
7	Redesign process and plan launching	1/2/13	1/10/13	9			█	█	█	█	█	█	█	█	█																				
8	Educate staff	1/2/13	2/1/13	28			█	█	█	█	█	█	█	█	█	█	█	█	█	█	█	█	█	█	█	█	█	█	█	█	█	█	█	█	█	█
9	Execute	1/25/13	2/9/13	13																									█	█	█	█	█	█	█
10	Provide support and evaluate	2/9/13	3/1/13	21																															
11	Close project and celebrate	3/1/13	3/1/13	5																															

Team project — February / March

Number	Task	Start	End	Duration	% complete	1	2	3	4	5	6	7	8	9	10	11	12	13	14	15	16	17	18	19	20	21	22	23	24	25	26	27	28	1	2
1	Assemble team	12/5/12	12/8/12	4																															
2	Define project scope	12/5/12	12/8/12	4																															
3	Meet with stakeholders	12/5/12	12/15/12	11																															
4	Kick-off meeting	12/16/12	12/16/12	1																															
5	Decide on software product	12/16/12	12/30/12	15																															
6	Delivery of software	1/12/13	1/13/13	2																															
7	Redesign process and plan launching	1/2/13	1/10/13	9																															
8	Educate staff	1/2/13	2/1/13	28		█																													
9	Execute	1/25/13	2/9/13	13		█	█	█	█	█	█	█	█	█																					
10	Provide support and evaluate	2/9/13	3/1/13	21										█	█	█	█	█	█	█	█	█	█	█	█	█	█	█	█	█	█	█	█	█	
11	Close project and celebrate	3/1/13	3/1/13	5																														█	█

Execution risk: The risk that specific work will not be done correctly.

Integration risk: Failure of all the work in a project to come together at a specific time (i.e., the end of the project).

Scope creep: Deviation from a project plan after it is designed and formalized so as to deal with problems that arise, with these events being used as an opportunity to include additional work in the deliverables.

You can then estimate the duration of the project. Keep in mind that scope creep—when the unexpected occurs and causes a delay—is likely (more about that shortly).

Every good project plan includes contingency plans—that is, plans for issues that may arise during the course of the project. Team brainstorming can help the team in anticipating the various types of problems that may occur and then plan for their resolution. Such problems can include things totally out of the team's control, such as the new equipment failing to arrive at the designated hour or the team leader being called away for a family emergency. Planning ahead for the unexpected assures that the project keeps moving forward. Conversely, failure to identify risks and proactively address them can cause the project to fail.

Some of the risks that can arise are execution risks. An **execution risk** is the risk that specific work will not be done correctly. At the end of the project, all the work needs to come together at a specific time. If this fails to occur, it is called **integration risk**. If the potential for this risk is not identified early in the project, it will cause the project to fail. Another risk that can cause the project to fail is failure to identify required activities at the beginning of the project (Matta & Ashkenas, 2003).

Scope creep is a term used to describe another set of risks. Frequently the work of the project uncovers much more work that needs to be done. After the plan is designed and formalized, problems may arise, with these events being used as an opportunity to include additional work in the deliverables. If you deviate from the focused goal, however, it may cost time, money, and resources. These problems should be set aside for the future.

As an example, a team was given the charge of painting the oncology medication room in the infusion center. The medication room was used to service both the inpatient and outpatient units. The inpatient unit functioned 24 hours a day, 7 days a week, so this task qualified as a project (rather than a process). In their desire to have excellent outcomes, and because of the cries of some team members, the team decided to add the task of redesigning and updating the room to the original project. This extended project took on a life of its own and ended up being both far over budget and late. The room was finally painted and the renovation was tabled for a future date when funding would be available. As this example demonstrates, scope creep can lead to extra (and unexpected) expense, extra time, or extra resources to complete the project. Keeping the team's eye on the deliverables is a challenge that is a key part of project management.

Some teams tend to process too much information and so deviate from the goal. Still others keep asking, "Can't we make this better?" The project manager needs to be alert to these deviations from the project plan and close the discussion so that the project can move forward.

Planning the Team

The roles and specific responsibilities of each team member need to be clear. Team members should be selected for their skills. All teams need members who are good communicators, have excellent interpersonal skills, have effective problem-solving skills, and are able to think creatively. Not all team members need to have the expertise or knowledge in the area of the project scope. Some members bring specific needed skills. Having some team members with no knowledge of the specific work will allow pointed questions to be raised, such as "Why are you doing the work that way?" Aside from contributing the knowledge that he or she brings to the table, each team member is given an assignment. The assignments should be congruent with the members' skills. For example, a member with a knowledge of quality control should become the quality control manager of the project. The financial expert on the team should manage the budget. There might need to be a technical manager. During the planning phase, the team leader should ensure the team includes members with all the required skills and expertise. All team members should be clear on why they were selected and their role and responsibility. **FIGURE 13-2** represents the various members to be included in a project management team.

Although the team needs the expertise of many people, the larger the team, the more difficult it is for the team to move rapidly. An option in this circumstance is to have a smaller team and bring in some experts as needed to be consultants to the team. For example, when planning to paint the oncology day infusion center, the infection control expert can attend the planning meeting and advise on infection control principles; he or she may review the plan before it is implemented, but does not attend the other meetings.

Planning for Quality

The overall plan for the project should include a quality plan. What are the accepted criteria for each deliverable? How is quality measured? Be specific and clearly define what success will look like, how it will be measured, and when it will be delivered. Establish the metrics. Establishing the quality parameters early in the planning phase provides a framework for the overall plan. Team members and stakeholders will then be able to monitor the progress of the project and to evaluate its success. In addition, the team leader will be able to better manage and control the project if the plan is specific.

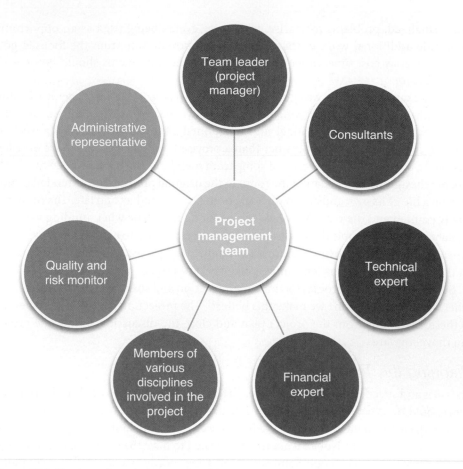

Figure 13-2 Members of a project management team.

Plan for Securing Resources

At this point in the planning phase, the needed resources should be determined. The resources include people: Do you have all the appropriate people on the team? Are the team members able to be released from their regular work to attend the team's meetings and perform the team's work? Other resources include financial resources necessary to do the work: Does the team need to travel to another site to view work of another institution? Does the team need any special tools or equipment? Do you have the space and facility necessary to meet and be productive? If you need computer access and a large viewing screen, now is the time to identify that need. Then acquire the resources before the next phase.

Communication Plans

If there is one most important part of the overall project plan, it is the communication plan. Sufficient time must be devoted to making sure this part of the plan is successful, and one team member needs to be assigned to oversee this plan. All the stakeholders need to be kept informed of the team's progress and any major decisions that are made. All stakeholders should be kept on high alert when it comes to the work of the team. Usually, successful teams take on a life of their own and move with healthy momentum toward project completion. This is why team projects are successful—but the team cannot lose sight of the communication plan as it moves. A good rule is to communicate in multiple forums. For example, the chief executive officer (CEO) might need bullet points to be updated, the chief financial officer (CFO) may need finance reports, and the employees may need an overview of the progress and goals. Certainly any delays or unexpected events need to be addressed with the team sponsor immediately.

At the end of the planning phase, ask yourself whether you have answered all the questions. Has the plan been reviewed and approved by the sponsor? Does the plan have the appropriate sign-off? Without a well-designed plan, some things will be missing at the end of the project. When a project fails to deliver the expected results, it is very possible that this shortcoming was the fault of the plan, not the concept itself.

Projects can fail because the plan fails. The importance of a clear and agreed-upon plan is crucial. The initial meeting of the team is the time to ensure that the planning phase will happen properly. Spend time on developing the plan and defining the deliverables, and get everyone's input while you do so. It is far better to spend extra time on this phase and have everyone in alignment, even if it means changing the plan.

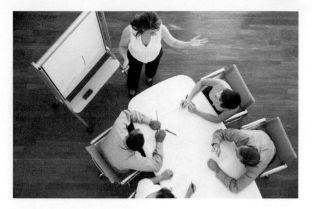

© Monkey Business Images/Shutterstock.com

The Role of the Project Manager

Effective project managers (PMs) are visionaries. The PM is able to lead the team by example and be a motivator. As a leader, this person generates both enthusiasm and a sense of urgency about the project. Ideally, the PM is decisive, competent, and a good communicator. The PM supports team members, standing up to the organization's executives when necessary to promote the work and needs of the team. To perform this role, the PM needs to have skills as an organizer, planner, leader, quartermaster, facilitator, persuader, coach, problem-solver, and taskmaster, all while encouraging team members to present new ideas. Perhaps finding this mix of skills seems impossible, but it is necessary because the project moves rapidly—that is, the work is intensive but time limited.

As a planner, the leader should ensure that the project is well defined and all stakeholders are engaged. In this role, the PM confirms that all processes are in place to manage the project. As an organizer, the PM oversees the work breakdown and determines who will do the work, in what time, and at what cost; he or she organizes the proper sequence of the work to ensure that the work is done on time. Moreover, the PM serves as the central person for all communication. In the quartermaster role, the PM works to ensure that all resources are available when they are needed. As a facilitator, the PM makes sure all team members understand one another and work together as a cohesive team to accomplish the goals. The PM as persuader gains agreement from stakeholders, manages stakeholder expectations, and manages competing demands on time, cost, and quality.

In the problem-solver role, the PM uses experiential knowledge and takes advantage of the knowledge and technical skills of team members. Root-cause analysis skills are also used to take corrective action when issues emerge. As a coach, the PM motivates and provides constructive feedback to team members to help them improve their skills and learn from experience. There are also opportunities to educate the team about project management and role expectations.

The PM serves as a protector for team members, shielding them from political issues surrounding the project so that they can stay focused. For example, team members chosen from the workforce because of their potential skills may face petty jealousy from their coworkers; the PM is in a position to mentor and help team members deal with this problem so it does not interfere with the team's work. The final role is to be a taskmaster: The PM follows up to make sure all work commitments are completed, and issues are resolved.

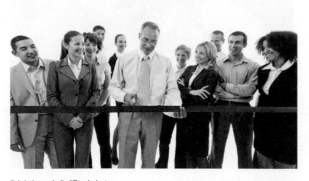

© kristian sekulic/iStockphoto

The Execution Phase

Projects get off to a quick start when team members come prepared to the meetings. Before the first meeting, it is a good idea to provide each member of the team with a copy of the team's project plan. Members should be clear on the deliverables and the time frame for the project. In some cases a teleconference may be helpful to address any potential conflicts or problems. A sense of urgency should be instilled so that the progress occurs quickly and team members are eager to arrive on time and not miss meetings (a difficult accomplishment). At the first team meeting, ground rules need to be set—for example, use of phones and pagers, respect for the speaker, and starting and finishing on time. The team should also decide how to handle conflict.

Another issue to address is how to handle issues that arise that are peripheral to the project. During this initial meeting, the leader should assess for any disagreements or confusion related to the project plan and the team members' responsibilities and roles. Now is the time to be very clear and flush out concerns and conflicts about the project's deliverables. The leader should also get a sense of the team's ability to work together at the initial meeting.

The team should than be ready to brainstorm about the deliverables and the work needed to get to the end point. It is important to identify milestones along the way that indicate the plan is on track. For example, an important milestone might be the arrival of a software program or the ground-breaking ceremony for the new senior citizens center. These milestones help with the ongoing monitoring necessary to keep the project on track and on time. After all, it is easier to make adjustments if you know where you are at all times. These points along the project's path should be reviewed and celebrated at each meeting.

During the execution phase, the PM has the responsibility to control the course of the project. The PM uses facilitation skills to manage the meetings and monitor the work of each team member. As part of the PM's role, he or she constantly evaluates individual performance and team performance, and is always on guard for discontent among the members. Team members need support and clarification of work expectations periodically. Members who have never functioned on a team need more mentoring. When the progress is monitored and measured constantly and carefully, deviations from the plan may be detected early, which in turn can save time and money. Over the course of the project's execution, the PM remains in communication with the sponsor and stakeholders to advise them of any risks to the plan schedule.

The Closing Phase

When a project is completed, a plan is needed for a smooth transition. It is helpful to use a checklist to make sure the transition is complete. There are usually reports to write, finances to reconcile, and records to be completed and properly stored. The sponsor signs off on the deliverables; the team is dismantled. This final phase of every project is a very important part of the project's overall life—specifically, it is a valuable time to review and evaluate the work. The team should review the questions in **Table 13-2**, and answers should be generated by all team members. The answers represent lessons learned that may be applied to future projects.

If the project failed in any way, it should be analyzed and discussed. Learning about the failure of one project may enable another project to be successful in the future. Instead of looking at the outcome as a failure, it should be viewed as an opportunity to

TABLE 13-2
Review and Evaluation of Work: Questions and Answers

Questions	Answers
Was the project successful?	
Did you come in on time and on budget?	
What lessons have you learned?	
Where are the opportunities to have done this project better?	
What were the challenges or roadblocks, and how could the team have managed them differently or avoided them?	

learn. All lessons are valuable. The information learned may be useful to develop more cohesive teams, for example, or to change the allotment of resources needed for success.

At the end of the project, the team should celebrate. Official recognition of the work and the team's accomplishments is an important part of project management. It helps with closure for the team members and leaves them with good feelings about being valued by the organization.

Challenges of Project Management

Change

A project represents a change, going into uncharted waters. It can be seen as either exciting or threatening. Some employees welcome change and see it as a positive force indicating that the organization is alive and well. Others perceive it as a threat to their comfort zone or fear change in the organization's mission and goals. In either case, many projects create anxiety.

Often project management interacts with other ongoing projects. This can be an issue if team members are participating in more than one project. In such a situation, competing priorities and demands become a challenge to manage, and coordination is required to ensure the project's success.

Another challenge is the multiple expectations of the stakeholders. The chief financial officer may be desirous of a more cost-effective outcome, while the quality manager may be seeking improved client outcomes and the staff may be envisioning a better work environment. While everyone's main concern is the care of the client, each person will view the project from his or her own vantage point and hear the communication about the project filtered through his or her own biases.

This raft of expectations creates the ongoing challenge of communication. No matter how many ways you say something, there will always be some people who fail to hear the message.

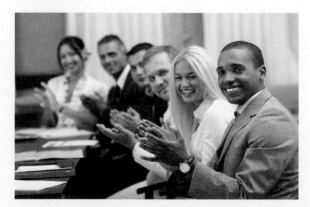

© Vadym Drobot/ShutterStock, Inc.

Why Projects Fail

Projects can fail because the plan fails. A clear and agreed-upon plan is crucial because ambiguity is one of the major reasons why projects fail. The initial meeting of the team is the time to avoid this kind of confusion. Spend time hammering out the plan and the deliverables, and get everyone's input. Spending the extra time is worth it to have everyone in alignment, even if it means changing the plan. Uncertainty can lead to missed deadlines, poor utilization of resources, and failure to adhere to the budget.

Summary

Using project management to coordinate community program development represents an attempt to foster a lasting change that is viable—that will survive. Project management gives life to ideas, nurturing and developing them until they can become part of standard operating procedures. This chapter examined the usefulness of project management as a tool for implementing viable change in community program development. The phases of project management include concept development, a planning phase, an execution phase, and a closing phase.

The planning phase encompasses developing a plan for quality, use of resources, and communication. These elements are critical aspects of the overall plan for the success of the project manager as well as the project itself. The construction and compatibility of the project management team is also key to the viability of the project, and to the process of lasting change. Community health nurses working in the community are potentially key players in the process of project management, because of their special relationship as advocates for their clients in the community.

REFERENCES

Elbeik, S., & Thomas, M. (1998). *Project skills*. Oxford, UK: Butterworth-Heinemann.

Harvard Business Essentials. (2004). *Managing projects large and small*. Boston, MA: Harvard Business School Press.

Healthy people 2020: Improving the health of Americans. (n.d.). Retrieved from http://www.healthypeople.gov/2020/default.aspx

Houston, S., & Bove, L. (2007). *Project management for healthcare informatics*. New York, NY: Springer.

Martin, V. (2002). *Managing projects in health and social care*. New York, NY: Routledge.

Matta, N., & Ashkenas, R. (2003, September). Why good projects fail anyway. *Harvard Business Review*, 109–114.

Meredith., R., & and Mantel, S. J. (2011). *Project management: A managerial approach* (8th ed.). Hoboken, NJ: John Wiley & Sons.

Overgaard, P. (2010, June). Get the keys to successful project management. *Nursing Management*, 53–54.

United States national physical activity plan. (n.d.). Retrieved from http://www.physicalactivityplan.org/theplan.php

Wysocki, R. (2006). *Effective project management* (4th ed.). Indianapolis, IN: John Wiley & Sons.

ADDITIONAL RESOURCES

A guide to the project management body of knowledge (PMBOK Guide) (4th ed.). (2008). Troy, MI: Project Management Institute. Retrieved from http://www.pmi.org/PMBOK-Guide-and-Standards/Standards-Library-of-PMI-Global-Standards-Projects.aspx

Labrosse, M. (2010, September/October). A fruitful project launch. *Industrial Management*, 19–24.

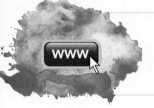

For a full suite of assignments and additional learning activities, use the access code located in the front of your book to visit the exclusive website: http://go.jblearning.com/Holzemer/. If you do not have an access code, you can obtain one at the site.

LEARNING ACTIVITIES   www

1. Which of the following describes a project that a community health nurse might undertake?

    A. A plan that requires an outside expert
    B. A task that is not part of daily operations
    C. Any assignment outside of the CHN's department
    D. An idea that requires a substantial outlay of money

2. Which of the following is an example of a project that a CHN might initiate with other team members?

    A. Implementing the use of electronic medical records
    B. Reducing the number of falls in the homes of clients
    C. Coordinating influenza inoculations for elderly persons in the community
    D. Hiring a nutritionist to educate clients in a community center

3. In most settings, what would be a definition of project management?

    A. An organization run by outside consultants that seeks to improve care delivery
    B. The concept of managing an activity that has a well-defined set of outcomes
    C. A method of solving financial problems
    D. A method of streamlining daily operations

4. What are the basic elements of a project that need to be incorporated into all of the project activities?

    A. Stakeholders, clients, and staff
    B. The budget, the plan, and the leader
    C. The project manager, stakeholders, and the budget director
    D. The task, the resources, and time

5. How would a CHN answer the question, "Who is a stakeholder?"

    A. The person whose idea it was to start the project
    B. A key executive in the organization
    C. Anyone who will be affected by the project
    D. The person chosen to lead the project

6. Which of the following roles are needed to manage a project? Choose all that apply.

    A. Technical experts
    B. Project manager
    C. Financial experts
    D. Clients
    E. Family members

7. A CHN is working on a project and helps to develop a Gantt chart. What is the purpose of this chart?

    A. To isolate problems
    B. To manage finances
    C. To monitor project progress
    D. To perform a formative evaluation

8. Which of the following concepts relates to the statement, "This project needs to be completed in 18 months."?

    A. Projects have life cycles.
    B. Projects are expensive.
    C. Projects depend on leader input.
    D. Projects have non-negotiable goals.

ADDITIONAL QUESTIONS FOR STUDY

Read the following case study and decide how a similar program could be developed as part of the community where you live.

Establishing a Physical Activity Project for Community Women of Childbearing Age

The local community nurse association and the local community center administrator were brainstorming about how they could help educate women regarding inactivity and obesity. They knew from past experiences that they would need an approach that meets the needs of the community.

In reviewing the *Healthy People 2020* website, they discovered an approach that recommends a multidisciplinary focus to promote physical activity. The recommendation is to include both traditional partnerships and nontraditional partnerships. The traditional partnerships would include health care and education, while the nontraditional partnerships would include transportation, urban planning, and recreation (http://www.healthypeople.gov/2020). The website led them to the U.S. National Physical Activity Plan, a series of national guidelines for physical activity. The National Physical Activity Plan's Strategy 1 calls for the development of programs where people work, learn, live, play, and worship, so as to provide easy access to safe and affordable physical activity opportunities (http://www.physicalactivityplan.org/parks_st1.php). This strategy excited the group and encouraged them to pursue the idea of helping the women in their underserved, low-income community. Their idea was taking form, and the group was excited.

The next step was to find a champion who would support their plan. After much debate, the local congressman was identified as an advocate for women. Over the course of several meetings with the congressman, the decision was made to establish a project team to accomplish the work. With the help of the congressman, the scope of the project was outlined and team members were identified.

The scope of the project included establishing an educational and physical activity program at a yet to be determined site. The program would be based on the *Physical Activities Guidelines for Americans* (PAG), which was published in 2008. The congressman allocated $10,000 from his budget to initiate the project and an annual budget of $80,000 to maintain the project.

Deciding on the project team members was the next step. It was important to identify a project manager. One of the nurses had experience working on projects and was eager to lead the team; she was also passionate about the project. It was agreed that some of the funds would be used for a consultant to assist the leader and keep the team on track. With the help of the consultant and the sponsor (the congressman), the group went about deciding on team members. They needed a community nurse education expert, an exercise expert, a nutritionist, a finance expert, an administrator with knowledge of legal implications and local laws, and a woman from the community who would know the needs of the women and any barriers to success. They also needed to identify other experts whom they could call upon as needed—for example, someone with knowledge of child care regulations and child care facilities whom they could engage as a partner, and someone from the local department of transportation.

After much debate and negotiation, a team was formed. One of the criteria for team member selection was involvement in the community. It was felt that this attribute was as important as specific expertise. The final team consisted of the PM, two community nurses, an exercise physiologist, a nutritionist, two community members, an accountant from the community center, a local clergy member, and a local political leader with knowledge of local laws and regulations. In total, there were 10 team members including the PM. The consultant agreed to work closely with the PM.

The first team meeting was held in the community center, and expectations were high. A week before the meeting, the PM distributed to each member an agenda and a short account of the project scope. The members were informed that this scope would be the issue highlighted in the meeting. The first agenda item was setting the terms of engagement. Group norms were identified such as that cell phones were to be turned off, the meeting would start and end on time, and everyone's opinion was of value. It was also decided that if something came up that was not within the scope of the project, a list of ideas for future work would be kept.

The PM explained the importance of keeping on track. There would be eight weeks of meetings, and everyone was expected to attend all meetings. The PM let the members know that she was available to support members who had to negotiate time off to attend the meetings. The PM understood the importance of supporting members, as it was essential that members attend all meetings and be prepared if the project was to come in on time and on target.

The main agenda item was discussion of the project, and time was allowed for idea sharing. This effort allowed the team to define the project scope: The project was to design a community education and exercise program for community women of childbearing age. The program would last 12 weeks and include nutrition counseling, personal training assessment, and a twice-weekly group exercise program. Child care would be provided during the program. Twenty women would be enrolled in the initial program. It was decided that the community center was the appropriate site for the

program; it had adequate space and was available at no cost to the program.

Each team member was assigned a role and responsibility that was congruent with the member's area of expertise. The roles included communication, quality management, risk assessment, and management of the budget. The women from the community were assigned to solicit feedback from other women in the community. The local clergy member promised to meet with community clergy and explain the project, and to get feedback before the next meeting. The local political leader agreed to identify potential liability. The nurse educator, the nutritionist, and the exercise physiologist promised to work together before the next meeting to draft a curriculum.

In addition, the team discussed possible barriers to success and possible risks. One serious concern was the child care issue. It was decided to invite the director of the child care center to the next meeting. At the end of the meeting, the team discussed the agenda for the next meeting.

At the next meeting, the PM, the project management consultant, and the rest of the team worked on identifying all the tasks and work necessary to complete the project. The work was then broken down into manageable parts—a step identified as a work breakdown in the project management literature (Meredith & Mantel, 2011). The PM and consultant agreed to develop a Gantt chart based on the work that needed to be accomplished in the next five weeks. Also at this meeting, the child care expert identified concerns about the staff needed to manage additional children during the program—a potential barrier to success. The child care director promised to return to the next meeting with potential solutions. The local political leader planned to look at the Department of Health's most recent census to estimate the number of children not in school who would need care for the hours of

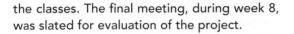

the classes. The final meeting, during week 8, was slated for evaluation of the project.

During the project, the team member in charge of communication used multiple methods to keep all stakeholders informed. Flyers were posted on the community bulletin board in the community center, a newsletter was designed with weekly updates of decisions and project progress, talking points were developed for team members, and the clergy were given news updates to share with their congregations. The PM kept the project sponsor informed.

One of the things that the team identified was outcome measures or deliverables. What would the project team deliver? How would success be measured? The PM knew that it was important for everyone to be clear on the charge of the team. For this team, success would be measured by the successful initiation of the program. Recall that a project ends, in this case with the program being transferred to the community center as process to manage and maintain. Therefore the deliverable for this team was a viable program that would meet the needs of the community women.

The team functioned well because the plan was clear and the PM stayed focused and was able to keep all the members on track. By week 7, the group had a well-developed program plan to provide education and exercise to 20 community women. Child care would be provided on-site and transportation vouchers were being donated by the community clergy group. The women were recruited through announcements at the churches, flyers at the community center, and recommendations from the nurses in the mother–baby clinic. The first 20 women who applied and committed to attend were selected.

Because the community center did not charge additional fees for the use of the space, the annual budget would cover the salaries of the nutritionist, the exercise physiologist, and the child care professionals. In addition, the CHNs would be available to assist with blood pressure screening on the first day, and that cost would be billed to the program. Part of the community center administrative assistant's salary would be paid by the program as well. She would be required to maintain records and write a monthly report on the project; she would also oversee the recruitment and selection of the next group of women.

In week 8, the group met to plan for the transition of the work to the community center. The plan was in place, the sponsor approved the plan, and the community center was ready to accept the responsibility for the daily operations of the program. The group discussed their accomplishment but also discussed opportunities that would improve the process. The issue of child care almost delayed the project; the team agreed that the child care representative should have been included in the team from the beginning. On another measure of success, the team came in on budget.

One final task awaited the team: It was now time to celebrate!

Questions

1. How do you think a similar program could be developed as part of the community where you live?

2. Using the roles identified in Figure 13-2, how would you assign tasks of this project to team members?

3. What are the benefits of debriefing after a project like the one described in this case study?

OBJECTIVES

www

1. Explain the importance of staying alert to the potential of emergency situations that would include the resources of community health nursing.

2. Describe the use of triage in meeting the needs of a community in crisis.

3. Explain the role of the nurse in the phases of disaster management.

4. Develop a plan for personal safety in the event of a local and/or national disaster.

KEY TERMS

www

Alternate care facilities (ACFs)

Anthropogenic

Emergency/relief/ isolation phase (of a disaster)

"Griage"

Impact (of a disaster)

Nondisaster/ interdisaster phase (of a disaster)

Points of dispensing (points of distribution) (PODs)

Predisaster/warning phase (of a disaster)

Reconstruction/ rehabilitation phase (of a disaster)

START (Simple Triage and Rapid Treatment)

Triage

Worried-well patients

CHAPTER 14

Staying Alert as the Key to Emergency and Disaster Management

Kenneth C. Rondello

ALERTNESS

I beg you take courage; the brave soul can mend even disaster.

—Catherine II (1729–1796)

Introduction

This chapter examines the role of the nurse in emergency and disaster management. Disasters and emergency conditions have many causes: Some are natural, some are human-made and accidental, and still others are purposeful or intentional. Nurses play a vital role in engaging both the threat and the reality of disasters, including those that are caused by terrorism. A method of triage used in disasters is discussed in this chapter, as is the way nurses can protect and prepare themselves so they can participate in disaster recovery. The chapter also provides information from the U.S. Department of Homeland Security related to the Ready Campaign, which encourages the public to secure emergency supplies, make a plan, and stay informed about disaster management.

The Importance of Staying Alert in Community Health Nursing

Nurses in the community are traditionally alert to emergency situations that might affect their clients. Community health nurses (CHNs) are educated to identify and react to actual and potential changes in the condition of their clients, so as to provide optimal care. In the same way, it is the CHN's responsibility to anticipate, prepare for, and respond to disasters that might occur. To best do so, nurses must have an awareness of the most commonly expected types of emergencies, have a plan to protect themselves and their families in the event of an emergency, and be prepared to utilize their knowledge and expertise in a disaster recovery effort.

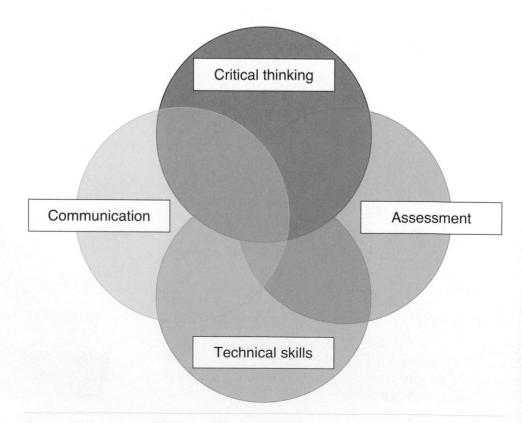

Figure 14-1 The core competencies for entry-level registered nurses related to mass-casualty incidents.

TABLE 14-1
Classification of Disasters

Natural
Floods
Hurricanes/cyclones
Tornadoes
Earthquakes
Volcanic eruptions
Tsunamis/typhoons
Avalanches
Drought/famine
Blizzards (can be sudden impact or slow onset)
Human-Made: Accidental
Industrial/technological
Transportation/vehicular
Environmental/deforestation
Complex emergencies (e.g., war, civil strife)
Human-Made: Intentional
Terrorism: biochemical terrorism
Direct contact (airborne)
Water and food contamination
Droplet or blood contact
Nuclear terrorism

Regardless of the nurse's clinical role, the importance of staying alert to the possibility of emergency situations and disaster events is central to core nursing values and principles when caring for clients in the community. Competencies for entry-level registered nurses related to mass-casualty incidents were developed by the Nursing Emergency Preparedness Education Coalition in 2003/2007. **FIGURE 14-1** depicts the interrelated competencies as critical thinking, assessment, technical skills, and communication.

Emergency Situations and Disaster Management

Disaster situations can be either anticipated or unexpected. Common emergency situations can escalate into full-fledged disasters when the number of people involved exceeds the capacity of the usual care providers, or the systems of care management are insufficient or inadequate to care for the ill and injured. **Table 14-1** classifies disasters as natural, human-made accidental, and human-made intentional and cites examples of each type. Although any of the three types of disasters may be catastrophic, intentional human-made disasters are most difficult to comprehend and to anticipate by establishing a state of readiness.

The Disaster Cycle

Disasters unfold in a series of phases that can be viewed as a five-stage cycle. These five phases occur in a continuous time sequence and always follow the same order—no phase can ever be skipped. The duration of each phase, however, can vary widely depending on the type of disaster; phases may last years, months, weeks, or even just a few seconds. Nurses have a critical role in each phase of the disaster cycle, and success in the disaster response is often contingent upon the preparation of the nurse as a care provider and, more importantly, as a member of society. The disaster cycle is illustrated in **FIGURE 14-2**.

Nondisaster/Interdisaster

Nondisaster/interdisaster phase (of a disaster): The period between disaster events, which is an important time for developing and operationalizing prevention and preparedness measures.

The **nondisaster/interdisaster phase** is often viewed as the period between disaster events and is an important time for developing and operationalizing prevention and preparedness measures. During this phase, disaster professionals conduct training and education programs for both emergency personnel and the community at large. Potential disaster locations are mapped, vulnerability analyses are conducted, and risk assessments are made. This phase provides an opportunity to inventory existing re-

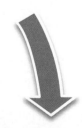

1. Nondisaster/
interdisaster

2. Predisaster/
warning

3. Impact

4. Emergency/
relief/
isolation

5. Reconstruction/
rehabilitation

Figure 14-2 The disaster cycle.

sources (e.g., medications, medical material, personnel) and enhance communication and cooperation among emergency responders—a vital characteristic in a real disaster.

Predisaster/Warning

In the **predisaster/warning phase**, emergency professionals have become aware that a disaster is imminent. It may be weeks away (as in a riverine flood), days away (as in a hurricane or cyclone), minutes away (as in a tornado), or mere seconds away (as in an earthquake). Depending on the nature of the pending disaster and the time frame allotted, this is the phase during which a warning is made to the public, protective actions such as evacuation are implemented, and emergency plans are activated. All emergency services, whether they be municipal or volunteer, are placed on heightened alert and readied for the next phase.

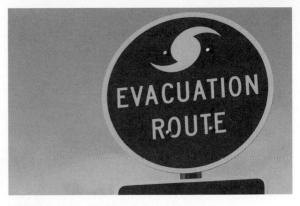

© CHRISTOPHER MAMPE/ShutterStock, Inc.

Impact

Simply put, **impact** is the period during which the destruction, injury, and death actually occur. Like the predisaster/warning phase, it can last anywhere from several weeks to just a few seconds. The magnitude of the impact can also vary widely and depends on its suddenness (how long the predisaster/warning phase was), the population density of the area affected, the community's level of preparation, the climate and environmental conditions, and the area's predisaster status and degree of organization.

Emergency/Relief/Isolation

During the **emergency/relief/isolation phase**, relief and assistance are provided to victims of the disaster. Search and rescue operations for the survivors take place, and emergency medical care is rendered. In addition, the basic infrastructure, such as transportation, communication, and power, is restored. While some additional morbidity and mortality may occur during this phase, most of the damage has been done and rescue operations are under way. Evacuation may be continued, depending on the condition of the community. Health surveillance begins, so that trends in illness and injury can be tracked.

Reconstruction/Rehabilitation

In the **reconstruction/rehabilitation phase**, the affected region is ready to restore its community to the condition it was in before the disaster occurred. Normal health services are reestablished, buildings and facilities are reconstructed, and life returns to normal. Importantly, this is the phase during which disaster responders and emergency professionals examine the "lessons learned" from the event, critically analyzing what happened, what went well, and what could be improved before disaster strikes again.

Predisaster/warning phase (of a disaster): The period in which emergency professionals have become aware that a disaster is imminent.

Impact (of a disaster): The period during which the destruction, injury, and death actually occur.

Emergency/relief/isolation phase (of a disaster): The period during which relief and assistance are provided to victims of the disaster.

Reconstruction/rehabilitation phase (of a disaster): The period during which the affected region is ready to restore its community to the condition it was in before the disaster occurred.

Steps in Disaster Management

Another way to view disaster management is as a process with steps, from beginning to resolution. **FIGURE 14-3** shows how the prevention of a disaster begins the process, which ends with lessons learned about disaster management. In a disaster, the CHN and other providers make every effort to provide needed care while minimizing the risk to others and compounding the disaster (Bostick et al., 2008; Veenema, 2009).

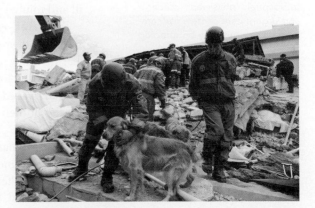

© fotostory/Shutterstock.com

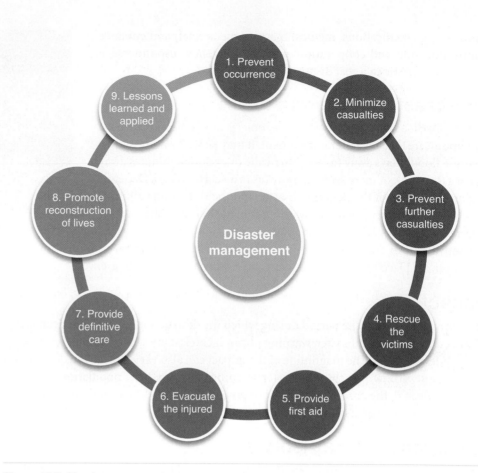

Figure 14-3 Disaster management.

Engagement in the Reality of a Disaster Threat

Virtually all disasters, whether they are natural or **anthropogenic**, require health services as part of the initial response and continuing recovery. Public health agencies, hospitals, physicians' offices, emergency medical services, and other healthcare entities are integral components of disaster response. In disasters of a significant magnitude, these medical agencies are likely to become quickly overwhelmed, not only by acutely ill and injured persons but also by the "worried well."

Worried-well patients are those individuals who clinically have no malady, yet self-refer themselves to hospitals, physicians' offices, and urgent care centers for care in fear that they may be affected by a disaster. This is particularly true in events involving chemical, biological, and/or radiological agents, as exposure may not be able to be readily determined. The screening and triage of these worried-well patients often creates a greater burden on the healthcare system than caring for those victims who are actually ill or injured.

To best manage casualties—both real and worried-well—who cannot be accommodated by inundated healthcare facilities, emergency managers are likely to establish temporary alternate care sites to treat the victims of disaster. These **alternate care facilities (ACFs)** may be established in a variety of locations under numerous conditions. Nevertheless, they all share one thing in common: They are nonmedical sites (e.g.,

Anthropogenic: Human-made.

Worried-well patients: Those individuals who clinically have no malady, yet self-refer themselves to hospitals, physicians' offices, and urgent care centers for care in fear that they may be affected by a disaster.

Alternate care facilities (ACFs): Nonmedical sites that are temporarily adapted to render health care in times of disaster.

schools, churches, municipal buildings, sports arenas) that are temporarily adapted to render health care in times of disaster.

In some disaster circumstances, such as the intentional release of a biological weapon or the spread of a preventable communicable illness, healthcare facilities are not likely to be overwhelmed with the ill and injured requiring medical treatment. Instead, what will engulf the facility will be citizens requiring prophylaxis for potential exposure to a virulent pathogen. In these cases, temporary care sites must be established *not* for the treatment of traumatic injuries or medical conditions, but rather for the administration of protective oral antimicrobials or vaccines. The nonmedical sites temporarily adapted to render health care are referred to as **points of dispensing** or **points of distribution (PODs)**.

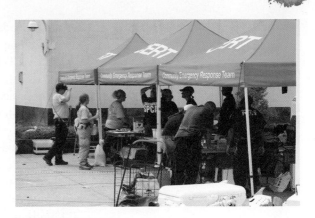

© Frontpage/Shutterstock.com

Certainly, CHNs and emergency department nurses will be called upon to staff this effort; however, the availability of these personnel will be severely limited in a disaster. As a consequence, nurses from the community with all types of training and expertise will be called upon to assist in the management and functioning of these alternate care sites. Accordingly, it is important for all nurses to have a basic understanding of these facilities' purpose, structure, and function. While some of these considerations (such as size and location) may be intuitive, many more factors must be carefully assessed before a site is ultimately chosen.

Points of dispensing (points of distribution) (PODs): During a disaster, nonmedical sites that are temporarily adapted to render health care in the form of protective oral antimicrobials or vaccines.

"Griage": The combined operations of greeting and triage at an alternate care site during a disaster.

Logistical Site Issues

Size

Initially, when tasked with selecting a location for the establishment of an ACF or a POD, a disaster official may simply consider choosing a site with adequate space (square footage) to accommodate the operation. While sufficient size is certainly a vital concern, it is only one of several logistical issues that must be contemplated before a site is chosen. Of course, the principal purpose of an ACF/POD is to ultimately provide clinical care in one form or another. Thus the site must have adequate space to accommodate **"griage"** (greeting and triage), patient registration, initial patient education (if necessary, such as indicating why a vaccine is necessary or how the flow of patients through the facility will be conducted), health screening and evaluation, medical treatment, and postcare instruction (if necessary, such as how to care for a wound or the conditions under which a patient should return for further care).

Depending on the arrangement of the facility, clinical space may also be required for patient holding/waiting prior to evaluation/treatment, for continuing treatment (such as for those requiring long duration transfusions of medications or treatments such as dialysis), and for patients who have been treated but must be observed (such as for vaccine reaction) prior to release.

In addition to the square footage that must be allocated for these clinical issues, space must be made available for ACF/POD administration, including not only office space, but also areas for storage of medical and nonmedical supplies. Some of these supply areas will need to be securable (e.g., those holding narcotics, vaccines, or expensive office equipment), while other storage will not require this level of safeguarding (e.g., those holding forms and paperwork, routinely used bandages, and standard desk supplies). Regardless of whether the ACF/POD will be staffed continuously, areas must be set aside for nutrition and hydration of the personnel working at the facility. These nutrition/hydration areas should be continuously stocked (even if with light snacks during certain periods of the day or night) and available to personnel at any time the ACF/POD is in operation.

If the ACF/POD is being designed to allow for continuous operation (24 hours/day, 7 days/week), appropriate sleeping quarters must be made available for the off-duty staff. These sleeping accommodations may be as sophisticated as actual beds with linens or as austere as athletic mats with blankets, depending on the availability of space and supplies, the origin of the personnel, and the duration of the mission. Even if the ACF/POD is designed to operate noncontinuously (such as 12 hours on, 12 hours off), space must be set aside away from clinical care and administrative areas where staff can briefly retire to for periodic quiet mental health breaks. Such breaks are essential for the psychological well-being of ACF/POD personnel.

Finally, an area must be purposefully designated for the media. A media staging area is created for several reasons. First, messages communicated to the public should come from a single source. Having an assigned media area allows the public information officer (PIO) to address all media outlets at once, thereby ensuring the delivery of a clear, consistent message. Second, experience has shown that when made aware of the existence of an ACF or POD, media outlets will attempt to gain access to clinical care, administrative, and other "restricted" areas by any means necessary. This not only poses a problem by adding unnecessary congestion to vital operational areas, but also may pose a security risk, as inaccurate or inappropriate information may be disseminated to the public. Having a specified media area, to which the media are fully restricted, helps alleviate these concerns.

Security and Safety

ACFs and PODs can be chaotic undertakings. Emotions run high, misinformation and frustration may occur due to long waiting periods, and anxiety levels of both the emergency workers and the patients using the facilities can rise quickly. Furthermore, the ACF/POD may serve as the repository of a life-saving vaccine or a limited supply of critical medications that must be secured and protected. Therefore, these facilities must have a plan for adequate security. Such consideration is intended to ensure the protection of both personnel and supplies and to maintain a general state of order. Additionally, a location chosen for an ACF/POD was likely not designed to accommodate large numbers of people in various states of health and mobility. Dangerous ramps, staircases, and walkways may exist. Escape routes, fire suppression plans, and other general safety concerns must be identified and addressed before the ACF/POD is opened for operation.

Utility Support

The sheer number of people working (and, in some cases, living) at the ACF/POD site will put an exceptional demand on the utility infrastructure of the facility. There will be a greater draw on electrical service, which may need to be supplemented with the use of commercial portable generators. Comfortable environmental ambient temperatures must be maintained during the operational hours of the ACF/POD—a factor that may put additional demand on the existing heating/cooling systems of the facility, requiring a greater than average power draw and/or fuel supply (such as No. 2 heating oil). Managers must take this increased demand into consideration, as well as the heat that will be generated simply through the increased flow of human traffic. Additional deliveries of fuel oil or natural gas may be required or supplemental power may be needed simply to support climate control.

Water will also be in great demand, both for hydration and for hygiene. Accordingly, emergency managers must ensure that the municipal water feed into the ACF/POD

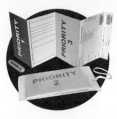

continues to be both potable and available. This may require supplementation by water trucks ("water buffalos").

Likewise, ACF/POD managers must have a plan to deal with an increased volume of waste, which comes in the form of rubbish, infectious waste, human excreta and gray water. Even if the ACF/POD site has toilet facilities, it is unlikely that they will be adequate to support the increased usage. Therefore, planners might consider the installation of latrines. Rubbish can be compacted and later removed by a waste management company, provided that adequate space for storage is available. If space is limited, or if disposal/removal services are not operational, this trash may be burned safely at a location removed from the ACF/POD.

Gray (used) water may be channeled into existing sewer lines if they are operational; if not, it would permissible to discharge gray water environmentally. This action should be seen as a last resort, however, and as soon as municipal sewer systems become available, gray water should be channeled back into them.

Infectious waste should be stored separately from noninfectious rubbish. If it cannot be removed by an appropriate disposal service (one that specializes in the removal of infectious materials), it should be stored in tightly sealed containers for the duration of the ACF/POD operation. Burning or burying infectious material should be considered only in the event that there is no other option and ACF/POD operation is likely to continue for a long time to come.

Fatality management must also be considered. If an ACF is established to help manage an incident that involves high mortality, a plan must be in place to address a large number of fatalities. Ideally, these casualties would be placed in specially designed bags, labeled appropriately, and stored in a refrigerated location. While a newly deceased fatality poses no immediate health threat (assuming the casualty died of a noninfectious cause), if long-term storage of fatalities is necessary, refrigeration must be considered for both hygienic and forensic reasons. If such a situation is likely, emergency managers might consider dispatching refrigerated trucks or large storage containers to the ACF to store the fatalities until they can be removed by the local medical examiner's office.

Finally, in terms of utility support, the ACF/POD must have appropriate communications with other ACF/PODs; local, state, and federal agencies; and other parties operating outside of the facility. This communication demand may include landline telephones (plain old telephone service [POTS] lines), cellular telephones, satellite telephones, fax capability, Internet connection, commercial terrestrial broadcast radio and television, and emergency services radios (i.e., VHF or 800-MHz radio systems). The number of each of these communication adjuncts will depend on the size of the ACF/POD and the nature of the incident. At a minimum, they must be adequate to support all functions of the ACF/POD's emergency operations center.

Triage Systems

In an emergency room, the **triage** of patients follows a specific methodology designed to optimize available resources by treating those patients in most dire need before those who are less acutely ill or injured. A similar strategy is employed in disaster conditions. It is meant to be entirely objective, so that the burden of determining who receives care in a disaster is not left to any single member of the rescue team.

The most common model of disaster triage is known as **START (Simple Triage and Rapid Treatment)**. Its primary objective is to quickly group patients by the severity of their condition so that they can receive treatment in as efficient a manner as possible, thereby allowing rescue workers to maximize the efficacy of their efforts by treating those who are most critical first. The START process begins by simply ascertaining which patients can self-ambulate. Those who can are classified as having minor injuries (and

Triage: A specific methodology for categorizing patients that is designed to optimize available resources by treating those patients in most dire need before those who are less acutely ill or injured.

START (Simple Triage and Rapid Treatment): A triage method that classifies patients into four groups: (1) those having minor injuries, (2) those for whom treatment can be delayed, (3) those who require immediate treatment, and (4) deceased victims.

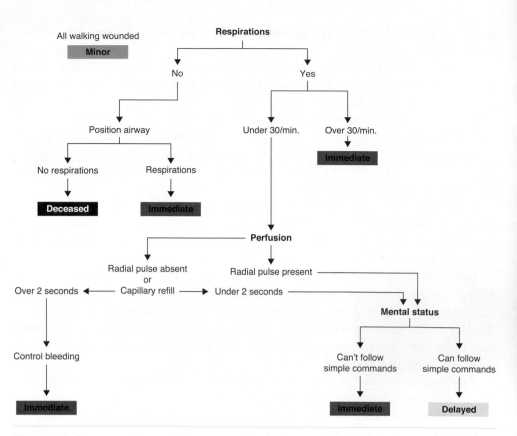

Figure 14-4 Decision tree for care of casualties of a disaster.

color-coded green). Next, those patients who cannot self-ambulate are quickly assessed on three parameters: their respirations, their degree of tissue perfusion, and their level of consciousness. Based on these findings, the nonambulatory patients are classified as appropriate for delayed treatment (color-coded yellow), necessitating immediate treatment (color-coded red), or deceased (color-coded black). A decision tree is used to assist the provider in using staff and material supplies wisely (**FIGURE 14-4**).

Once this classification is made, the patient is provided with a triage tag (**FIGURE 14-5**), documenting their status, certain vital signs, and other important information. It is important to note that a patient's level of severity (and associated START triage classification) may change over time; thus patients must be regularly reassessed to determine if their deterioration or improvement warrants reclassification (Kapucu, 2008; Wineman et al., 2007).

Protecting Yourself and Your Family

All disaster preparedness begins at home, and the most important preparation for any disaster consists of protecting yourself and your family. Only after you and your loved ones are healthy, safe, and secure will you be able to participate in a communal disaster recovery effort. Therefore, it is essential that all individuals who may be called upon to aid in a disaster response—particularly nurses and other professional caregivers—take measures to prepare themselves and their families for the myriad of disasters that may occur. Through several campaigns, the federal government has provided guidelines and advice to all Americans on how to prepare for and cope with a disaster.

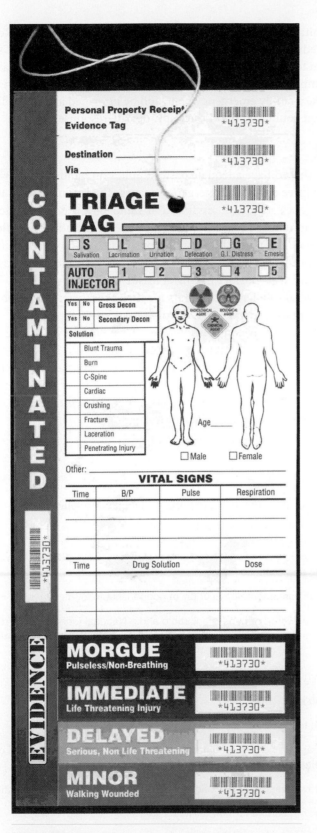

Figure 14-5 Triage tag for casualties of a disaster.

Source: Copyright © 2004, Steve Mann.

One such initiative is the U.S. Department of Homeland Security's Ready Campaign, which aims to educate and empower Americans to take several simple steps to prepare for and respond to any potential emergency, from a natural disaster to a terrorist attack. The Ready Campaign suggests that individuals do three key things: get an emergency supply kit, make a family emergency plan, and be informed about the different types of emergencies that could occur and their appropriate responses.

Get a Kit

All Americans should have adequate basic supplies on hand such that they could survive for at least three days if an emergency occurs. The recommended items to include in a basic emergency supply kit are found in **Table 14-2**. Additional items that should be considered for a more extensive emergency kit are included in **Table 14-3**. It is important that individuals tailor these lists as appropriate to their geographic location, the most commonly expected disasters in their region, and the unique needs of their family. Individuals should also consider having at least two emergency supply kits: one full kit at home and several smaller portable kits for their workplace, their vehicle(s), and any other places where they spend a significant amount of time.

You may need to survive on your own after an emergency. This means having your own food, water, and other supplies in sufficient quantity to last for at least three days. Local officials and relief workers will be on the scene after a disaster, but they cannot reach everyone immediately. You could get help in hours, or it might take days. In addition, basic services such as electricity, gas, water, sewage treatment, and telephones may be cut off for days, or even a week or longer.

TABLE 14-2
Recommended Items to Include in a Basic Emergency Supply Kit

- Water—one gallon of water per person per day for at least three days, for drinking and sanitation
- Food—at least a three-day supply of nonperishable food
- Battery-powered or hand crank radio and a National Oceanic and Atmospheric Administration (NOAA) weather radio with tone alert and extra batteries for both
- Flashlight and extra batteries
- First-aid kit
- Whistle to signal for help
- Dust mask (to help filter contaminated air) and plastic sheeting and duct tape (to shelter in place)
- Moist towelettes, garbage bags, and plastic ties for personal sanitation
- Wrench or pliers to turn off utilities
- Can opener for food (if the kit contains canned food)
- Local maps
- Cell phone with chargers, inverters, or solar chargers

TABLE 14-3
Additional Items to Consider Adding to an Emergency Supply Kit

- Prescription medications and glasses.

- Infant formula and diapers.

- Pet food and extra water for your pet.

- Cash or traveler's checks and change.

- Important family documents such as copies of insurance policies, identification and bank account records in a waterproof, portable container. (You can use the Emergency Financial First Aid Kit developed by Operation Hope, FEMA, and Citizen Corps to help you organize your information.)

- Emergency reference material such as a first aid book or information from www.ready.gov.

- Sleeping bag or warm blanket for each person. Consider additional bedding if you live in a cold-weather climate.

- Complete change of clothing, including a long-sleeved shirt, long pants, and sturdy shoes. Consider additional clothing if you live in a cold-weather climate.

- Household chlorine bleach and medicine dropper. When diluted nine parts water to one part bleach, bleach can be used as a disinfectant. In an emergency, you can also use it to treat water by using 16 drops of regular household liquid bleach per gallon of water. Do not use scented bleach, color-safe bleach, or bleach with added cleaners.

- Fire extinguisher.

- Matches in a waterproof container.

- Feminine supplies and personal hygiene items.

- Mess kits, paper cups, plates, and plastic utensils, paper towels.

- Paper and pencil.

- Books, games, puzzles, or other activities for children.

Make a Plan

Your family may not be together when disaster strikes, so it is important to plan in advance how you will contact one another, how you will get back together, and what you will do in different situations. **Table 14-4** provides guidelines for constructing a family plan of action.

Depending on your circumstances and the nature of the emergency, the first important decision is whether you will stay where you are or evacuate. You should understand and plan for both possibilities. Use common sense and available information, including what you are learning here, to determine if there is an immediate danger. In any emergency, local authorities may or may not immediately be able to provide information on what is happening and what you should do. In any case, you should watch TV, listen to

TABLE 14-4
Constructing a Family Emergency Plan

1. Identify an **out-of town contact.** It may be easier to make a long-distance phone call than to call across town, so an **out-of-town contact** may be in a better position to communicate among separated family members.

2. Be sure every member of your family **knows the phone number** and has a cell phone, **coins,** or a **prepaid phone card** to call the emergency contact. If you have a cell phone, program that person(s) as "ICE" ("In Case of Emergency") in your phone. If you are in an accident, emergency personnel will often check your ICE listings to get a hold of someone you know. Make sure to tell your family and friends that you have listed them as emergency contacts.

3. Teach family members how to use text messaging (also known as Short Message Service [SMS]). Text messages can often get around network disruptions when a phone call might not be able to get through.

4. Subscribe to **alert services**. Many communities now have systems that will send instant text alerts or emails to let you know about bad weather, road closings, local emergencies, and other conditions. Sign up by visiting your local Office of Emergency Management website.

5. Consider your options for contingency care of pets or domestic animals.

the radio, or check the Internet often for information or official instruction as it becomes available, including further information on staying put or sheltering in place.

Find out what kinds of disasters, both natural and human-made, are most likely to occur in your area and how you will be notified. Methods of getting your attention vary from community to community. One common method is to broadcast via emergency radio and TV broadcasts. You might hear a special siren, or get a telephone call, or emergency workers may go door-to-door. Use the Online Family Emergency Planning Tool created by the Ready Campaign in conjunction with the Ad Council to prepare a printable comprehensive family emergency plan. Use the Quick Share application to help your family in assembling a quick reference list of contact information for your family and identifying a meeting place for emergency situations.

You may also want to inquire about emergency plans at places where your family spends time—for example, work, day care, and school. If no plans exist, consider volunteering to help create one. Talk to your neighbors about how you can work together in the event of an emergency. You will be better prepared to safely reunite your family and loved ones during an emergency if you think ahead and communicate with others in advance.

Be Informed

Some of the things you can do to prepare for the unexpected, such as making an emergency supply kit and developing a family communication plan, are the same for both a natural or human-made emergency. Important differences among potential emergencies, however, may affect the decisions you make and the actions you take. Learn more about the potential emergencies that could happen where you live and the appropriate ways to respond to them. In addition, learn about the emergency plans that have been established in your area by your state and local government.

Emergency preparedness is no longer the sole concern of residents of earthquake-prone California and those who live in the part of the United States known as "Tornado Alley." For Americans, preparedness must now account for human-made disasters as well as natural ones. Knowing what to do during an emergency is an important part of being prepared and may make all the difference when seconds count.

Protecting Your Community

The CHN can work with small groups in the community to discuss and demystify the process of emergency preparedness. Working with other providers, the CHN can assist groups of people in the community to discuss and prepare to respond to emergency and disaster situations. Group discussions can occur at the workplace, as well as at schools, houses of worship, and recreational facilities. The CHN should use the nursing process in identifying the role of the nurse in disaster management. **Table 14-5** outlines the stages of the nursing process and links them with the phases of a disaster.

TABLE 14-5
Examples of Each Disaster Phase Linked to the Steps of the Nursing Process

Disaster Phase	Definition	Assessment	Planning	Implementation	Evaluation
Mitigation	Prevent a disaster or emergency; minimize vulnerability to effects of an event.	Assess a group of elderly citizens for their awareness about preventing heat stroke.	Develop community education plan to increase awareness about preventing heat stroke.	Conduct community education activities to increase awareness about preventing heat stroke.	Evaluate community education activities on preventing heat stroke.
Preparedness	Assure capacity to respond effectively to disasters and emergencies.	Assess the populations at risk for special needs during a disaster.	Develop plans to care for special-needs populations during a disaster.	Conduct training, drills, and exercises related to care of special-needs persons.	Evaluate plans for serving populations with special needs.
Response	Provide support to persons and communities affected by disasters and emergencies.	Serve on a response team to determine the impact and specific health needs of hurricane survivors. Triage victims.	Develop plans to rotate staff on response teams to prevent stress and burnout among responders.	Deploy staff to shelters after a hurricane, in accordance with local and/or state emergency response plans.	Participate in after-action reviews and/or debriefings to evaluate the quality of health services provided and lessons learned.
Recovery	Restore systems to functional level.	Serve on a team to assess community assets and potential for recovery from a recent flood.	Collaborate with partners and community leaders to plan long-term recovery priorities after a flood.	Participate in restoring community services after a flood.	Serve on team to evaluate long-term impact on persons displaced by a flood.

Source: Reprinted with permission from the Association of State and Territorial Directors of Nursing. (2007). *The role of public health nurses in emergency preparedness and response.* Retrieved from http://www.astdn.org/downloadablefiles/ASTDN%20EP%20Paper%20final%2010%2029%2007.pdf

Each disaster is unique. In some instances, nurses must be deployed rapidly to emerging disaster conditions such as mass-casualty events, infectious disease outbreaks, or environmental disasters. During all phases of the disaster cycle, collaboration among healthcare providers is necessary to improve the emergency response infrastructure at local, regional, state, and national levels. It is important to remember that greater distance from a disaster does not necessarily protect a community from the effects of a disaster (Hsu et al., 2006; Veenema, 2009). As examples, consider the more than 1 million people of the Gulf Coast who were displaced to shelters, mobile homes, hotels, cruise ships, and arenas in Georgia, Louisiana, Texas, and Tennessee after Hurricane Katrina in 2005, as well as the thousands of people who were evacuated from their homes following the 2011 nuclear disaster in Japan, the result of an earthquake and tsunami.

Summary

Disasters and emergency conditions may occur as the result of natural, human-made and accidental, or purposeful or intentional causes. This chapter examined how disasters unfold, and how nurses can participate in their resolution. Nurses play a vital role in engaging both the threat and the reality of disasters, including those that are caused by terrorism. A method of triage used in a disaster was discussed in this chapter, as was the way nurses can protect and prepare themselves so they can participate in disaster recovery. This chapter also provided information from the U.S. Department of Homeland Security related to the Ready Campaign, which encourages the public to secure emergency supplies, make a plan, and stay informed about disaster management.

REFERENCES

Alcabes, P. (2009). *Dread: How fear and fantasy have fueled epidemics from the Black Death to avian flu*. New York, NY: Public Affairs.

Association of State and Territorial Directors of Nursing. (2007). The role of public health nurses in emergency preparedness and response. Retrieved from http://www.astdn.org/downloadable-files/ASTDN%20EP%20Paper%20final%2010%2029%2007.pdf

Bostick, N. A., Subbarao, I., Burkle, F. M., Hsu, E. B., Armstrong, J. H., & James, J. J. (2008). Disaster triage systems for large-scale catastrophic events. *Disaster Medicine and Public Health Preparedness, 2*(suppl 1), S35–S39.

Hsu, E. B., Thomas, T. L., Bass, E. B., Whyne, D., Kelen, G. D., & Green, G. B. (2006, March 20). Healthcare worker competencies for disaster training. *BMCMedical Education, 6*, 19.

Kapucu, N. (2008). Collaborative emergency management: Better community organizing, better public preparedness and response. *Disasters, 32*(2), 239–262.

Veenema, T. G. (2009). *ReadyRN: Handbook for disaster nursing and emergency preparedness* (2nd ed.). St. Louis, MO: Mosby Elsevier.

Wineman, N. V., Braun, B. I., Barbera, J. A., & Loeb, J. M. (2007). Assessing the integration of health center and community emergency preparedness and response planning. *Disaster Medicine and Public Health Preparedness, 1*(2), 96–105.

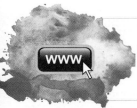

For a full suite of assignments and additional learning activities, use the access code located in the front of your book to visit the exclusive website: http://go.jblearning.com/Holzemer/. If you do not have an access code, you can obtain one at the site.

LEARNING ACTIVITIES

1. A CHN is helping a family identify an adult contact person to use in the event of a disaster situation. Which of the following persons should serve as an emergency contact?

    A. An adult in the epicenter of a disaster
    B. A family member or friend not living near the disaster
    C. A member of the family on a disaster response team
    D. An adult who has previous experience with disaster situations

2. A client with moderate congestive heart failure (CHF) has to relocate to a shelter due to serious flooding. Which of the following items would be most important for the client to have on hand at the time of the evacuation?

    A. Food for three days
    B. Water in reusable containers
    C. Multiple changes of socks to keep the feet warm and dry
    D. A week's supply of prescribed medications

3. What is the purpose of emergency workers having an opportunity for debriefing after a disaster occurs?

    A. Provide comprehensive psychiatric counseling
    B. Discuss plans for improving response activities
    C. Discipline staff who did not follow the plan of action
    D. Prevent future emergencies from occurring

4. Which of the following is the most important part of a family emergency plan?

    A. Securing first-aid supplies for travel
    B. Possessing an automatic teller machine (bank) card
    C. Having a second set of house and car keys
    D. Deciding on a place to meet when it is safe to gather

5. An earthquake necessitates the evacuation of a public health clinic. Which of the following statements is true about when it is safe for the CHN to reenter the building?

    A. Do not enter until the building structure is deemed safe.
    B. Do not enter if you need to use the elevator to return to the clinic.
    C. Enter the site only if someone from building security escorts you.
    D. Enter the site only if you have completed advanced life-support training.

ADDITIONAL QUESTIONS FOR STUDY

1. Triage decision-making models suggest that the CHN treat patients in the following order: (1) most urgent—critical, then (2) urgent—delayed, then (3) minor—walking wounded. People who are designated non-salvageable (but alive) are not treated. What is your response to this model?

2. Why are people who are designated as "chemically contaminated" not treated until the decontamination process is complete, even if that means that they die waiting for care?

3. Contact the closest Citizen Corps facility to where you live.

   ## Citizen Corps

   Get involved in preparing your community. Citizen Corps, the Federal Emergency Management Agency's grassroots effort, localizes preparedness messages and provides opportunities for citizens to get emergency response training; participate in community exercises; and volunteer to support local first responders. To learn more and to get involved, contact your nearest Citizen Corps Council by visiting www.citizencorps.gov.

   Describe your interest in becoming involved with this group.

4. Use the Online Family Emergency Planning Tool created by the Ready Campaign in conjunction with the Ad Council to prepare a comprehensive family emergency plan.

The Future of
Community Health

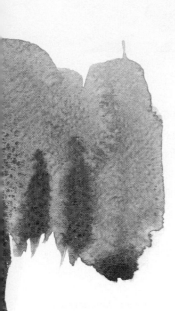

SECTION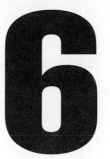

CHAPTER OUTLINE

- ▶ Introduction
- ▶ Responsibility and Larger Community Health Concerns
- ▶ Interstate, International, and Global Community Health Concerns
  - Disasters
  - Healthcare Disparities
  - Medical Tourism
- ▶ Creating Interstate and National Responsibility
  - Response to Disasters
  - Robert T. Stafford Disaster Relief and Emergency Assistance Act
- ▶ National Incident Management System
  - Incident Command System
  - Medical Disaster Relief Networks
  - National Disaster Medical System
  - Disaster Medical Assistance Teams
  - Medical Reserve Corps
- ▶ The Contributions of the Nursing Profession to National, International, and Global Health Concerns

- U.S. Public Health Service Commissioned Corps
- Association of Community Health Nursing Educators
- Association of State and Territorial Directors of Nursing
- ▶ Legal and Practice Barriers During Disasters and Interstate Practice
  - Nurse Licensure Compact
  - Civil Liability Concerns During Disasters and Interstate Practice
  - Interstate Travel Nursing
- ▶ Global Community Health Responsibility and International Organizations
  - Cultural Concerns
  - Safety Concerns
  - United Nations
  - Nongovernmental Organizations
- ▶ Summary

OBJECTIVES

1. Explain the relationship between local, international, and global health needs.

2. Define the role of national agencies and organizations in planning for a healthier global community.

3. Explore the legal and ethical potentials and limitations of interstate practice in meeting the needs of the community.

4. Identify the role of the nurse in meeting the Millennium Development Goals of the United Nations.

KEY TERMS

Disaster

Disaster Medical Assistance Teams (DMATs)

Emergency System for Advance Registration of Volunteer Health Professionals (ESAR-VHP)

Good Samaritan laws

Incident Command System (ICS)

Medical Reserve Corps (MRC)

Medical tourism

Millennium Development Goals (MDGs)

National Disaster Medical System (NDMS)

National Incident Management System (NIMS)

Nongovernmental organizations (NGOs)

Nurse Licensure Compact (NLC)

Telehealth nursing

U.S. Public Health Service Commissioned Corps

CHAPTER 15

Responsibility and Interstate, International, and Global Community Health Concerns

Andrea McCrink

Today, more than ever before, life must be characterized by a sense of universal responsibility, not only nation to nation and human to human, but also human to other forms of life.

—Dalai Lama (1935–)

Introduction

The world, as we know it, is complex, due to social, political, cultural, religious, and economic issues. And yet, at the same time, it is simple. The world is a community made up of individuals who strive for collective health and well-being in their family, group, and community structures. This chapter examines health concerns of the larger community. According to the World Health Organization (WHO), health is a basic human need, one that is essential to human welfare and sustained economic and social development. The achievement of the highest level of health possible is a fundamental human right (WHO, 2010a, 2010b). Community health nurses (CHNs) are called upon to develop a sense of responsibility to foster health and well-being at the local, regional, state, national, and international levels.

Through social action, nurses have an unprecedented opportunity to significantly and positively affect the health and well-being of individuals, families, groups, and communities around the world. To aid them in this quest, this chapter identifies health concerns confronting CHNs nationally and internationally and points out opportunities for nurses to create social responsibility to improve the health and well-being of people in both developed and underdeveloped countries.

Responsibility and Larger Community Health Concerns

Nurses around the world share a common and global responsibility to promote the health and well-being of individuals, families, groups, and communities. In the United States, through a variety of opportunities, CHNs can readily promote and achieve optimal client outcomes on interstate and national levels. In taking on the mantle of social responsibility, the CHN plays an integral role in shaping the healthcare outcomes of people around the world by addressing the health issues and policies that affect the health and well-being of people in developed and underdeveloped societies. The nursing profession is not one of isolation; rather, it is a profession that shares a global responsibility to decrease healthcare disparities around the world, in conjunction with other professions.

Interstate, International, and Global Community Health Concerns

Global health concerns reflect issues that affect the entire world. As a consequence of globalization, disasters, epidemics, armed conflict, social inequities, poor economic conditions, and migration patterns are no longer viewed as isolated occurrences that affect the health and well-being of isolated people and local communities. Likewise, the health of nations can no longer be viewed in isolation, especially in times of mass-casualty disasters and epidemics. The consequences of epidemics, social inequities, and disasters know no boundaries.

Our global community is becoming smaller. Around the world, CHNs recognize the importance of a basic human need: the right to health and well-being. The health of a nation and its people is influenced by a variety of issues, including the availability of sustainable health care, food sources, basic sanitation, and safe drinking water. Many social inequities and healthcare disparities around the world negatively affect the overall health and well-being of a nation and its people. Additionally, poor, underdeveloped

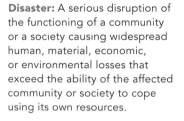

countries disproportionally share the burden of disaster and disease. When the infrastructure of a country fails to provide basic human rights and a mass-casualty event occurs, tragedy is the outcome.

There are more than 11 million nurses worldwide, including the more than 2.6 million nurses in the United States. The knowledge, skill, and expertise of CHNs are immensely valuable when it comes to meeting the healthcare needs of people around the world. Nurses, in particular, appreciate the "wholeness" of a person and what it means to be a human being. Therefore, all nurses, including CHNs, should be integral participants in improving world health, whether in response to national or international disasters or by using their skills to decrease social inequities around the world.

Disasters

According to WHO (2010c), a **disaster** is a serious disruption of the functioning of a community or a society causing widespread human, material, economic, or environmental losses that exceed the ability of the affected community or society to cope using its own resources. A disaster can also be described as a destructive event that threatens a population or community.

Disaster: A serious disruption of the functioning of a community or a society causing widespread human, material, economic, or environmental losses that exceed the ability of the affected community or society to cope using its own resources.

According to the *Annual Disaster Statistical Review* (Centre for Research on the Epidemiology of Disasters, 2010), 335 worldwide disasters in 2009 killed 10,655 people and cost more than $41.3 billion. The overall impact from disasters in 2009 was relatively small compared to the toll exacted in previous years. Consider the Indian Ocean earthquake in 2004, which generated a tsunami that killed more than 280,000 people, and the catastrophic Haiti earthquake in 2010, which killed more than 200,000 people. In 2011, the magnitude 9.0 earthquake in Japan and the subsequent tsunami and nuclear crisis resulted in significant loss of life and ensuing community burdens that included concerns about physical and psychological health and well-being as well as concerns about food safety and security—the most basic of human needs.

When disaster strikes, CHNs are often front and center in responding to those in need. The caring and compassionate legacy of the nursing profession shows that nurses traditionally respond in large numbers to rescue and aid people in times of a public health threat. As the largest population of healthcare providers in the United States, nurses have the ability to play significant roles in community response to natural disasters (earthquakes, floods, heat waves, hurricanes, tornadoes), human-made disasters (terrorist attacks, industrial chemical accidents), and infectious epidemics (influenza, Legionnaires' disease) (Bureau of Labor Statistics, U.S. Department of Labor, 2010).

In recent years, nurses have responded nationally to a variety of disasters, including the Oklahoma City bombing in 1995, the devastation caused by Hurricanes Katrina and Rita on the Gulf Coast in 2005, and the terrorist attacks in 2001 on the World Trade Center in New York City, on the Pentagon near Washington, D.C., and in Shanksville, Pennsylvania. On an international scale, CHNs from the United States have mobilized response efforts to care for people during the devastation caused by the Asian tsunami of 2004, the catastrophic Haiti earthquake of 2010, and the nuclear and environmental disaster of 2011 in Japan. Each of these events required nurses who played key roles during all phases of the disaster cycle.

Community health nurses are competent to step into "mass care voids" during times of disasters, "to render public health, population based services" (Polivka, Stanley, Gordon, Taulbee, Kieffer, & McCrokle, 2008, p. 159). Through the delivery of specific skills in times of disaster, CHNs serve as integral members in "emergency operations and command centers, in leadership and management roles and . . . in

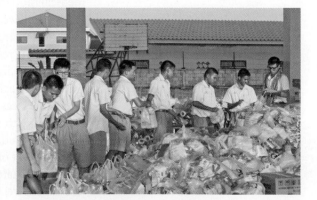

© Yuttasak Jannarong/Shutterstock.com

the field where they provide frontline disaster health and core public health services" (Jakeway, LaRosa, & Schoenfisch, 2008, p. 354).

Healthcare Disparities

Healthcare disparities are differences in the incidence, prevalence, and morbidity and mortality rates among racial, ethnic, socioeconomic, and geographic groups that exist as part of populations around the world. They occur in developed nations as well as underdeveloped nations. No one is immune when differences exist among people of the world. The elimination of healthcare disparities has become a major worldwide public health objective.

Globally, people around the world may be disenfranchised and suffer healthcare disparities due to religious or cultural beliefs and gender. A specific example is the high maternal and neonatal morbidity and mortality rates found around the world. According to WHO (2010c), approximately 1,000 women die each day due to postpartum hemorrhage, infections, pregnancy-induced hypertension, and unsafe abortions. Around the world and even in the United States, healthcare disparities result in missed opportunities to administer immunizations, screen and treat cardiac disease, decrease death rates from cancer, and provide education on smoking cessation and nutrition.

In the United States, the Agency for Healthcare Research and Quality (AHRQ) states that healthcare disparities are a national problem that affects people at "all points in the process, at all sites of care, and for all medical conditions" (AHRQ, 2004, para. 21). Healthcare disparities are felt to a disproportionate degree by many racial and ethnic minorities and by people of lower socioeconomic status. The lack of healthcare insurance further widens the gap associated with healthcare disparities (AHRQ, 2004).

According to the U.S. Census Bureau (2010), the number of people without health insurance coverage rose from 46.3 million in 2008 to 50.7 million in 2009. One specific response related to healthcare costs and lack of insurance is the recent rise and growth of medical tourism. The lure of this practice is the ability of uninsured and underinsured people to obtain relatively cheap healthcare services. With the cost of medical services climbing in the United States, people, even those individuals with insurance may "shop" around the world for a variety of healthcare services.

Medical Tourism

Medical tourism: The practice of some clients seeking low-cost healthcare services in countries other than their own.

Medical tourism is a recent healthcare trend that bears close scrutiny by CHNs. This practice, which involves clients seeking low-cost healthcare services in countries other than their own, is on the rise. In the United States, both the increasing cost of healthcare services and the affordability of international travel are driving forces in the expansion of medical tourism around the world. Additionally, recent advances in technology around the world have increased the prevalence of medical tourism; no longer do Americans view healthcare facilities in the United States as the sole sources of clinical excellence. The growing recognition that healthcare services constitutes big business has raised the estimated annual global healthcare expenditures on medical tourism to more than $3 trillion per year (Kassim, 2009).

The services provided include both nonelective and elective procedures, and are often packaged with sightseeing and travel tours (Smith, 2006). Central and South America, India, Thailand, Malaysia, and Israel are popular medical tourism destinations. In Costa Rica, the cost of healthcare services is approximately 30% to 40% less expensive than in the United States; in Brazil, the cost of healthcare services is approximately 40% to 50% less expensive. People flock to these countries for dental and cosmetic procedures due to their proximity to the United States. Common procedures sought by clients include elective cosmetic surgery, joint replacement surgery, cardiac surgery, infertility treatments, and dental care. The low cost of health care in countries other than the United States is a primary driving force behind this movement, especially among people who lack adequate healthcare insurance.

To further promote the healthcare services provided in countries other than the United States, many hospitals around the world have sought and obtained Joint Commission International (JCI) accreditation. More than 250 JCI-accredited hospitals now offer a variety of healthcare services to the public. Other companies and services have also emerged to create a seamless healthcare experience for those interested in finding international healthcare services. Consumer packages are often created and described as exotic vacations associated with healthcare services, which can include spa-like recovery services. By 2012, according to the Deloitte Center for Health Solutions (2008), more than 10 million people were expected to travel abroad for healthcare services.

Questions have been raised about the safety and appropriateness of care received by individuals who use medical tourism as a means of achieving health and well-being (Ben-Natan, Ben-Sefer, & Ehrenfeld, 2009). These issues include questions about the quality of such care and the lack of regulatory policies governing it, especially in hospitals that do not hold JCI accreditation. Caution is needed, especially given that international standards and Joint Commission standards in the United States differ. Moreover, outcome statistics from hospitals outside the United States are difficult to find, making it problematic to compare outcomes following procedures in the various countries.

The lack of adequate client follow-up is also important to consider. Practitioners in the United States may be hesitant to provide care to a client following an international procedure, specifically in the case of a postoperative complication. Additionally, postoperative travel in itself may pose an increased risk for complications such as deep vein thrombosis and respiratory complications. The lack of legal remedies for malpractice may leave a patient with inadequate resources to mitigate any postoperative complication. Owing to all of these factors, CHNs must be able to help clients with their decision to seek care outside to the United States—that is, they must help clients to compare and contrast domestic and international options for care with regard to cost and quality of services provided.

Creating Interstate and National Responsibility

Response to Disasters

Effective management of a large-scale national disaster requires the coordination, collaboration, and integration of activities from multiple community systems, including emergency response teams, acute care health settings, and community/public health venues (Association of Community Health Nursing Educators, 2008). The only way to effectively respond to and manage health concerns, including public health emergencies, is through the coordination of personnel and community resources with support from local, state, and federal agencies. In the United States, multiple resources are available to CHNs. It is important, therefore, for nurses preparing for interstate population-based practice to know and understand the laws, regulations, systems, and organizations in place that will influence the care they give to patients, especially in times of public health emergencies.

During natural disasters, disease pandemics, terrorist attacks, and other public health emergencies, the health system must be prepared to accommodate a surge in the number of individuals seeking medical help. For the health community, a primary concern is how to provide care to individuals during such periods of high demand, when the health system's resources are exhausted and there are more patients than the system can accommodate (Institute of Medicine, 2010).

Robert T. Stafford Disaster Relief and Emergency Assistance Act

The Robert T. Stafford Disaster Relief and Emergency Assistance Act was passed by the U.S. Congress in 1988 and amended in 2000. It allows the federal government to provide assistance through response activities to local and state governments during times of emergencies and major disasters. In addition, it designates the Federal Emergency Management Agency (FEMA) as being responsible to coordinate government-wide relief efforts in times of disaster within the United States. Disaster situations may include chemical emergencies, dam failure, earthquake, fire, flood, hazardous material, heat, hurricane, landslide, nuclear power plant emergency, terrorism, thunderstorm, tornado, tsunami, volcano, wildfire, and winter storm.

National Incident Management System (NIMS): A U.S. government-created management system that integrates communication, equipment, facilities, personnel, and procedures to ensure effective and efficient management of disasters within the United States.

Incident Command System (ICS): A standardized, on-scene, all-hazards incident management effort that is a significant component of the National Incident Management System, and is used by local, state, federal, and tribal agencies.

National Incident Management System

The **National Incident Management System (NIMS)** was created by FEMA to provide a systematic, proactive approach to prevent, protect against, respond to, recover from, and mitigate the effects of incidents, regardless of cause, size, location, or complexity, so as to reduce the loss of life and property and harm to the environment. This management system integrates communication, equipment, facilities, personnel, and procedures to ensure effective and efficient management of disasters within the United States (NIMS, 2010). A significant component of NIMS, used by local, state, federal, and tribal agencies, is the Incident Command System.

Incident Command System

The **Incident Command System (ICS)** is a standardized, on-scene, all-hazards incident management effort that meets the following aims:

- Allows for the integration of facilities, equipment, personnel, procedures, and communications operating within a common organizational structure
- Enables a coordinated response among various jurisdictions and functional agencies, both public and private
- Establishes common processes for planning and managing resources (FEMA, 2010)

During times of disaster, interdisciplinary response skills of all healthcare providers, including CHNs, are needed to deal with the event (Gebbie & Qureshi, 2006). Community health nurses can readily serve within the ICS. The knowledge and expertise they possess make them integral participants in all aspects of emergency preparedness, planning, and response. Their specialized skill sets allow them to serve as first responders in many disasters—to journey into scenes of disaster while others flee. The cadre of CHNs embraces a population-based vision that allows them to "enhance the emergency response infrastructure at the local, regional, state, national and global levels" (Jakeway et al., 2008, p. 354). Examples include the nurses who responded to the terrorist attacks of September 11, 2001, and who remained on duty in New Orleans, Louisiana, during Hurricane Katrina.

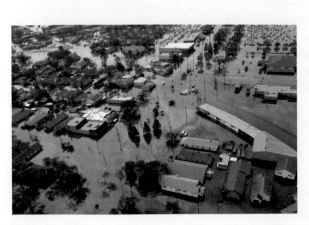

Courtesy of Jocelyn Augustino/FEMA.

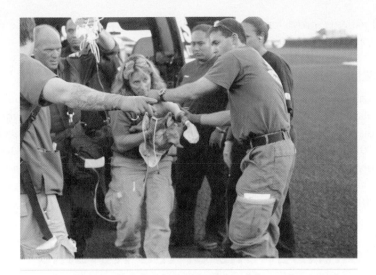

Members of a Disaster Medical Assistance Team (DMAT) in American Samoa rush an infant onto a Coast Guard plane that will evacuate the infant to Hawaii. (2009)

FEMA/Casey Deshong

Medical Disaster Relief Networks

Following the tragic events of September 11, 2001, the U.S. Congress passed the Public Health Security and Bioterrorism Preparedness and Response Act (2002) to enhance national readiness and response capabilities to public health emergencies. One section of the act calls for the coordination of volunteers who would be available to respond to public health emergencies within the United States. The **Emergency System for Advance Registration of Volunteer Health Professionals (ESAR-VHP)** was implemented in all 50 states to facilitate volunteer response readiness throughout the United States through the verification of individual professional credentials. These state-based registries maintain a comprehensive list of qualified volunteers, verify their credentials prior to a disaster to facilitate response time, and provide disaster response educational training opportunities (Litchfield, 2010).

National Disaster Medical System

When a disaster or public health concern overwhelms local resources, federal assistance may be requested by the state governor. One measure of assistance may come from the **National Disaster Medical System (NDMS)**, a national organization of rapid response teams designed to deliver quality medical care to the victims of, and responders to, a domestic disaster (U.S. Department of Health and Human Services, Public Health and Medical Services Support, National Disaster Medical System, 2010). Through the NDMS, state-of-the-art medical care is available at a disaster site, in transit from the disaster area, and in participating care facilities. One important component of the NDMS is the Disaster Medical Assistance Team.

Disaster Medical Assistance Teams

Disaster Medical Assistance Teams (DMATs), under the direction of the NDMS of the U.S. Department of Health and Human Services, are teams of healthcare volunteers, including nurses, who are ready to provide rapid response emergency care during a national disaster or event. Responsibilities of the rapid response team include the

Emergency System for Advance Registration of Volunteer Health Professionals (ESAR-VHP): A system of state-based registries that facilitate volunteer response readiness throughout the United States through verification of individual professional credentials. The registries maintain a comprehensive list of qualified volunteers, verify their credentials prior to a disaster to facilitate response time, and provide disaster response educational training opportunities.

National Disaster Medical System (NDMS): A national organization of rapid response teams designed to deliver quality medical care to the victims of, and responders to, a domestic disaster in the United States.

Disaster Medical Assistance Teams (DMATs): As a component of the National Disaster Medical System, these teams of healthcare volunteers (including nurses) provide rapid response emergency care during a national disaster or event.

Medical Reserve Corps (MRC): A network of community-based public health professionals, including community/public health nurses and physicians, who respond to natural disasters and emergencies to support community health and medical resources.

U.S. Public Health Service Commissioned Corps: A team of public health professionals, including nurses, who are trained and equipped to respond to public health crises and national emergencies.

triaging of patients, provision of ongoing health care to patients in adverse or austere conditions, and the evacuation of patients as needed (Litchfield, 2010).

Medical Reserve Corps

The **Medical Reserve Corps (MRC)** is a network of community-based public health professionals, including community/public health nurses and physicians, who respond to natural disasters and emergencies to support community health and medical resources (MRC, 2010). The mission of the MRC is specific and specialized; it is to establish teams of local volunteer medical and public health professionals who can contribute their skills and expertise throughout the year and during times of community need (MRC, 2010).

The Contributions of the Nursing Profession to National, International, and Global Health Concerns

U.S. Public Health Service Commissioned Corps

The **U.S. Public Health Service Commissioned Corps** is a team of public health professionals, including nurses, who are trained and equipped to respond to public health crises and national emergencies (U.S. Public Health Service Commissioned Corps, 2010). The mission of the Commissioned Corps (2010) is to protect, promote, and advance the health and safety of the United States through rapid and effective response to public health needs. The core values of leadership, service, integrity, and excellence demonstrate the corps' commitment to public health.

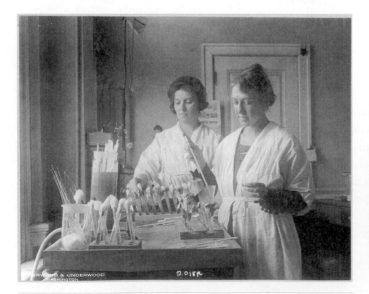

Testing antipneumoccus serum for potency. The Public Health Service keeps a close check on the commercial production of serums, vaccines, and analogous products so that physicans and patients may be assured of a safe remedy. Hygienic labratory. Doctor Ella Eulows (right) and laboratory assistant Sadie Carlin (left) making the tests. (1920)

U.S. National Archives and Records Administration; Underwood & Underwood, Photographer.

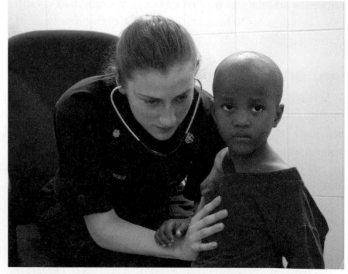

U.S. Public Health Service Lt. Cmdr. Sandra Bender, attached to Military Sealift Command hospital ship USNS Comfort (T-AH 20), listens to the lungs of a patient at Centre Hospitalier Eliazar Germain in Pétion-Ville, Haiti. (2007)

U.S. Navy photo by Mass Communication Specialist 1st Class John Fields.

In the United States, rapid response corps teams aided victims of the terrorist attacks in 2001, Hurricane Katrina in 2005, the earthquake in Hawaii in 2006, Hurricanes Gustav and Ike in 2008, and the Deepwater Horizon oil spill in 2010. Officers in the corps also provide mental health services using a public health model based on building resilience and facilitating recovery for people with or at risk for mental illness or substance use disorders. Additionally, the corps responds to international public health needs. Corp members have been deployed to America Samoa, Haiti, Indonesia, and Panama.

Association of Community Health Nursing Educators

The Association of Community Health Nursing Educators (ACHNE, 2008) recognizes the social responsibility CHNs have in times of disasters. However, the ability of nurses, including CHNs, to respond to "sudden and emerging health trends from natural, intentional, or technological disasters" can be challenging (ACHNE, 2008, p. 3). The safety of self and that of all team members is one of the most important things a first responder must ensure. Secure perimeters, especially during terrorist attacks, to control access to and from the site of the disaster are very important. Therefore, disaster preparedness requires an organized approach that is based on the ability of CHNs to "function safely, effectively, and with a commitment to contribute to a disaster response" through the use of knowledge, skills, and abilities (ACHNE, 2008, p. 4).

Association of State and Territorial Directors of Nursing

The Association of State and Territorial Directors of Nursing (ASTDN, 2007) has described an ideal world in which every individual, family, and community has a comprehensive emergency preparedness plan that minimizes the consequences of disasters. The goal of ASTDN is to protect and promote the health and safety of the public through public policy efforts, leadership development, and advocacy for the preparation, practice, and role of the CHN (ASTDN, 2010). One significant accomplishment of ASTDN has been the provision of guidelines for all CHNs in the United States and its territories regarding emergency preparedness and response. These guidelines describe the roles and actions that CHNs must take to protect the health and safety of individuals, families, and communities during times of disasters (**Table 15-1**).

TABLE 15-1
Association of State and Territorial Directors of Nursing's Guidelines to Protect the Health and Safety of Individuals, Families, and Communities in a Disaster

1. Nursing roles in emergency preparedness must be consistent with the scope of practice for the specialty or area of nursing practice.

2. The nursing process must be used in all areas of emergency preparedness.

3. Competencies are necessary to provide a framework for defining nursing roles and actions. These competencies are linked to education, training, and practice events.

4. Leadership, policy, planning, and practice expertise are essential nursing skills used during emergency preparedness and response.

TABLE 15-2

Association of State and Territorial Directors of Nursing's Emergency Core Competencies for Community/Public Health Nurses

1. Know and describe prior to an emergency their role during an emergency
2. Understand and describe the chain of command during an emergency
3. Identify and locate their agency's emergency response plan before an emergency occurs
4. Define and describe functional roles and responsibilities during an emergency
5. Demonstrate the correct use of the equipment and skills needed during an emergency
6. Demonstrate the correct use of all emergency communication devices used by their agency
7. Describe communication role(s) used during an emergency.
8. Identify self-limitations regarding knowledge, skills, and authority and identify appropriate resources available for matters that exceed these limits
9. Use creative problem-solving skills, given that each disaster is unique
10. Recognize deviations from the norm through assessment skills
11. Participate in continuing education to maintain current knowledge in relevant areas
12. Participate in planning, exercising, and evaluating drills

To protect the health and safety of individuals, families, and communities during times of disasters, ASTDN (2007) has identified 12 specific core competencies for community/public health nurses (**Table 15-2**). All of these competencies address the need for CHNs to be competent and prepared. Therefore, it is important to know and understand the four phases of emergency preparedness (these phases, and the specifics of local disaster management, were discussed in the "Staying Alert as the Key to Emergency and Disaster Management" chapter).

Legal and Practice Barriers During Disasters and Interstate Practice

Community health nurses who respond to a public health crisis must be qualified and competent. Unfortunately, legal and practice barriers may exist for CHNs who could be deployed to national disaster areas due to a lack of licensure and credentialing information. This could potentially slow down and hamper interstate rescue efforts (McHugh, 2007). During the attacks on September 11, 2001, in New York, Washington, D.C., and Pennsylvania, countless interstate volunteers, including nurses, reported to healthcare facilities; unfortunately, the inability to rapidly confirm their licensure, credentials, skill sets, and scope of practice resulted in many of them being turned away (Hodge, Gable, & Calves, 2005).

Nurse licensure and practice regulation is the responsibility of individual states, and each state has established a different scope and standards of nursing practice. Consequently, nurses cannot readily transfer their nursing practice to other states, even in times of disasters. To alleviate this problem, the declaration of a state of emergency is a vital governmental tool that would allow nurses to provide interstate nursing care. Additionally, emergency power acts of the federal government may allow nurses to practice in other states during times of mass-casualty events and national disasters. Therefore, it is important that nurses know and understand the provisions of their individual state Nurse Practice Acts.

Nurse Licensure Compact

The need for a licensure system that would facilitate interstate nursing practice, especially during a disaster, was recognized by the National Council of State Boards of Nursing (NCSBN) in 1997. The goal of NCSBN was to create a common professional nursing license that would be "recognized nationally and enforced locally" (NCSBN, 1997, p. 1). The process of creating a **Nurse Licensure Compact (NLC)** agreement began with the primary goal of allowing nurses to practice the profession of nursing in multiple states without the need to obtain additional state licenses. This coordination of activities associated with nursing licensure would reduce multiple and duplicate state requirements and create a mechanism to share disciplinary action information between states.

The overriding purpose of the NLC was to increase the access individuals, families, and groups in the United States have to nursing care by removing regulatory barriers. In 1998, the NCSBN adopted a plan for multistate licensure that would allow a nurse (registered nurse and licensed practical/vocational nurse) to hold a multistate license in a primary (home) state of residence and practice in person or electronically in other compact (remote) states.

As of this book's writing, 24 states had enacted legislation or regulations that allow for nurse participation in the NLC (**Table 15-3**). These state boards of nursing have entered into an interstate compact agreement that is governed by Nurse Licensure Compact Administrators (NLCA) in each participating state. This agreement creates a legal contract between states that allows nurses to practice across state lines. Individual nurses remain accountable for their nursing practice in the state where the patient resides at the time care is provided. The compact agreement does not alter an individual state's Nurse Practice Act. A national database called Nursys maintains license and disciplinary action information contributed by participating states on all nurses. Nurses who reside in non-NLC states are not eligible for nurse compact licensure.

Proponents of the NLC note that geography has become less of a barrier in the delivery of nursing care and that legislation is needed to facilitate recent healthcare trends—especially the transportation of patients across state lines, the integration of healthcare systems or managed care organizations that operate in multiple states, and the use of **telehealth nursing**, which is the use of telecommunication and information technology to provide nursing care when large distances exist between patient and nurse. Advocates of the NLC maintain that the requirement of nurses to hold multiple state nursing licenses is impractical, costly, and inefficient. One of the most significant aspects of the NLC may be the ability of nurses to respond to mass-casualty events at the very time when qualified nursing services are needed most.

Critics of the NLC warn that individual states could lose their authority to regulate nurses, as license requirements would be set by a nurse's primary state of residence and

Nurse Licensure Compact (NLC): An agreement that allows nurses to practice the profession of nursing in multiple states without the need to obtain additional state licenses.

Telehealth nursing: The use of telecommunication and information technology to provide nursing care when large distances exist between patient and nurse.

TABLE 15-3
Nursing Compact Licensure States

Arizona	New Hampshire
Arkansas	New Mexico
Colorado	North Carolina
Delaware	North Dakota
Idaho	Rhode Island
Iowa	South Carolina
Kentucky	South Dakota
Maine	Tennessee
Maryland	Texas
Mississippi	Utah
Missouri	Virginia
Nebraska	Wisconsin

not by the remote state of practice. Additionally, nurses who hold an interstate license may be susceptible to multiple disciplinary actions by state boards of nursing, should the nurse become involved in an adverse patient outcome. Some critics warn that confidentiality, in the form of licensure information and certain issues such as history of substance abuse treatment and judicial actions, may be breached. According to Crotty (2007), the major beneficiaries of interstate licensure are not nurses, but rather the insurance companies and multistate healthcare organizations that want to promote telenursing. Another concern raised is the potential for increased cost of liability premiums to nurses. Critics of the NLC also warn that collective bargaining efforts in labor disputes may be weakened, thereby making it easier for healthcare facilities to hire nurses from other states.

Civil Liability Concerns During Disasters and Interstate Practice

Mass-casualty events, where healthcare providers are overwhelmed by the number and severity of casualties during a disaster, are often chaotic and unpredictable. Because even the best planning efforts cannot always lessen the impact of disasters, it must be recognized that people may be harmed during emergency responses and that responders to mass-casualty events may not be able to achieve optimal patient outcomes (Hodge et al., 2005). In turn, CHNs who respond in times of disasters could be vulnerable to civil litigation for injuries a person may experience at the time of the emergency response (McHugh, 2007), including charges of negligence and a breach of privacy and duty. **Good Samaritan laws**, which provide liability protection to nurses in emergency situations, may be in effect in many individual states. In addition, the NLC and state and federal laws and regulations may provide protection and immunity from civil liability to mass-casualty volunteers.

Good Samaritan laws: Laws that provide liability protection to nurses and other healthcare providers in emergency situations.

Interstate Travel Nursing

Another opportunity open to nurses who want to foster social responsibility within the United States is travel nursing. Although the impetus in the development and growth of travel nursing and the travel nursing industry was, in part, national nursing shortages, nurses may choose to use travel nursing as a venue to alleviate community health needs by bringing skilled nursing care to impoverished areas of the United States. Qualified travel nurses can work at temporary, short-term (average of 13 weeks) assignments across the United States. They are frequently offered incentives such as relocation assistance, furnished housing, higher wages, healthcare benefits, and sign-on bonuses.

Additionally, travel nursing offers opportunities for professional growth and development and personal adventure. With more than 350 travel agencies in the United States, qualified nurses have a variety of assignments from which to choose, including community health settings (Travel Nurse Companies Allied Health Agencies Web Directory, 2009). Minimum qualifications include one year of clinical experience, licensure in the state of employment, and demonstrated knowledge and proficiency in the nurse's area of expertise. The CHN would need to study the Nurse Practice Act in the state(s) to be visited, so as to ensure that safe and effective nursing practice can be maintained.

One concern about travel nursing relates to the practice of some companies that focus on replacing nurses involved in unionized job actions. Some travel nursing companies may negotiate with institutions to replace nurses on strike for potentially unfair labor practices. Nurses working for travel companies have the right to investigate why a potential work setting needs replacement nurses before accepting an assignment. Most travel nurse assignments, however, are not related to any unusual employment conditions.

Global Community Health Responsibility and International Organizations

Nurses recognize that health is a global issue. As a consequence, many nurses, including CHNs, often feel the pull to work as humanitarian aid volunteers to improve the health and well-being of people in developing countries. This can be accomplished in the form of short-term humanitarian efforts in response to a disaster or as long-term national or international developmental work. Globally, specific healthcare issues and conditions exist that are not seen in the United States, are rarely seen in the United States, or present themselves very differently than they do in the United States. For example, outbreaks of cholera, dengue fever, malaria, avian (bird) flu, and Ebola (hemorrhagic fever) are endemic to nations and regions other than the United States. Globally, by the end of 2008, 33.4 million people were living with HIV infection, with two-thirds of these individuals residing in sub-Saharan Africa (WHO, 2010c). Malaria is a disease that kills nearly 1 million people a year, most of them children in Africa younger than the age of five years (WHO, 2010c).

Cultural Concerns

Working in countries other than the United States requires unique skill sets that are essential during global humanitarian aid efforts. Volunteers must have the ability and interpersonal skills to work with people who speak different languages and are of diverse cultures and nationalities; culture includes the values, beliefs, and practices shared by a group of people. International volunteers must recognize and appreciate the similarities and differences among people around the world if they are to create an atmosphere of mutual respect and acceptance. Some volunteers may work in very isolated areas, which requires them to be extremely flexible and resourceful. The standards of care so readily accepted in the United States may not be available in other countries due to lack of resources and knowledge. Additionally, international group dynamics among healthcare providers from various nations will certainly be different.

Safety Concerns

Safety is something that needs to be considered when working in other countries. While many developing countries enjoy political stability but lack significant resources to adequately respond to local healthcare needs and mass-casualty events, other countries are involved in ongoing political upheaval and armed conflict that could significantly and negatively impact humanitarian relief efforts. Healthcare workers, including CHNs, are encouraged to keep in close contact with official international organizations or the regional U.S. Consulate. These international organizations support the work of providers like the CHN to foster social responsibility. Several international organizations are in existence to foster international peace, improve global health, decrease global healthcare disparities, reduce global poverty, advance human rights, and promote social responsibility; they are discussed next.

United Nations

The United Nations (UN) is an international organization committed to maintaining international peace and security, developing friendly relations among nations, and promoting social progress, better living standards, and human rights. In 2000, the UN adopted objectives for the global community called the **Millennium Development Goals (MDGs)**. Through this global action plan, the United Nations hopes to achieve significant positive outcomes that will promote the health and well-being of people around the world. The purpose of the eight MDGs is to reduce poverty, improve global health, and focus on worldwide educational and environmental concerns (**Table 15-4**). These eight anti-poverty goals have a target date of 2015; in 2010, a United Nations Summit provided an update on the goals.

In 2010, the UN announced that pledges in excess of $40 billion have been received to support the MDGs; these pledges have the potential of saving the lives of more than 16 million women and children, preventing 33 million unwanted pregnancies, protecting

Millennium Development Goals (MDGs): A global action plan developed by the United Nations that is designed to promote the health and well-being of people around the world. The purpose of the eight MDGs is to reduce poverty, improve global health, and focus on worldwide educational and environmental concerns.

TABLE 15-4

2000–2010 Millennium Development Goals

Goal 1: Eradicate Extreme Poverty and Hunger
The goal is to halve, between 1990 and 2015, the proportion of people whose income is less than $1 per day and the proportion of people who suffer from hunger. Between 1990 and 2005, the number of people living under the international poverty line of $1.25 per day declined from 1.8 billion to 1.4 billion. Overall, the poverty rate decreased from 46% in 1990 to 27% in 2005 in developing regions. The greatest achievements to date have been mainly in East Asia. Unfortunately, the recent economic crisis was expected to push an estimated 64 more million people into extreme poverty in 2010. The proportion of people suffering from hunger has declined, but according to the UN, the pace is unsatisfactory. According to the Food and Agricultural Organization of the UN, more than 925 million people were expected to suffer chronic hunger in the year 2010.

TABLE 15-4
2000–2010 Millennium Development Goals *(Continued)*

Goal 2: Achieve Universal Primary Education

The goal is to ensure that by 2015, children around the world—boys and girls alike—are able to complete a full course of primary schooling. In 2008, the enrollment in primary education in developing regions reached 89%, up from 83% in 2000. However, approximately 69 million school-age children are not in school; almost half of them are in sub-Saharan Africa (enrollment increased by only 18%) and more than one-fourth of them are in Southern Asia (enrollment increased by only 11%). The summit noted that the pace of progress is insufficient.

Goal 3: Promote Gender Equality and Empower Women

The goal was to eliminate gender disparity in primary and secondary education by 2005 and in all levels of education by 2015. While gender gaps in access to education around the world have narrowed, disparities remain in university-level education, with large inequality gaps primarily in sub-Saharan Africa and Western Asia. Men continue to outnumber women in paid employment. Even when women are employed, they are typically paid less and have less job security than men.

Goal 4: Reduce Child Mortality

The goal was to reduce by two-thirds, between 1990 and 2010, the mortality rate of children younger than the age of five years. While the number of child deaths is falling (it decreased by 28% from 100 to 72 deaths per 1,000 live births), almost 9 million children still die every year before they reach the age of five. The highest child mortality rates continue to be found in sub-Saharan Africa, where one in seven children dies before the age of five.

Goal 5: Improve Maternal Health

The goal is to reduce by three-fourths the maternal mortality rate and achieve universal access to reproductive health care. The maternal mortality rate remains unacceptably high, with more than 350,000 women dying annually from pregnancy complications such as postpartum hemorrhage, hypertension, obstructed labor, and infection. In sub-Saharan Africa, the maternal mortality risk is 1 in 30, compared to 1 in 5,600 in developed regions around the world. While contraceptive use has increased since 2000, funding for reproductive services has not kept pace with demand. It is estimated that meeting the needs for contraceptive services alone would decrease by one-third the overall maternal mortality rates around the world.

Goal 6: Combat HIV/AIDS, Malaria, and Other Diseases

The goal is to halt and even reverse by 2015 the spread of HIV/AIDS and the incidence of malaria and other major diseases around the world. The summit reported "tangible progress" toward this goal. The number of new HIV infections decreased from 3.5 million in 1996 to 2.7 million in 2008. The number of deaths from AIDS-related illnesses decreased from 2.2 million in 2004 to 2 million in 2008. Unfortunately, more than 14.1 million children in sub-Saharan Africa have lost one or both parents to AIDS. The increased global production of mosquito nets between 2004 and 2009 and the increased availability of antimalarial medication in countries around the world have reduced the overall rate of malaria. Even so, approximately 243 million cases of malaria occurred in 2008, causing 863,000 deaths (89% of them in Africa).

Goal 7: Ensure Environmental Stability

The goal is to integrate principles of sustainable development into national policies and programs to reverse the loss of environmental resources and reduce by half the number of populations without access to safe drinking water and sanitation. It is estimated that the world will meet or even exceed the drinking water target by 2015. To date, four regions—Northern Africa, Latin America and the Caribbean, Eastern Asia, and Southeastern Asia—have met the target. That translates into 1.7 billion people who have gained access to safe drinking water since 1990. Unfortunately, 884 million people around the world still do not have access to safe drinking water, and 2.6 million people, primarily in sub-Saharan Africa and South Asia, lack basic sanitation equipment such as toilets or latrines.

Goal 8: Develop a Global Partnership for Development

The goal is to develop an open, rule-based, predictable, nondiscriminatory trading and financial system to address the needs of the least developed countries, landlocked countries, and small island developing nations. While developing countries are gaining access to markets of developed countries, aid to underdeveloped nations, specifically in Africa, remains well below the target set by the United Nations.

120 million children from pneumonia and 88 million children from stunting, advancing the control of deadly diseases such as malaria and HIV/AIDS, and ensuring access for women and children to quality facilities and skilled health workers. Three of these goals—the reduction of child mortality, the improvement of maternal health, and the fight against HIV/AIDS, malaria, and other diseases—can be directly addressed by the work of CHNs.

United Nations Children's Fund

The United Nations Children's Fund (UNICEF) is an organization whose sole purpose is to build a world where the rights of every child are realized. UNICEF was created in December 1946 by the UN to provide food, clothing, and health care to children after World War II. In 1953, it became a permanent part of the UN. In 1959, the UN General Assembly adopted the Declaration of the Rights of the Child, which defined children's rights to protection, education, health care, shelter, and good nutrition. UNICEF has global authority to influence the health and well-being of children around the world and believes that nurturing and caring for children are the "cornerstones of human progress" (UNICEF, 2010, para. 2).

This organization is dedicated to improving the lives of children around the world on a daily basis through the promotion of education, immunizations, and measures that give children the best opportunities to realize optimal health and well-being. Promoting the health and well-being of children by the achievement of growth and development milestones is a global imperative that will result in healthy global communities.

TABLE 15-5
World Health Organization Agenda Items

1. Health development through activities that promote health outcomes in poor, disadvantaged, or vulnerable groups. This directive is driven by the ethical principle of equity: Life-saving or health-promoting interventions should not be denied for unfair reasons, including those with economic or social roots.

2. Health security through collective action to decrease the shared vulnerability of emerging and epidemic-prone diseases, which may be partially due to rapid urbanization, environmental mismanagement, the way food is produced and traded, and the way antibiotics are used and misused.

3. Using research, information, and evidence to set priorities, define strategies, and measure results.

4. Strengthening of global health systems to reach poor and underserved populations. Areas being addressed include adequate numbers of healthcare providers, sufficient financial funding, systems for the collection of vital statistics, and access to technology including essential medications.

5. Enhanced partnerships with other United Nations agencies, international organizations, donors, and private organizations to implement programs.

6. Improved performance in its efficiency and effectiveness through ongoing reforms.

World Health Organization

The World Health Organization is the directing and coordinating authority for health within the UN system. Its overall goal is to improve world health by "providing leadership on global health matters, shaping the health research agenda, setting norms and standards, articulating evidence-based policy options, providing technical support to countries and monitoring and assessing health trends" (WHO, 2010a, 2010b). Four key words describe this mission: prevention, promotion, treatment, and rehabilitation. The WHO objectives are met through the provision of leadership on matters critical to health and the development of partnerships when joint action is needed. One example is the role WHO played following the 2011 earthquake and subsequent tsunami and nuclear crisis in Japan. **Table 15-5** identifies the WHO Agenda Items and their contribution to global health.

Pan American Health Organization

The Pan American Health Organization (PAHO) is an international public health organization that works to improve health and living standards of the countries of the Americas. It is the regional office for the Americas of the World Health Organization. This organization focuses on health needs of the Americas through health surveillance, disease prevention and control, emergency preparedness, and disaster relief. Recent programs undertaken by PAHO have included immunization clinics, family and community health education, and chronic disease prevention and control.

Nongovernmental Organizations

Nongovernmental organizations (NGOs) are independent, legal organizations that have no governmental status. The World Bank (2010) defines NGOs as "private organizations that pursue activities to relieve suffering, promote the interests of the poor, protect the environment, provide basic social services, or undertake community development" (para. 1). Each has a mission and philosophy. Some are secular and independent, some are faith-based, and some are affiliated with political organizations. Given this multiplicity of possible motivations, it is important for volunteers to carefully research an NGO before becoming part of a humanitarian effort. Many nurses have joined NGOs to deliver much need care around the world.

> **Nongovernmental organizations (NGOs):** Independent, legal organizations that have no governmental status; "private organizations that pursue activities to relieve suffering, promote the interests of the poor, protect the environment, provide basic social services, or undertake community development" (World Bank, 2010, para. 1).

One example of an NGO that has attracted healthcare volunteers is the International Medical Corps (IMC, 2010), a "global, humanitarian, nonprofit organization dedicated to saving lives and relieving suffering through health care training and relief and development programs" (para. 1). IMC was established in 1984 by volunteer doctors and nurses as a private, voluntary, nonpolitical, nonsectarian organization with the mission to improve the quality of life through health interventions and related activities that build local capacity in underserved communities worldwide.

Another example is the Health Volunteer Organization (HVO, 2010), which is a network of healthcare professionals, organizations, corporations, and donors united in a common commitment to improving global health through education. Nurses in HVO have provided education to nurses in Cambodia, India, Tanzania, and Uganda, with the goal of developing and expanding clinical expertise to improve the overall health and well-being of people in designated countries.

Summary

Community health nurses play a vital role in interstate, international, and global community health concerns. Through the nursing process, all nurses, and particularly CHNs, can readily and significantly influence the overall health and well-being of people around the world. According to Litchfield (2010), the most effective way for nurses to volunteer during a disaster is to respond as a member of an organized response team. This approach may include affiliations with organizations whose primary responsibility is emergency response to disasters or with organizations that focus on ongoing programs to improve the health and well-being of a population nationally or internationally.

REFERENCES

Agency for Healthcare Research and Quality (AHRQ). (2004). *National healthcare disparities report, 2003.* Retrieved from http://www.ahrq.gov/qual/nhdr03/nhdrsum03.htm

Association of Community Health Nurses Educators (ACHNE). (2008). *Disaster preparedness white paper for community/public health nursing educators.* Retrieved on from http://www.achne.org/files/public/DisasterPreparednessWhitePaper.pdf

Association of State and Territorial Directors of Nursing (ASTDN). (2007). *The role of public health nurses in emergency preparedness and response.* Retrieved from http://www.astdn.org/downloadablefiles/ASTDN%20EP%20Paper%20final%2010%2029%2007.pdf

Association of State and Territorial Directors of Nursing (ASTDN). (2010). Retrieved from http://www.astdn.org/ASTDN-Mission-Values-Goals-History-new.htm

Ben-Natan, M., Ben-Sefer, E., & Ehrenfeld, M. (2009). Medical tourism: A new role for nursing? *Online Journal of Issues in Nursing, 14*(8). Retrieved from http://web.ebscohost.com.libproxy.adelphi.edu:2048/ehost/detail?vid=5&hid=13&sid=3d1d3789-6114-4e76-9991 ed3f3a204 b31%40sessionmgr15&bdata=JnNpdGU9ZWhvc3QtbGl2ZSSzzY29wZT1zaXRl#db=rzh& AN=2010587446

Bureau of Labor Statistics, U.S. Department of Labor. (2010). Registered nurses. In *Occupational outlook handbook 2010–2011 edition.* Retrieved from http://www.bls.gov/oco/ocos083.htm

Centre for Research on the Epidemiology of Disasters. (2010). *Annual disaster statistical review.* Retrieved from http://www.preventionweb.net/files/14382_ADSR2009.pdf

Crotty, M. (2007). Interstate licensure of nurses. Important information about proposed compact licensure. *Massachusetts Nurse Advocate, 76*(10), 12–13.

Dalai Lama. (n.d.). BrainyQuote.com. Retrieved from http://www.brainyquote.com/quotes/quotes/d/dalailama139179.html

Deloitte Center for Health Solutions. (2008). *Medical tourism: Consumers in search of value.* Retrieved from http://www.deloitte.com/assets/Dcom-UnitedStates/Local%20Assets/Documents/us_chs_MedicalTourismStudy%283%29.pdf

Federal Emergency Management Agency (FEMA). (2010) Retrieved from http://www.fema.gov/emergency/nims/IncidentCommandSystem.shtm

Gebbie, K., & Qureshi, K. (2006). A historical challenge: Nurses and emergencies. *Online Journal of Nursing Issues, 11*(3). Retrieved from http://www.nursingworld.org/MainMenuCategories/ANAMarketplace/ANAPeriodicals/OJIN/TableofContents/Volume112006/No3Sept06/NURSESANDEMERGENCIES.aspx

Health Volunteers Overseas (HVO). (2010). Retrieved from http://www.hvousa.org/whereWeWork/index.shtml

Hodge, J. G., Gable, L. A., & Calves, S. H. (2005). The legal framework for meeting surge capacity through the use of volunteer health professionals during public health emergencies and other disasters. *Journal of Contemporary Health Law & Policy, 22,* 5–72.

Institute of Medicine. (2010). *Medical surge capacity: Workshop summary.* Retrieved from http://iom.edu/Reports/2010/Medical-Surge-Capacity-Workshop-Summary.aspx

International Medical Corps (IMC). (2010). Retrieved from http://www.internationalmedicalcorps.org/

Jakeway, C. C., LaRosa, G., & Schoenfisch, S. (2008). The role of public health nurses in emergency preparedness and response: A position paper of the association of state and territorial directors of nursing. *Public Health Nursing, 25*(4), 353–361.

Kassim, P. N. J. (2009). Medicine beyond borders: The legal and ethical challenges. *Medicine and Law, 28*, 439–450.

Litchfield, S. M. (2010).How to help when disaster strikes. *American Association of Occupational Health Nurses, 58*(3), 85–87.

McHugh, M. D. (2007). The legal context of nurses volunteering in mass casualty events. *Pennsylvania Nurse, 62*(2), 14–15.

Medical Reserve Corps (MRC). (2010). Retrieved from http://www.medicalreservecorps.gov/HomePage

National Council of State Boards of Nursing. (1997). Boards of nursing adopt revolutionary change for nursing regulations. *Issues, 18*(3), 1.

National Incident Management System (NIMS). (2010). Retrieved from http://www.fema.gov/emergency/nims/AboutNIMS.shtm

Polivka, B. J., Stanley, S. A., Gordon, D., Taulbee, K., Kieffer, G., & McCrokle, S. M. (2008). Public health nursing competencies for public health surge events. *Public Health Nursing, 25*(2), 159–165.

Smith, G. H. (2006). *The globalization of health care: Can medial tourism reduce care costs?* (U.S. Senate hearing, Serial No. 109 26). Washington, DC: U.S. Government Printing Office.

Travel Nurse Companies Allied Health Agencies Web Directory. (2009). Retrieved from http://trav.nurse.googlepages.com/Travel-Nurse-Companies.html

United Nations (UN). (2010). *UN at a glance.* Retrieved from http://www.un.org/en/aboutun/index.shtml

United Nations Children's Fund (UNICEF). (2010). *About UNICEF: Who we are.* Retrieved from http://www.unicef.org/about/who/index_introduction.html

United Nations Summit. (2010). Millennium goals. Retrieved from http://www.un.org/en/mdg/summit2010

U. S. Census Bureau. (2010). Retrieved from http://www.census.gov/newsroom/releases/archives/income_wealth/cb10-144.html

U.S. Department of Health and Human Services, Health Resources and Services Administration, Bureau of Health Professionals, National Center for Workforce Analysis. (n.d.). *Projected supply, demand, and shortage of registered nurses: 2000–2010.* Retrieved from http://www.ahcancal.org/research_data/staffing/Documents/Registered_Nurse_Supply_Demand.pdf

U.S. Department of Health and Human Services, Public Health and Medical Services Support, National Disaster Medical System. (2010). Retrieved from http://www.phe.gov/preparedness/support/medicalassistance/Pages/default.aspx#ndms

U.S. Public Health Service Commissioned Corps. (2010). Retrieved on from http://www.usphs.gov/

World Bank. (2010). Retrieved from http://web.worldbank.org/WBSITE/EXTERNAL/TOPICS/EXTSOCIALDEV/0,,contentMDK:21154393~menuPK:3291389~pagePK:64168445~piPK:64168309~theSitePK:3177395,00.html#N

World Health Organization (WHO). (2010a). Retrieved from http://www.who.int/about/en/

World Health Organization (WHO). (2010b). Retrieved from http://www.who.int/whr/en/index.html

World Health Organization (WHO). (2010c). Retrieved from http://www.who.int/topics/millennium_development_goals/diseases/en/index.html

ADDITIONAL RESOURCES

Klug, N. (2001). Interstate licensure: Nursing beyond your state borders. *Nursing 2001, 31*(2), 51.

Weeks, S. M. (2007). Mobilization of a nursing community after a disaster. *Perspectives in Psychiatric Care, 43*(1), 22–29.

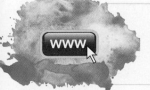

For a full suite of assignments and additional learning activities, use the access code located in the front of your book to visit the exclusive website: http://go.jblearning.com/Holzemer/. If you do not have an access code, you can obtain one at the site.

LEARNING ACTIVITIES

1. The Millennium Development Goals are intended to apply to all age groups. Which age group would be most dramatically affected if all of these goals were met?

   A. Infants
   B. Adolescents
   C. Adults
   D. Older adults

2. The primary goal of creating social responsibility within the nursing profession relates to which of the following?

   A. Ensure equal rights among all people regarding health policy and their right to vote
   B. Improve the health and well-being of people in developed and underdeveloped countries
   C. Develop policies regarding incident command centers within the context of disaster management
   D. Protect the health and safety of individuals, families, and communities during times of disaster

3. According the U.S. Census Bureau, how many people in the United States currently lack healthcare insurance?

   A. 10 million
   B. 30 million
   C. 50 million
   D. 70 million

4. Which of the following best describes medical tourism?

   A. The practice of physicians setting up medical clinics in countries other than their own country of primary licensure
   B. The practice of people having elective cosmetic surgery in countries other than their own
   C. The practice of physicians accompanying patients to international countries to ensure quality patient care
   D. The practice of people seeking low-cost healthcare services in countries other than their own

5. What is the name of the standardized, on-scene, all-hazards management system that allows for coordinated responses among jurisdictions and agencies during a disaster?

   A. Medical Disaster Relief Network
   B. Incident Command System
   C. Disaster Medical Team
   D. Emergency Response Squad

ADDITIONAL QUESTIONS FOR STUDY

1. Visit the United Nations website. Go to *one* of the two information areas and identify *one* of the topics listed. Review the topic and reflect on the significance of this topic from a global level. Coordinate the topics with classmates, if appropriate, so that, as a group, you investigate different topics.

Information area 1: http://www.un.org/rights

Topics:

Peace and Security

Economic and Social Development

Human Rights

Humanitarian Affairs

International Law

Information area 2: http://www.un.org/works

Topics:

Children	HIV/AIDS
Education	Human Rights
Poverty	Climate Change
Peace	Emergencies
Health	Women

CHAPTER OUTLINE

▸ Introduction
▸ Permission to Act in the Various Community Health Nursing Roles
▸ The Institute of Medicine 2011 Report
  • Key Messages of the Report
  • Recommendations of the Report
▸ Quality and Safety Education for Nurses Prelicensure Competencies
▸ Developing a New Skill Set to Create the Future of Community Health Nursing
▸ Question 1: What Will Be the Guiding Principles and Theoretical Orientation for Community Health Nursing in the Future?
  • Reflective Practice
  • Respect
  • Vision
  • Relatedness
  • Clarity
  • Using Reflective Practice, Respect, Vision, Relatedness, and Clarity in Community Health Nursing of the Future
▸ Question 2: What Will Be the Meaning Behind the Assessment and Diagnosis of the Voice of the Client by the Nurse in the Future?
  • Courage
  • Compassion
  • Using Courage and Compassion in Assessment and Diagnosis in the Future
▸ Question 3: How Will the Nurse Approach Assessment and Diagnosis of Community-Based Needs in the Future?
  • Inquisitiveness

• Validity/Reliability
• Using Inquisitiveness and Validity/Reliability to Understand Community-Based Needs in the Future
▸ Question 4: How Will the Nurse Approach Assessment and Diagnosis of the Effectiveness of Systems of Care Management and Needed Resource Allocation Solutions in the Future?
  • Flexibility
  • Justice
  • Using Flexibility and Justice to Understand Systems of Care Management and Resource Allocation Solutions in the Future
▸ Question 5: What Will Be the Meaning of Community Health Program Planning, Implementation, Evaluation, and Termination in the Future?
  • Precision
  • Viability
  • Alertness
  • Using the Concepts of Precision, Viability, and Alertness to Understand Program Planning, Implementation, Evaluation, and Termination in the Future
▸ Question 6: What Is the Future of Community Health Nursing?
  • Responsibility
  • Evidence-Based Future
  • Using the Concepts of Responsibility and Securing an Evidence-Based Future for Ongoing Community Health Nursing Care Delivery, Education, and Research
▸ Summary

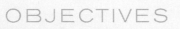

OBJECTIVES

1. Identify how the recommendations from the IOM report, and the QSEN competencies can be used to improve the practice of community health nursing.

2. Evaluate the six chapter questions intended to reflect the scope of community health nursing practice.

3. Explain the usefulness of the 17 concepts identified throughout the textbook, when fostering change in nursing care delivery, education, and research in the community.

4. Link the local challenges of community health nursing to the national concerns of health care delivery.

KEY TERMS

Advanced practice registered nurses (APRNs)   Residency programs

CHAPTER 16

Creating an Evidence-Based Future in Community Health Nursing

Marilyn Klainberg
Stephen Paul Holzemer

EVIDENCE-BASED FUTURE

I touch the future. I teach.

—Christa McAuliffe (1948–1986)

Introduction

The future of community health nursing is now. Changes in the methods by which care is being delivered and expectations for care by the public are complex issues needing the attention of any healthcare discipline expecting a place in the future of health care. This chapter explores the possibilities associated with creating an evidence-based future in community health nursing. The chapter begins with an examination of how the American Nurses Association's (ANA) Social Policy Statement, the recommendations of the Institute of Medicine (IOM) 2011 report, and the Quality and Safety Education for Nurses (QSEN) prelicensure competencies can be incorporated into the development of an evidence-based future in community health nursing.

This chapter also revisits the concepts and questions designed to promote the development of a contemporary skill set for working in the community. The community health nurse (CHN) of the future will need to use the concepts of reflective practice, respect, vision, relatedness, clarity, courage, compassion, inquisitiveness, validity/reliability, flexibility, justice, precision, viability, alertness, and responsibility to create an evidence-based future. The skill to act by employing any and all of these concepts will take the dedication nurses usually reserve for mastery of expert technical skills and procedures.

Permission to Act in the Various Community Health Nursing Roles

Nurses secure permission to act in a variety of nursing roles from society. Nursing serves at the pleasure of society; nursing exists within the context of a special relationship with society to provide nursing care (ANA, 2003, 2010a, 2010b). Through state regulations, standards, and laws, individuals meet social, legal, and professional expectations and become nurses. In the example of CHNs, society allows these nurses to focus, for the most part, on the needs and concerns of populations and communities. This role would necessarily include creating an evidence-based future in community health nursing. Instead of viewing nursing as a discipline as "being owned by society," the nursing profession needs to "own" its future, in the service to society (ANA, 2003, 2010a, 2010b).

The Institute of Medicine 2011 Report

Key Messages of the Report

An evidence-based future in community health nursing will become a reality, in part, when four key messages of the IOM's 2011 report are considered. These messages serve as the foundation for the eight recommendations of the same report, as they focus on the nursing profession's contribution to health care in the future:

1. Nurses should practice to the full extent of their education and training.
2. Nurses should achieve higher levels of education and training through an improved education system that promotes seamless academic progression.
3. Nurses should be full partners with physicians and other health professionals in redesigning health care in the United States.
4. Effective workforce planning and policy making require better data collection and an improved information infrastructure.

Recommendations of the Report

Although the IOM made eight recommendations (**Table 16-1**), only four are examined here; these four statements relate directly to undergraduate community health nursing education. All of these recommendations follow from the consensus agreement on the need for all nurses to be able to practice to the full extent of their education and training.

TABLE 16-1
Eight Recommendations of the Institute of Medicine 2011 Report

1. **Remove scope-of-practice barriers.** Advanced practice registered nurses should be able to practice to the full extent of their education and training.

2. **Expand opportunities for nurses to lead and diffuse collaborative improvement efforts.** Private and public funders, healthcare organizations, nursing education programs, and nursing associations should expand opportunities for nurses to lead and manage collaborative efforts with physicians and other members of the healthcare team to conduct research and to redesign and improve practice environments and health systems. These entities should also provide opportunities for nurses to diffuse successful practices.

3. **Implement nurse residency programs.** State boards of nursing, accrediting bodies, the federal government, and healthcare organizations should take actions to support nurses' completion of a transition-to-practice program (nurse residency) after they have completed a prelicensure or advanced practice degree program or when they are transitioning into new clinical practice areas.

4. **Increase the proportion of nurses with a baccalaureate degree to 80% by 2020.** Academic nurse leaders across all schools of nursing should work together to increase the proportion of nurses with a baccalaureate degree from 50% to 80% by 2020. These leaders should partner with education accrediting bodies, private and public funders, and employers to ensure funding, monitor progress, and increase the diversity of students to create a workforce prepared to meet the demands of diverse populations across the life span.

5. **Double the number of nurses with a doctorate by 2020.** Schools of nursing, with support from private and public funders, academic administrators and university trustees, and accrediting bodies, should double the number of nurses with a doctorate by 2020 to add to the cadre of nurse faculty and researchers, with attention to increasing diversity.

6. **Ensure that nurses engage in lifelong learning.** Accrediting bodies, schools of nursing, healthcare organizations, and continuing competency educators from multiple health professions should collaborate to ensure that nurses and nursing students and faculty continue their education and engage in lifelong learning to gain the competencies needed to provide care for diverse populations across the life span.

7. **Prepare and enable nurses to lead change to advance health.** Nurses, nursing education programs, and nursing associations should prepare the nursing workforce to assume leadership positions across all levels, while public, private, and governmental healthcare decision makers should ensure that leadership positions are available to and filled by nurses.

8. **Build an infrastructure for the collection and analysis of interprofessional healthcare workforce data.** The National Health Care Workforce Commission, with oversight from the Government Accountability Office and the Health Resources and Services Administration, should lead a collaborative effort to improve research and the collection and analysis of data on healthcare workforce requirements. The Workforce Commission and the Health Resources and Services Administration should collaborate with state licensing boards, state nursing workforce centers, and the Department of Labor in this effort to ensure that the data are timely and publicly accessible.

Recommendations that relate to changes in the workforce and changing the numbers of providers are not identified as recommendations central to this discussion. System changes and complex operational changes are best approached by students in graduate programs in nursing (Recommendations 2, 4, 5, and 7).

Recommendation 1

Recommendation 1: Remove scope-of-practice barriers. Advanced practice registered nurses should be able to practice to the full extent of their education and training.

Advanced practice registered nurses (APRNs): Clinical specialists in public and community health, as well as nurse practitioners.

Although Recommendation 1 refers to **advanced practice registered nurses (APRNs)**—who include clinical specialists in public and community health, as well as nurse practitioners—as their scope of practice grows, so will the practice of (general practice) registered nurses (RNs) working as CHNs. The practice of CHNs will likely change as additional providers begin managing care in the community. As APRNs practice to the full extent of their education, CHNs will increasingly receive guidance in providing care from them as well as from physicians. Advanced practice registered nurses will be responsible for creating plans of care for clients, just as physicians and other providers do.

Recommendation 3

Recommendation 3: Implement nurse residency programs. State boards of nursing, accrediting bodies, the federal government, and healthcare organizations should take actions to support nurses' completion of a transition-to-practice program (nurse residency) after they have completed a prelicensure or advanced practice degree program or when they are transitioning into new clinical practice areas.

Residency programs: Transition-to-practice programs for nurses who have completed a prelicensure or advanced practice degree program or are transitioning into new clinical practice areas.

Recommendation 3 refers to **residency programs** that will become the norm for nurses entering acute care and community-based nursing environments. The role of CHNs will change as they are more involved in the comprehensive education of nurses entering the workforce. Although some institutions have established formal preceptorships and residency programs, this recommendation calls for specific transition-to-practice programs that will be managed by CHNs and APRNs to assure a smooth movement into practice following graduation from the school of nursing. The Visiting Nurse Service of New York (VNSNY; http://www.vnsny.org/careers/internships) provides such a model program, thereby fostering the development of new graduates.

Another opportunity will be to encourage some students to secure placement with community-based agencies in their "end-of-program" course before graduation. Many programs desire to place students in skill-rich, hospital-based programs, which may provide limited skill development in the care of aggregates and communities. End-of-aca-

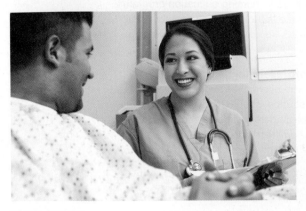

© Creatas/Thinkstock

demic-program experiences, often using clinical preceptors, can be designed to better prepare graduate nurses to be successful in residency programs.

Recommendation 6

> **Recommendation 6: Ensure that nurses engage in lifelong learning.**
> Accrediting bodies, schools of nursing, healthcare organizations, and continuing competency educators from multiple health professions should collaborate to ensure that nurses and nursing students and faculty continue their education and engage in lifelong learning to gain the competencies needed to provide care for diverse populations across the life span.

The nursing profession speaks of being devoted to lifelong learning, but in many states and institutions, continuing education remains optional. This failure to continue with nursing education is obviously problematic because the outcome includes having a number of CHNs who are not current in best practices. Advanced formal education—that is, education resulting in the award of an advanced academic degree—is also not available or of interest to some CHNs. Nurses "in the field" need to embrace continuing education, whether job specific or more formal in nature. The Internet can serve as a portal to quality education programs for CHNs in any location.

The CHNs of the future will work in environments that value continuing education and make the personal sacrifices necessary to continue their education as they address Recommendation 6. The American Nurses Association, the National League for Nursing, and the American Public Health Association have all established continuing education and certification programs to support the continuing education needs of CHNs. Community health nurses need to take responsibility for remaining clinically competent in a rapidly changing community environment. Rapid and somewhat recent changes in knowledge related to bioterrorism, social problems, and behavioral problems such as methamphetamine addiction, for example, have all contributed to the changing landscape of community health nursing concerns.

Recommendation 8

> **Recommendation 8: Build an infrastructure for the collection and analysis of interprofessional healthcare workforce data.** The National Health Care Workforce Commission, with oversight from the Government Accountability Office and the Health Resources and Services Administration, should lead a collaborative effort to improve research and the collection and analysis of data on healthcare workforce requirements. The Workforce Commission and the Health Resources and Services Administration should collaborate with state licensing boards, state nursing workforce centers, and the Department of Labor in this effort to ensure that the data are timely and publicly accessible.

Central to Recommendation 8 is the process of developing and sustaining interprofessional relationships. Nursing care is not a solo activity. Instead, the meaningfulness of nursing care in the community is found in how it complements the work of physicians,

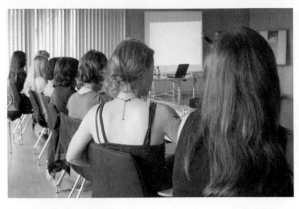

© Marc Dietrich/ShutterStock, Inc.

epidemiologists, health educators, and others. Both new and seasoned CHNs can seek out the expertise of other disciplines in creating interdisciplinary approaches to care. Nurses should not wait to be invited to the table of innovative practice, but rather should actively invite others to the table to create improvements in nursing practice.

This recommendation will also require CHNs who are eager to "improve research and the collection and analysis of data on health care workforce requirements" to expand their skill set in research and data management, even at the beginning practitioner level. Although research and aggregate data management needs advanced education and preparation to direct activities, entry-level CHNs must become increasingly skilled in discussing these issues and concerns as they relate to their practice. Success in meeting Recommendations 1 and 3 is contingent on CHNs becoming skilled in research and the collection and analysis of data on healthcare workforce requirements—that is, providing care to those in need of community-based care. Recommendation 8 can also be realized by engaging with another document—the QSEN competencies.

Quality and Safety Education for Nurses Prelicensure Competencies

The QSEN prelicensure knowledge–skills–attitudes (KSA) competencies include six elements: (1) patient-centered care; (2) teamwork and collaboration; (3) evidence-based practice (EBP); (4) quality improvement (QI); (5) safety; and (6) informatics (Cronenwett et. al., 2007). The KSAs related to these competencies are needed for the ongoing practice of any specialty in nursing, such as community health.

A focus on patient (client) safety provides common ground for various health-related disciplines to focus attention on creating "best practices." An emphasis on safety provides a common language through which diverse disciplines can center their efforts to foster better healthcare outcomes.

Using the IOM and QSEN materials offers at least five benefits:
- The guidelines are nursing centered but not nursing exclusive.
- They are national in scope.
- They are related to the practice of nursing by both novice and experienced nurses.
- They offer an opportunity to engage in activities that will enable the profession to serve as a viable force in change.
- They present an opportunity to encourage ownership of professional roles in future healthcare delivery, education, and research.

Table 16-2 shows a relationship between the IOM recommendations and the QSEN competencies. This relationship ties the future concerns of the IOM with the six competencies that nursing values in quality and safety, in an effort to provide a blueprint for the future concerns of the practice of community health nursing.

Developing a New Skill Set to Create the Future of Community Health Nursing

At the beginning of this text, the reader was invited to consider ways to develop a new skill set for community health nursing. As previously stated, nurses working in the com-

TABLE 16-2

Relationship Between the Quality and Safety Education for Nurses (QSEN) Prelicensure Knowledge–Skills–Attitudes (KSA) Competencies and the Institute of Medicine (IOM) Recommendations

Six QSEN Competencies (plus Reflection)	Nurses should practice to the full extent of their education and training.	Nurses should achieve higher levels of education and training through an improved education system that promotes seamless academic progression.	Nurses should be full partners with physicians and other health professionals in redesigning health care in the United States.	Effective workforce planning and policy making require better data collection and an improved information infrastructure.
Patient-Centered Care	X		X	
Teamwork and Collaboration	X	X	X	X
Evidence-Based Practice (EBP)	X	X	X	X
Quality Improvement (QI)	X		X	
Safety	X		X	
Informatics	X	X	X	X
Reflection	X	X	X	X

munity need an additional skill set, sometimes the same as, but often different from, that of nurses working in acute care settings. With the exception of home care and subacute care settings in the community, the focus on prevention of illness as the goal of practice requires the CHN to approach nursing care differently.

The chapters in this textbook were written to foster different ways of thinking (cognitive), feeling (affective), and performing (psychomotor) the work of nursing in the community. The goal was to assist the nurse in developing a new skill set. This skill set was introduced by examining 17 different, but related concepts—reflective practice, respect, vision, relatedness, clarity, courage, compassion, inquisitiveness, validity/reliability, flexibility, justice, precision, viability, alertness, responsibility, and evidence-based future. It was suggested by the authors that the mastery of this skill set was critical for creating an evidence-based future in community health nursing.

These concepts were initially presented as a way to help answer six questions that reveal the scope of community health nursing practice in the present. Here, answering these questions is considered as a means to reveal the scope of community health nursing practice in the future. **FIGURE 16-1** suggests that all of these concepts have a place in the creation of an evidence-based future for community health nursing.

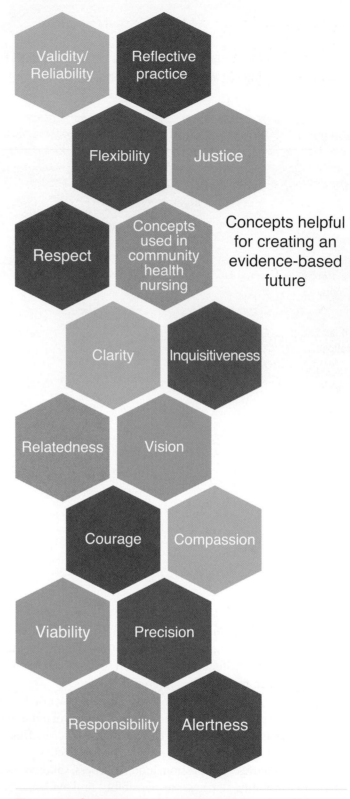

Figure 16-1 Concepts helpful for creating an evidence-based future.

Question 1: What Will Be the Guiding Principles and Theoretical Orientation for Community Health Nursing in the Future?

The concepts that may help answer this question are reflective practice, respect, vision, relatedness, and clarity (**FIGURE 16-2**). These concepts allow the nurse to prepare for the thinking, feeling, and performing aspects of work in the community in the future. These principles will continue to assist the nurse to care for others safely, or refer the work to a provider with a better skill match for problem resolution.

Reflective Practice

Reflecting on nursing practice allows the nurse to commit to the plan of care, and make changes in the plan of care in a timely and efficient manner. Through reflection, the nurse accepts personal and professional responsibility for the creation of a safe and productive client–nurse relationship. The nurse reflects on current practice, with a historical understanding of former practice, to create ideas about best practice for the future. Future practice will necessarily be more interdisciplinary in focus, and more directed toward the public health responsibilities of the CHN.

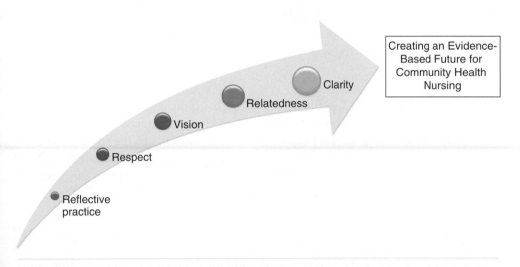

Figure 16-2 Moving toward answering the question: What will be the guiding principles and theoretical orientation for community health nursing in the future?

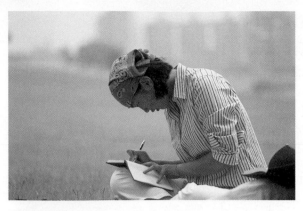

© Photos.com

Respect

Respect for the ethical beliefs and the cultural experience of the client is the core of a successful nurse–client relationship. When caregivers lack an ethical–cultural awareness of the client, the client remains invisible. As communities become more culturally diverse in the future, and as persons of various cultures increase their presence in health professions as providers, respect for the similarities and differences of providers and care recipients will become more important for the CHN to understand.

Vision

Having a vision of the potential for a well-developed client–nurse relationship allows for the client and the nurse to address specific concerns within the healthcare delivery system, and to create new models of care in the future. As previously identified, conceptual models will emerge to assist the nurse in developing a clearer understanding of the integration between community-based needs, the systems of care management, and the resource allocation strategies required to meet these needs. The vision of community assessment needs to evolve into a more interdisciplinary process, with all providers contributing to the process of visionary assessment.

The Alliance for Health Model is one model that represents the integration of community-based needs, systems of care management, and resource allocation as a means to promote the vision of providing comprehensive health services to clients in the community. Future development of this model will continue to expand upon the role of social or distributive justice as central to the community assessment process, as well as drawing attention to the need for environmental protection and consideration of global health concerns on local communities.

Relatedness

The success of supporting healthy communities is intimately related to the progress of sound health policy and evidence-based quantitative and qualitative research. The community health nurse relates policy and research concerns to the specific needs of the community where practice is occurring. The ongoing growth of knowledge and its relatedness to policy formation and development will assist the CHN of the future in participating in best practices that clearly support the needs of people served by sound health policy.

Clarity

Clear intradisciplinary and interdisciplinary communication is key to information management and validating coordinated, successful health outcomes of clients. Clarity of communication between and among nurses and other healthcare providers allows for the support of best practices as well as the termination of practices that do not effect healthy client outcomes. The development of systems of care in the future, and the way in which the CHN communicates with them to meet client needs, will be transparent as long as clarity in communication is kept central to the process of care delivery.

Using Reflective Practice, Respect, Vision, Relatedness, and Clarity in Community Health Nursing of the Future

The CHN can use reflective practice, respect, vision, relatedness, and clarity to seek guiding principles and establish a theoretical orientation for community health nursing by devoting time and energy to refining interdisciplinary practice. Every CHN has an opportunity to embrace the knowledge and skill of other providers and the client seeking services. The aforementioned concepts have meaning only when the various health-related disciplines seek to care for individuals, families, other groups, and the community as a whole. Nurse-specific educational programs, for example, need to invite other-than-nursing professionals to the table to learn and grow in professional skills together.

Question 2: What Will Be the Meaning Behind the Assessment and Diagnosis of the Voice of the Client by the Nurse in the Future?

The concepts that may help answer this question are courage and compassion (**FIGURE 16-3**). These concepts describe the intimate relationship between the client and the nurse as they, for example, seek health solutions, or tolerate limitations of care delivery, both now and in the future. The language of courage and compassion will continue to eliminate the meaninglessness of "noncompliance" on the part of the client. The client and the nurse will work together for the answers to questions that the contemporary healthcare system may or may not address. Future care options, developed by both the client and by nurse (or other provider), will have the opportunity to be more meaningful when compassion and courage serve as their guides.

Courage

It takes courage for clients to navigate the healthcare system as they seek health, accept the limitations imposed by illness, and define their quality of life. The lived experience, or story of the client, must be heard in every client–nurse interaction. The uniqueness of every individual, family, group, aggregate, or community story takes courage to share. The CHN of the future will probably be instrumental in valuing the courage of the client in an increasingly technologically driven healthcare delivery system.

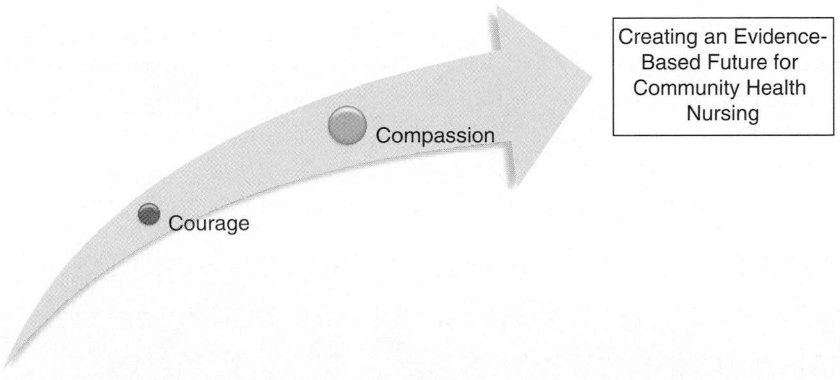

Creating an Evidence-Based Future for Community Health Nursing

Compassion

Courage

Figure 16-3 Moving toward answering the question: What will be the meaning behind the assessment and diagnosis of the voice of the client by the nurse in the future?

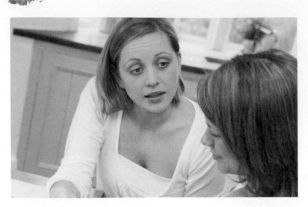

© Monkey Business Images/ShutterStock, Inc.

Compassion

Compassion for clients allows nurses to sustain their commitment to the client–nurse relationship. Compassion is an action that goes well beyond empathy; it requires an ongoing and informed commitment to act in a way that is present to the actual and potential needs of clients. The nurse needs to summon compassion to hear the uniqueness of every family, group, aggregate, or community story, and to act in a way that honors the client's experience.

Using Courage and Compassion in Assessment and Diagnosis in the Future

Having courage and compassion can assist the CHN in searching for the meaning behind the assessment and diagnosis of the voice of the client. One area in which the CHN could work with others in this search relates to the national problem of the infant mortality rate (IMR). It is unfathomable that the IMR in the United States is so high when the country's expenditures related to health care are the highest in the world. A multidisciplinary call to action will be necessary to reorganize the priorities in health care so that the IMR receives enough attention to promote real change. Nurses can use compassion to guide clients to share their stories with courage. Courage will be necessary on the part of clients as they learn to live with the realities of changing the allocation of resources to better care for infants and their parents.

Question 3: How Will the Nurse Approach Assessment and Diagnosis of Community-Based Needs in the Future?

The concepts that may help answer this question are inquisitiveness and validity/reliability (**FIGURE 16-4**). The value of these concepts in the future will apply equally to all aspects of the nursing process. The inner ability to seek meaningfulness in the nursing process will make each step purposeful and open to creative change. Investigation of health and illness patterns will instill the CHN with confidence that the data collected as part of the effort to improve health care are valid and reliable.

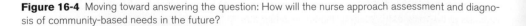

Creating an Evidence-Based Future for Community Health Nursing

Validity/Reliability

Inquisitiveness

Figure 16-4 Moving toward answering the question: How will the nurse approach assessment and diagnosis of community-based needs in the future?

Inquisitiveness

Inquisitiveness on the part of the nurse allows the nurse to develop skill in the assessment and diagnosis of community-based needs that may be met by the spectrum of health promotion, health maintenance, and health restoration services available to clients. Matching client needs with the services available becomes possible only after successful assessment and diagnosis. Best practices in health care and nursing are constantly emerging and undergoing revision. The CHN of the future can develop confidence in plans of care when they are repeatedly reviewed and reexamined with an inquisitive approach.

Validity/Reliability

Validity and reliability assist with the process of translating information from epidemiology and environmental health into an actual plan of care for the community. The use of scientific data that accurately portray what is known about the relationship between illness and the environment that supports it is the first step in problem resolution. Comfort with findings that are accurate in measurement and subject to replication of findings will support the choices of the models of healthcare delivery.

Using Inquisitiveness and Validity/Reliability to Understand Community-Based Needs in the Future

The CHN can use inquisitiveness and validity/reliability to approach assessment and diagnosis of community-based needs in the future. For example, the drug abuse problem, which is endemic in both urban and rural America, could be sensitive to these concepts. To date, a great deal of study has been conducted on drug-related problems, yet has produced few significant or lasting positive outcomes. An interdisciplinary approach involving the various levels of prevention with respect to drug use and abuse may be informed by continuous inquiry guided by inquisitiveness and validity/reliability. These concepts can be especially sensitive to the various influences, such as cultural differences, that are part of health-related problems that affect people of most ages and different socioeconomic and educational backgrounds.

Question 4: How Will the Nurse Approach Assessment and Diagnosis of the Effectiveness of Systems of Care Management and Needed Resource Allocation Solutions in the Future?

The concepts that may help answer this question are flexibility and justice (**FIGURE 16-5**). Systems of care management need to be flexible with respect to meeting client needs, yet consistent in meeting the needs of people fairly.

Flexibility

Creating systems of care management for families, groups, aggregates, and communities requires flexibility. This need arises because systems that are effective in one setting may fail in another setting. To be effective, systems of care management must adapt to changing community-based needs and the resources that are available to meet them.

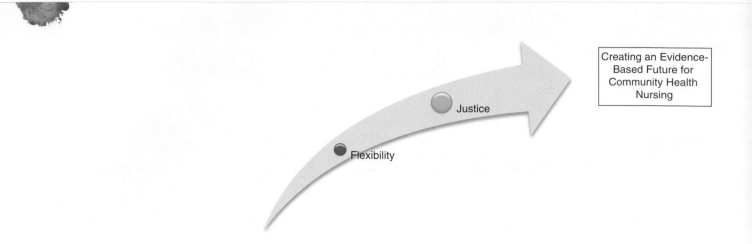

Figure 16-5 Moving toward answering the question: How will the nurse approach assessment and diagnosis of the effectiveness of systems of care management and needed resource allocation solutions in the future?

Future systems of care may well involve increased movement within and between care delivery settings. The CHN must move with the client as care is delivered to ensure the client's safety and responsible use of resources.

Justice

Resource allocation for families, groups, aggregates, and communities should be grounded in the ethical principle of justice. Justice as fairness promotes the meeting of community-based needs, with available resources, in a way that is acceptable to the community. The CHN can serve as an advocate for the community as decisions are made about the fair use of resources that are finite in nature. The CHN, working with other disciplines, can assist families, other groups, and communities in making difficult decisions about the allocation of resources in the future.

Using Flexibility and Justice to Understand Systems of Care Management and Resource Allocation Solutions in the Future

In the future, one area where flexibility and justice may inform the CHN in the assessment and diagnosis of the effectiveness of systems of care management and needed resource allocation solutions may be care of the aging population. As increasing numbers of people within the population enter old age, their many needs may be met by a flexible and just approach. The concepts of flexibility and justice can be beneficial in engaging clients to become empowered as active participants in creating useful healthcare delivery systems.

Question 5: What Will Be the Meaning of Community Health Program Planning, Implementation, Evaluation, and Termination in the Future?

The concepts that may help answer this question are precision, viability, and alertness (**FIGURE 16-6**).

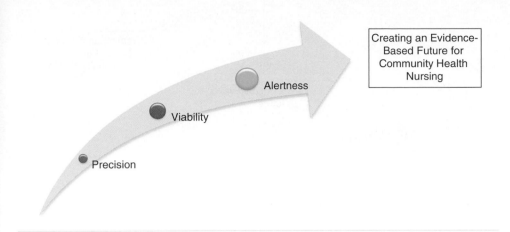

Figure 16-6 Moving toward answering the question: What will be the meaning of community health program planning, implementation, evaluation, and termination in the future?

Precision

Community health program planning, implementation, evaluation, and termination require precision to meet the needs of the community. The evolution of programs depends on the concept of precision to keep them relevant to the community. Questions of how to prioritize limited resources are answered, in part, by precise program development.

Viability

Coordinating community health program planning, implementation, evaluation, and termination through thoughtful project management fosters program viability in the community. Engaging in the process of the strategic use of material and personnel resources keeps programs functioning at an optimal level.

Alertness

Alertness to the realities of natural and human-made disasters in the community allows for the potential for adequate care to be delivered to the community if and when such events occur. The integrity of the community requires vigilance in avoiding, as well as preparing to cope with, threats that could destroy or cripple the status of health in the community.

Using the Concepts of Precision, Viability, and Alertness to Understand Program Planning, Implementation, Evaluation, and Termination in the Future

Using the concepts of precision, viability, and alertness may promote better community health program planning, implementation, evaluation, and termination in the future. These concepts have the potential to inform the CHN about how to keep program development transparent regarding the use of personal and material resources in an environment where resource limitations are real, and their use or misuse may be harmful.

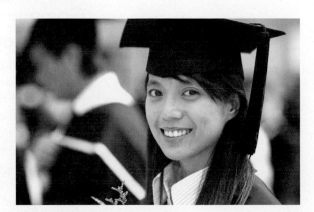

© leungchopan/ShutterStock, Inc.

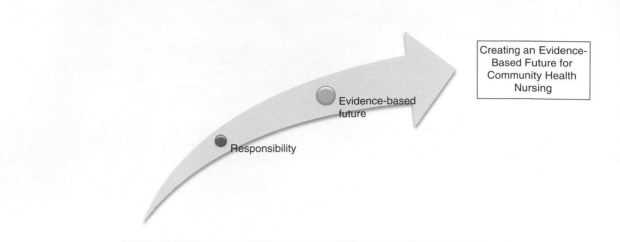

Figure 16-7 Moving toward answering the question: What is the future of community health nursing care delivery, education, and research?

Question 6: What Is the Future of Community Health Nursing?

The concepts that may help answer this question are responsibility and the evidence-based future of community health nursing care delivery, education, and research (**FIGURE 16-7**).

Responsibility

Attention to the impact of interstate, national, and global health concerns on local communities is a growing responsibility of community health nursing.

Evidence-Based Future

The nurse accepts personal and professional responsibility for the creation of models of care for a changing community through evidence-based care delivery, education, and research.

Using the Concepts of Responsibility and Securing an Evidence-Based Future for Ongoing Community Health Nursing Care Delivery, Education, and Research

Like the previously discussed concepts, the concepts of responsibility and securing an evidence-based future will surely be important for the future of community health nursing care delivery, education, and research. As noted earlier, one place for the CHN to focus on these concepts is via the QSEN competencies. **Table 16-3** outlines the fit between the questions asked about the future of community health nursing and the QSEN competencies. As suggested earlier, responsibility for the future of community health nursing should include attention to global health requirements as well as to local requirements. The QSEN competencies are applicable in any care delivery setting, whether global or local.

TABLE 16-3
The Quality and Safety Education for Nurses (QSEN) Prelicensure Knowledge–Skills–Attitudes (KSA) Competencies and Question 6: What Is the Future of Community Health Nursing?

Five Questions About the Future of Community Health Nursing / Six QSEN Competencies (plus Reflection)	Question 1: What will be the guiding principles and theoretical orientation for community health nursing in the future?	Question 2: What will be the meaning behind the assessment and diagnosis of the voice of the client, by the nurse, in the future?	Question 3: How will the nurse approach assessment and diagnosis of community-based needs in the future?	Question 4: How will the nurse approach assessment and diagnosis of the effectiveness of systems of care management and needed resource allocation solutions in the future?	Question 5: What will be the meaning of community health program planning, implementation, evaluation, and termination in the future?
Patient-Centered Care	X	X	X	X	X
Teamwork and Collaboration	X		X	X	X
Evidence-Based Practice (EBP)	X	X	X	X	X
Quality Improvement (QI)	X		X	X	X
Safety	X	X	X	X	X
Informatics	X		X	X	X
Reflection	X	X	X	X	X

Summary

This chapter considered the possibilities of creating an evidence-based future in community health nursing. It began with an examination of how the ANA Social Policy Statement, the recommendations in the Institute of Medicine's 2011 report, and the QSEN prelicensure competencies can be incorporated into the process of creating an evidence-based future in community health nursing. This chapter also revisited the concepts and questions designed to promote the development of a contemporary skill set for working in the community. The future of community health nursing is in the hands of the collective of CHNs who are willing to create care systems that reflect these key concepts, which make the skill set for working in the community contemporary.

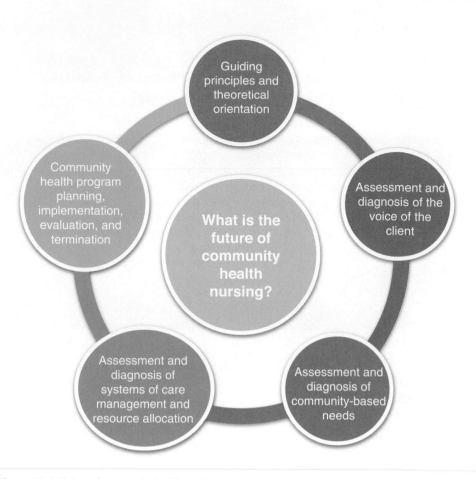

Figure 16-8 Future of community health nursing.

REFERENCES

American Nurses Association (ANA). (2003). *Nursing's social policy statement* (2nd ed.). Silver Spring, MD: Author.

American Nurses Association (ANA). (2010a). *Nursing: Scope and standards of practice* (3rd ed.). Silver Spring, MD: Author.

American Nurses Association (ANA). (2010b). *Nursing's social policy statement: The essence of the profession.* Silver Spring, MD: Author.

Cronenwett, L., Sherwood, G., Barnsteiner, J., Disch, J., Johnson, J., Mitchel, P., … Warren, J. (2007). Quality and safety education for nurses. *Nursing Outlook, 55*(3), 122–131.

Institute of Medicine (IOM). (2011). *The future of nursing: Leading change, advancing health.* Washington, DC: Author.

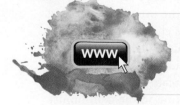

For a full suite of assignments and additional learning activities, use the access code located in the front of your book to visit the exclusive website: http://go.jblearning.com/Holzemer/. If you do not have an access code, you can obtain one at the site.

LEARNING ACTIVITIES

www.

1. Define the following terms, and identify how you can implement the use of these six QSEN competencies (plus reflection) in your work as a student, in both classroom and clinical settings:

> Patient-centered care
> Teamwork and collaboration
> Evidence-based practice
> Quality improvement
> Safety
> Informatics

2. Define the following terms, and identify how you can implement the use of these concepts to promote changes in thinking, feeling, and performing community health nursing in your work as a student, in both classroom and clinical settings:

> Reflective practice
> Respect
> Vision
> Relatedness
> Clarity
> Courage
> Compassion
> Inquisitiveness
> Validity
> Reliability
> Flexibility
> Justice
> Precision
> Viability
> Alertness
> Responsibility
> Evidence-based future

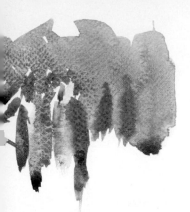

GLOSSARY

Accreditation: A voluntary process by which a healthcare organization is evaluated by an objective body of its peers on particular standards.

Advance medical directives: Legal orders that permit clients to choose in advance the type of healthcare treatment they want.

Advanced practice registered nurses (APRNs): Clinical specialists in public and community health, as well as nurse practitioners.

Advocacy: The act of pleading for another's cause.

Advocacy group: A type of special interest group that exists to assist less empowered groups to have a voice and get their needs met.

Aesthetics: Exposure to and participation in the fine arts, music, and spirituality, closely associated with one's cultural experience.

Affective skills: "Feeling" skills that describe the way people react emotionally or empathize with others.

Agent (in the disease process): A causative factor that contributes to health problems; it may be chemical, physical, biological, or a deficiency.

Age-specific death rate: The number of people in a defined age group who die each year (or during some other period of time).

Alliance for Health Model: A philosophy of nursing care—a template—to assist the nurse in focusing on the relationship between nursing and the community, so as to resolve problems within the scope of nursing practice. It consists of essential five components that represent areas of concern central to the three steps in the joint-venture process of seeking health by the community health nurse and the client.

Alternate care facilities (ACFs): Nonmedical sites that are temporarily adapted to render health care in times of disaster.

Analytical epidemiology: A branch of epidemiology that involves discovering and quantifying associations, testing hypotheses, and attempting to identify causes of health-related states of events.

Anthropogenic: Human-made.

Anticipatory guidance: The process of predicting which services may be needed for the client, and guiding the client in the use of those services.

Assessment: The community health nurse's practice of monitoring health status, investigating outcomes, and using the nursing process to diagnose and further explore problems and concerns in the community.

Assurance: Efforts directed at enhancing the public's perception that the providers of health care and the systems of care management are operating in their best interest.

Autonomy: Independence or self-determination.

Beneficence: A healthcare principle that mandates that the healthcare provider "do good for the client."

Client: The individual or collective of individuals who are the focus of community health nursing.

Clinical research: Research conducted to determine what the literature has concluded is the best practice in a specific area.

Code of ethics: The rules by which a profession is guided.

Cognitive skills: "Knowing" skills that encompass knowledge, critical thinking, and comprehension of particular topics.

Common morbidity rate: A measure of the incidence and prevalence of disease risk among populations.

Community: A collective of individuals that becomes a close, well-functioning group, and that may be described by geography, special interest, or special belief.

Community assessment: The process of searching for and validating relevant community-based data, according to a specified method, to learn about the interactions among the people, resources, and the environment.

Community-based organization (CBO): In health care, a local organization developed to augment care that is needed by the community in an other-than-hospital type of setting; such free-standing organizations may provide education, support, and a level of direct care.

Community diagnosis: A broad statement that represents a major concern in the community, made after the CHN (and other providers) collects and analyzes demographic data and other observed information related to the community, assesses the community's ability to respond to actual and potential threats, and determines how they can be resolved.

Community health nursing: The provision of nursing care for collectives of people, bound in relationships that are called families, other groups, aggregates, and communities.

Compassion fatigue: Exhaustion from the many demands of caregiving.

Competence: Having the capacity to function effectively as an individual and an organization to meet clients' needs.

Confidentiality: The obligation to uphold a client's privacy, maintain certain information in confidence, and respect the client's autonomy.

Control (in research): "The introduction of one or more constants (something that does not vary) into the experimental situation" (LoBiondo-Wood & Haber, 2010, p. 180).

Crude rate: A measure of the entire population in a designated geographic area in relationship to a condition that is being investigated.

Cultural competency: A set of behaviors, attitudes, and policies that come together in a system, agency, or professionals that allow for effective work in cross-cultural situations.

Cultural proficiency: The mastery by the individual nurse of the cognitive and affective phases of cultural development.

Culture: The integrated patterns of human behavior that include language, thoughts, communications, actions, customs, beliefs, values and institutions of racial, ethnic, religious, or social groups.

Curandero: A folk healer within Hispanic cultures.

Demographics: A way of describing a community statistically based on the community members' visible characteristics (e.g., age, race, gender, and location of housing) and invisible characteristics (e.g., level of education, income, and religion).

Descriptive epidemiology: A branch of epidemiology that involves characterizing the distribution of health- and disease-related events.

Determinants of health: Factors that collectively influence an individual's or population's health, such as biology, genetics, individual behavior, socioeconomic status, the physical environment, discrimination, racism, literacy levels, and legislative policies.

Disaster: A serious disruption of the functioning of a community or a society causing widespread human, material, economic, or environmental losses that exceed the ability of the affected community or society to cope using its own resources.

Disaster Medical Assistance Teams (DMATs): As a component of the National Disaster Medical System, these teams of healthcare volunteers (including nurses) provide rapid response emergency care during a national disaster or event.

Distributive justice: A system of justice based on the principle that benefits are distributed in the fairest way possible to all according to need.

"Do not resuscitate" (DNR) order: A medical order to abstain from cardiopulmonary resuscitation if the client's heart stops beating.

"Doughnut hole" (in Medicare): A coverage gap under Medicare Part D that occurs after a beneficiary reaches the initial coverage limit for prescription medications and becomes responsible for the total costs of all medications; when the next coverage limit is reached, the beneficiary becomes eligible for catastrophic coverage.

Egalitarian justice: A system of justice based on the principle that people are treated fairly; also known as equal justice.

Electronic health record (EHR): A digital medical record that is intended to allow access and updating of clients' medical records wherever they receive care and to make data available to the next healthcare team wherever the client seeks care.

Emergency/relief/isolation phase (of a disaster): The period during which relief and assistance are provided to victims of the disaster.

Emergency System for Advance Registration of Volunteer Health Professionals (ESAR-VHP): A system of state-based registries that facilitate volunteer response readiness throughout the United States through verification of individual professional credentials. The registries maintain a comprehensive list of qualified volunteers, verify their credentials prior to a disaster to facilitate response time, and provide disaster response educational training opportunities.

Endemic: "The habitual presence of disease or infectious agents in a defined geographical area or population" (Valanis, 1992, p. 428).

Environment (in the disease process): All external factors surrounding the host that might influence resistance to disease or injury, including biologic, physical, social, cultural, technological, educational, political, legal, demographic, sociological, and economic factors.

Environmental health: The freedom from illness or injury related to exposure to toxic agents and other environmental conditions that are potentially detrimental to human health.

Environmental press: The pressure brought upon individuals by a culture or society that produces specific behaviors.

Epidemic: A rate of disease that is at a significantly higher level than the usual frequency.

Epidemiology: The measurement of the distribution and determinants of states of health, illness, and accidents in human populations.

Ergonomics: The study of body mechanics and movement.

Ethical pluralism: The position that culturally diverse societies display multiple moral standards, which may lead to conflicting moral realities; also known as moral diversity.

Ethics: A system of moral principles, or the rules or guidelines of a particular group, culture, or society.

Evidence-based practice (EBP): Nursing that combines patient preferences with best practices that have been validated by evidence-based research and clinical expertise to formulate the plan of care for clients.

Execution risk: The risk that specific work will not be done correctly.

Experimental studies: Research studies that include randomization, control, and manipulation of at least one variable, and that produce Level 2 evidence; also known as randomized controlled trials.

Faith-based community (FBC): A group of people who find continuing connectedness, encouragement, hope, and love through a shared sense of faith.

Faith community nursing practice: Faith-based, parish, or congregational nursing directed toward "the intentional integration of the practice of faith with the practice of nursing so that people can achieve wholeness in, with, and through the community of faith in which parish nurses work" (American Nurses Association, 2005, p. 1).

Formative evaluation: A prospective assessment that reviews strengths and weaknesses of how a program is unfolding; it is used to help revise project direction and is ongoing.

Formulary: A list of drugs reimbursed by a healthcare insurance company.

Futile care: Interventions and treatments that cannot end dependency on intensive care and treatments and medical interventions that have no medical benefit.

Gantt chart: A tool used to build a project schedule and develop a work flow.

Global health: Health concerns of the international community (e.g., malaria eradication, vaccination programs, AIDS treatment) rather than individual nations' health issues.

Good Samaritan laws: Laws that provide liability protection to nurses and other healthcare providers in emergency situations.

"Griage": The combined operations of greeting and triage at an alternate care site during a disaster.

Health disparity: "A particular type of health difference that is closely linked with social, economic, and/or environmental disadvantage" (U.S. Department of Health and Human Services, 2010).

Health equity: The attainment of the highest level of health for all people.

Health Insurance Portability and Accountability Act (HIPAA): Federal legislation enacted in 1996 that identifies requirements for protection of confidentiality of information related to medical records and services. It protects information related to a person's health care, authorizes release of healthcare information by patients, and clarifies ownership of their health records.

Health ministry: A type of outreach that focuses on the health and healing needs of the members of a particular faith community and its extended community.

Health policy: Public policy that is concerned with the health of the public and the healthcare system that maintains it.

Health status: Age- and gender-specific morbidity and mortality, including patterns of disease.

Healthy People: A U.S. federal government initiative that has generated lists of objectives and desired outcomes of health care for the decades 2000, 2010, and 2020.

Healthy People 2020: The United States' national agenda for healthcare delivery; it strives to improve the health of all groups, with the goals of achieving health equity and eliminating disparities, to allow people to reach their health potential.

Home care services: Curative, restorative, or custodial/supportive services that are provided to individuals and families where they live.

Hospice: Care of the dying person; more formally, care of a person who has received a medical diagnosis and has an anticipated prognosis of less than six months to live.

Host (in the disease process): A susceptible human (or animal) who harbors and supports a disease-causing agent.

Huddle: To gather in a close packed group or to hold a consultation. In an acute care setting, it consists of a brief meeting, lasting 5 to 10 minutes, with all members of the healthcare team; in the community setting, it may involve a telephone conference call.

Impact (of a disaster): The period during which the destruction, injury, and death actually occur.

Incidence: The number of new cases identified in a measure of time.

Incident Command System (ICS): A standardized, on-scene, all-hazards incident management effort that is a significant component of the National Incident Management System, and is used by local, state, federal, and tribal agencies.

Inclusion/exclusion criteria: A means of controlling variables in research that aims to ensure that participating groups are as much alike as possible.

Infant mortality rate (IMR): The number of children younger than one year of age who die each year; a statistic used to measure the health of a community or nation.

Informatics: A multidisciplinary study of the application of information technology to any field.

Informed consent: A process in which a research subject is educated about the terms, procedures, and potential risks and benefits before agreeing to become involved in research.

Integration risk: Failure of all the work in a project to come together at a specific time (i.e., the end of the project).

Interdisciplinary plan of care (IPC): An action plan created and used by the various disciplines involved in the process of providing care that set minimal expectations for client outcomes or responses to care interventions.

ISBARR (identify–situation–background–assessment–recommendation–read back): The SBAR framework for communication between members of the healthcare team about a patient's condition, extended by a beginning stage in which the care provider identifies himself or herself, and an ending "read back," in which the care provider restates and clarifies instructions and expectations.

Justice: An ethical concept that suggests that there is a fair way to allocate resources.

Ladder of participation: Arnstein's method for measuring the participation of a community in eight steps, ranging from nonparticipation to citizen control.

Lobbying: The act of influencing the allocation of resources and the political decisions of public policy makers.

Lobbyist: A professional who represents the views of his or her client before lawmakers and tries to influence the outcome of legislation.

Medicaid: A state-administered healthcare program funded by federal statutes that is available to eligible low-income individuals and families recognized by federal and individual state law guidelines.

Medical Reserve Corps (MRC): A network of community-based public health professionals, including community/public health nurses and physicians, who respond to natural disasters and emergencies to support community health and medical resources.

Medical tourism: The practice of some clients seeking low-cost healthcare services in countries other than their own.

Medicare: A health insurance program managed by the U.S. federal government for people older than age 65, and younger individuals with disabilities and end-stage renal disease requiring dialysis or transplantation.

Millennium Development Goals (MDGs): A global action plan developed by the United Nations that is designed to promote the health and well-being of people around the world. The purpose of the eight MDGs is to reduce poverty, improve global health, and focus on worldwide educational and environmental concerns.

Morbidity: Illness.

Mortality: Death.

National Disaster Medical System (NDMS): A national organization of rapid response teams designed to deliver quality medical care to the victims of, and responders to, a domestic disaster in the United States.

National Incident Management System (NIMS): A U.S. government-created management system that integrates communication, equipment, facilities, personnel, and procedures to ensure effective and efficient management of disasters within the United States.

Natural history of disease: The process by which disease occurs and progresses in humans, involving the interaction of (at least) three different factors: host, agent, and environment.

Nondisaster/interdisaster phase (of a disaster): The period between disaster events, which is an important time for developing and operationalizing prevention and preparedness measures.

Nonexperimental studies: Research studies that usually lack randomization and manipulation of at least one variable, but do include control; they produce Level 4 evidence.

Nongovernmental organizations (NGOs): Independent, legal organizations that have no governmental status; "private organizations that pursue activities to relieve suffering, promote the interests of the poor, protect the environment, provide basic social services, or undertake community development" (World Bank, 2010, para. 1).

Nosocomial: Hospital acquired.

Not-for-profit (nonprofit) organization: An incorporated organization that exists for educational or charitable reasons, and from which its shareholders or trustees do not benefit financially.

Nurse Licensure Compact (NLC): An agreement that allows nurses to practice the profession of nursing in multiple states without the need to obtain additional state licenses.

Nursing: The protection, promotion, and optimization of health and abilities, prevention of illness and injury, alleviation of suffering through the diagnosis and treatment of human response, and advocacy in the care of individuals, families, communities, and populations.

Nursing of special interest: Provision of services to individuals, families, and groups in the community that are curative and restorative in nature.

Pandemic: A worldwide epidemic of a disease.

Phenomenological research method: An inductive, descriptive research method concerned with the investigation and description of all phenomena.

Planned change: A systematic, purposeful, collaborative effort to integrate change for health in a community, through the use of the agreed-upon actions or goals.

Points of dispensing (points of distribution) (PODs): During a disaster, nonmedical sites that are temporarily adapted to render health care in the form of protective oral antimicrobials or vaccines.

Policy: A "purposeful, overall plan of action or inaction developed to deal with a problem or a matter of concern in either the public or private sector" (Sudduth, 2008, p. 173).

Policy development: A process in which the community health nurse interacts with the community, mobilizes community partnerships for change, and molds policies and plans to support the evolution of healthy communities.

Policy process: The process of forming, influencing, and evaluating policy; it includes the steps of identification, formulation, adoption, implementation, and evaluation.

Political power: The ability to influence others to act or produce an effect.

Politics: "The process of influencing the allocation of scarce resources" (Mason, Leavitt, & Chaffee, 2007, p. 4).

Population health paradigm: Integrated care that focuses on health promotion, illness prevention, and chronic condition management but with a special emphasis on patient centeredness and engagement.

Power: "The ability to act or produce an effect" (Merriam Webster Online, n.d.).

Predisaster/warning phase (of a disaster): The period in which emergency professionals have become aware that a disaster is imminent.

Prepathogenesis: The period prior to illness.

Prevalence: The existing number of cases in a population at a given time or over time.

Primary prevention: Interventions implemented before disease occurs, during the prepathogenic stage of an illness; they include both health promotion behaviors and specific protection behaviors.

Procedure: A statement that explains the actual mechanics of how to do something.

Process: Continuing ongoing activity.

Project: A task that requires strategizing to get the work accomplished and is not part of the normal work day.

Project management: The concept of managing a one-time activity that has a well-defined set of outcomes, comprising the application of skills, knowledge, tools, and techniques to meet the requirements of a project.

Proportion: A specific type of ratio in which the numerator is included in the denominator, and the resultant value is expressed as a percentage.

Psychomotor skills: "Doing" skills that involve the physical ability to manipulate tools or instruments.

Public health nursing: "The practice of promoting and protecting the health of populations using knowledge from nursing, social, and public health sciences" (APHA, Public Health Nursing Section, 2007, p. 5.).

Public health nursing practice: A part of the healthcare system that responds to biological, cultural, environmental, economic, social, and political factors through working with the community to promote health and prevent disease, injury, and disability.

Public policy: Policy formed through a governmental body for the benefit of the public.

Qualitative studies: Research studies that explore the subjective experience of a phenomenon in an attempt to interpret it.

Quantitative studies: Research studies that use mathematical principles and statistics to measure phenomena or test hypotheses.

Quasi-experimental studies: Research studies that lack one of the three essential elements (randomization, control, and manipulation of at least one variable), usually randomization; they produce Level 3 evidence.

Randomization: A means of controlling variables in research that aims to ensure that any differences within the entire patient population in the study that existed before the intervention will be distributed evenly between the two groups and will not affect the outcome.

Rate: A statistic used for describing an event or occurrence; in epidemiology, the proportion of persons with a health problem among a population at risk.

Ratio: The relationship between two numbers expressed as a fraction; the value is obtained by dividing the numerator of the fraction by the denominator.

Reconstruction/rehabilitation phase (of a disaster): The period during which the affected region is ready to restore its community to the condition it was in before the disaster occurred.

Reflective practice: Practice in which the nurse considers how all parts of the nursing process relate to the care of individuals, families, other groups, and the community as a whole.

Relative risk: Exposure to risk factors across age groups.

Reliability: The demonstration of accuracy and consistency of information obtained over time—that is, repeated measurements agree and support each as being accurate.

Research: The systematic collection and analysis of data related to a particular problem or phenomenon.

Residency programs: Transition-to-practice programs for nurses who have completed a prelicensure or advanced practice degree program or are transitioning into new clinical practice areas.

Resource allocation: The way a community distributes its available funds among competing groups and programs.

Resource availability: The availability of socioeconomic and environmental resources including human capital, social connectedness, and social status as well as access to health care and quality of care.

SBAR (situation–background–assessment–recommendation): A framework for communication between members of the healthcare team about a patient's condition.

School nursing: A specialized practice of professional nursing that advances the well-being, academic success, and lifelong achievement and health of students.

Scientific research: Research accomplished for the purpose of generating knowledge.

Scope creep: Deviation from a project plan after it is designed and formalized so as to deal with problems that arise, with these events being used as an opportunity to include additional work in the deliverables.

Scope of practice: The legal limits of nursing practice within the community being served, as defined by state law and the Nurse Practice Act.

Secondary insurance: A type of insurance, from either a public or private source, that covers some costs that are not paid by the primary insurance policy.

Secondary prevention: Interventions are used during early pathogenesis—that is, after illness has occurred; they include early diagnosis, prompt treatment, and the limitation of disability.

Sentinel event: An unexpected event or occurrence involving death, or serious or permanent physical or psychological injury.

Social network sites: Online communities where people can meet, interact, and exchange information.

Special interest group: A group that uses its influence to get the services that its members want.

Sponsor: In Alcoholics Anonymous or similar programs, a fellow alcoholic or drug abuser who volunteers to assist the person with his or her recovery.

Stakeholder: Anyone who will be affected by a project.

START (Simple Triage and Rapid Treatment): A triage method that classifies patients into four groups: (1) those having minor injuries, (2) those for whom treatment can be delayed, (3) those who require immediate treatment, and (4) deceased victims.

Summative evaluation: A retrospective assessment that analyzes the outcomes and achievements of the project in a final way, at the end of the program.

Telehealth nursing: The use of telecommunication and information technology to provide nursing care when large distances exist between patient and nurse.

Tertiary prevention: Interventions used during later pathogenesis—specifically, the period of convalescence and rehabilitation; they include reeducation for the client and education of the public.

Third-party payment: A system in which a healthcare provider is paid by insurance companies for services rendered; that is, the fees for care are paid by the insurance provider rather than solely by the patient.

Third-party reimbursement: A healthcare funding mechanism in which the provider bills the insurance company and is paid directly for the services rendered to the client.

Triage: A specific methodology for categorizing patients that is designed to optimize available resources by treating those patients in most dire need before those who are less acutely ill or injured.

U.S. Public Health Service Commissioned Corps: A team of public health professionals, including nurses, who are trained and equipped to respond to public health crises and national emergencies.

Utilitarian justice: A system of justice based on the principle that benefits are first given to those who need them the most.

Validity: The idea that information is accurate and a reflection of reality—that is, the information is sound, unbiased, and well grounded.

Worried-well patients: Those individuals who clinically have no malady, yet self-refer themselves to hospitals, physicians' offices, and urgent care centers for care in fear that they may be affected by a disaster.

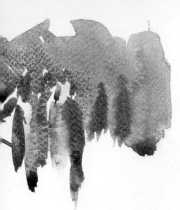

INDEX

Note: Page numbers in italics refer to figures or tables.